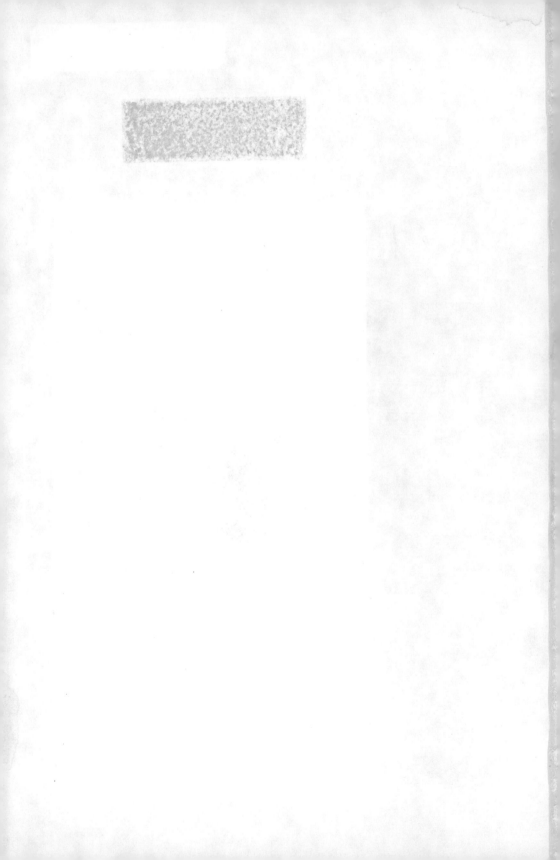

The Complete Book of Menopause

The Complete Book of Menopause

EVERY WOMAN'S GUIDE TO GOOD HEALTH

Carol Landau, Ph.D.
Michele G. Cyr, M.D.
Anne W. Moulton, M.D.

A GROSSET/PUTNAM BOOK
PUBLISHED BY G. P. PUTNAM'S SONS
NEW YORK

This book is meant to educate and should not be used as an alternative to appropriate medical care. The authors have made every effort to ensure that the information presented is accurate. In the light of ongoing research, however, it is possible that new findings may invalidate some of the data presented here.

A Grosset/Putnam Book
Published by G. P. Putnam's Sons
Publishers Since 1838
200 Madison Avenue
New York, NY 10016

Book design by H. Roberts

The authors gratefully acknowledge permission to reprint material from the following:
American Psychiatric Association: *Diagnostic and Statistical Manual of Mental Disorders, Third Edition, Revised,* Washington, DC, American Psychiatric Association, 1987.

Library of Congress Cataloging-in-Publication Data

Landau, Carol.
    The complete book of menopause : every woman's guide to good
  health / Carol Landau, Michele G. Cyr, Anne W. Moulton.
        p.   cm.
    "A Grosset/Putnam book."
    Includes bibliographical references and index.
    ISBN 0-399-13946-X (alk.paper)
    1. Menopause—Popular works. I. Cyr, Michele G. II. Moulton,
  Anne W. III. Title.
    [DNLM: 1. Menopause—popular works. 2. Women's Health—popular
  works. WP 580 L2528c 1994]
  RG186.L36 1994
  612.6'65—dc20   93-38651 CIP
  DNLM/DLC
  for Library of Congress

Printed in the United States of America

1 2 3 4 5 6 7 8 9 10

This book is printed on acid-free paper.
∞

ACKNOWLEDGMENTS

SOMETIMES YOU GET LUCKY. WE GOT LUCKY IN 1992. FIRST, COLLEEN Mohyde of The Doe Coover Agency telephoned us. Colleen had read our letter to the editor of *Vanity Fair,* in response to an article pointing out that menopause was not such a negative and symptomatic time for most women. One thing led to another. Colleen encouraged us to write a book and off we went. Colleen's editorial advice and guidance, as well as Doe's encouragement, have been invaluable.

Four months later, we got lucky again. A woman who was working part-time in our division offered to be our research assistant for the rapidly expanding book. Kathleen Jenkins is a junior at Brown University, as well as an accomplished playwright. She is a most talented writer, a diligent research assistant, and the voice of common sense. Kay has typed, annotated, edited and deciphered, and we are indebted to her.

As soon as we spoke to Jane Isay at Putnam's, we knew we were in good hands. Jane has been an enthusiastic, insightful and supportive editor. She has helped us maintain a positive outlook throughout the project and working with her has been a pleasure.

We would like to thank our consultants, Elizabeth Buechler,

M.D., Dorothy Bianco, Ph.D., Belinda Johnson, Ph.D., Douglas Kiel, M.D., Jacqueline Puhl, Ph.D., and Iris Shuey, M.D.

Steven A. Wartman, M.D., brought the three of us together when he was the Chief of the Division of General Internal Medicine at Rhode Island Hospital. We would like to thank all of the members of the division. Albert Most, M.D., our Chief of Medicine, has also been most supportive.

Laura Wald also helped us with research. Brenda Manchester and Helen O'Connor helped to type the manuscript.

We would also like to thank our colleagues at Women's Health Associates: Elaine Carlson, M.D., Sherri Fitts, Ph.D., Felise Milan, M.D., Karyn Montgomery, M.D., Laura Nevel, M.D., Karen Pevin, Norma Schorr, Jody Spencer, Ph.D., Mary-Anne Spizzirri, and Flora Treger, M.D.

Thank you to the staff of the Brown University Sciences Library, and to the Rhode Island Hospital Pharmacy Drug Information Service.

Other helpful colleagues and friends: David Abrams, Sally Ashworth, Kelly Brownell, Laura Brady, Richard Bump, Karen Carlson, Kenneth Coté, Elda Dawber, John DiOrio, Jr., Betty Fielder, Betty Wasielewski Harrington, Marcia Lawler, Jeannette Maynard, Barbara McCrady, Stephanie McKenna, Betsy Meyer, Bill Norman, Michael Norman, Patricia O'Sullivan, Olive Osborn, Lee Quattrucci, Judy Quattrucci, Melinda Small, Mark Smith, Michael Stein, Dominick Tammaro and Marion Wachtenheim.

The Wayland Collegium of Brown University provided initial support for our work. Professors Lucile Newman and Sally Zierler were especially helpful.

Ocean Coffee Roasters has been a relaxing "second office" for many of our meetings. We would like to thank Carol Grande in particular.

We thank our families, to whom this book is dedicated.

We have changed the names and identifying data of our patients; we would like to thank them, as well as other women who have shared their stories with us.

We dedicate this book to our families:

David A. Ames, John W. Ames and Robert Landau Ames
and
Alice and Henry Landau, Rosemarie Landau Helmbrecht
Richard J. Landau and Victoria J. Landau

Gregory J. Towne and Benjamin Cyr Towne
and
Nancy M. Cyr, Maureen C. Cyr and Mark G. Cyr
and
in memory of Francis J. Cyr

John, Katharine and Peter Murphy
and
Henry, Elizabeth, Sara and Peter Moulton

CONTENTS

✦ PREFACE

"WOMEN BEWARE! IF YOU'RE NOT MENOPAUSAL NOW, YOU WILL BE someday and you're sure to hate it!" This is the message that the three of us were hearing in 1992, and it motivated us to write this book. In numerous books, magazines, medical journals and conferences, we were being told that menopause is a difficult time and one to be feared. But this message did not match our experiences. Seven years ago, the three of us founded a women's health practice, Women's Health Associates, in conjunction with the Brown University School of Medicine's Department of General Internal Medicine at Rhode Island Hospital. We see adult women of all ages in our practice and have come to quite a different conclusion. Menopausal women may have special needs, but we are more impressed by their resourcefulness and strength. We do not see menopause as any type of pathology, but instead, as another creative stage of women's lives.

We created Women's Health Associates in response to the needs of many of our patients that we were seeing from other practices. We knew that women needed a place to come for their primary medical care. We knew that women today are among the most sophisticated health care consumers, who want to make their own decisions based on up-to-date information. We also knew that women needed comprehensive care to talk over concerns, be heard, and make informed treatment decisions. And we knew that women wanted to be able to come to a comfortable setting, where they would be free to focus on issues of prevention. Women want to maintain health, as well as to have a place to go when suffering from an illness.

We created an environment not only where women would be free to ask questions about their health, but where we would encourage their questions. We created an environment where primary care internists work side by side with clinical psychologists, gynecologists, nurse practitioners and nutritionists. We all work together and refuse to parcel out a woman's health by her organs. Our interest, then, is in the overall lives of women, not in their bodies alone. Our top priority at Women's Health is to maintain a setting where clinicians and patients can listen to each other and learn from each other. We have developed long-term relationships with many of our patients over the years, and they have shared their experiences with us, as well as their medical concerns.

When it comes to menopause, we have learned the most from our patients. Previously we had not known how frightened women are about menopause. When we started teaching and writing about menopause, many women who were *pre*menopausal would grimace and say, "Oh yuck!" Yet *post*menopausal women would often shrug and say, "No big deal." Since we have seen hundreds of women between the ages of forty-five and fifty-five, we have come to appreciate the individuality of each woman's experience, and we have come to understand the resourcefulness that women share.

Our primary goal is to share this philosophy—that each woman has an individualized experience at menopause, but shares many commonalities with other women. Women do not need a simplistic approach to their health care at menopause or at any other time of life. What they do need is the maximum amount of information and freedom to make these important health care decisions.

So we wrote this book because we had the opposite point of view from that which drums up fears about menopause. It is time to present a more comprehensive approach, one that emphasizes the power of women. Writing this book has been an education in itself. One of our first projects was to give seminars about menopause in a variety of community settings. Each time we offered a seminar, it would quickly become filled to capacity. At first, each of us would give a twenty-minute presentation and leave time for questions. However, after the first two sessions, we found that we could never leave the auditorium because we were surrounded by women asking more and more questions. Finally we came up with the concept of "menopause town meetings." In these sessions, we condensed our introductory remarks to a total of a half hour, and just let women ask questions. And did we get questions! We heard hours and hours of questions and shared experiences. These town meetings have been exciting and empowering experiences for all of us. We have enjoyed them so much, in part because they have provided us with a wealth of new stories about women's lives. We have recorded all these questions and included them for you in the back of the book as a second appendix. This allows you to find information quickly.

We have also included a glossary at the back of this book that explains medical and psychological terms. We believe that definitions are important so that we can share a vocabulary. In this book, we will use language that is easy to understand. Frequently, the three of us challenge one another to "Speak English!" when one of us becomes too technical. Learning a new vocabulary is important because it helps us counter the prevailing prejudices about menopause in our society. By being as specific as possible, we can regain access to the information ourselves and form more educated decisions about the next phase of our lives.

✦ HOW TO USE THIS BOOK

The Complete Book of Menopause is your comprehensive guide providing the most recent information. Armed with this knowledge, you can defeat the fear factor and make your own decisions. In each chapter, we will provide you with the information about the changes associated with the menopausal years.

We see menopause as a natural series of gradual changes. We know that by providing information, most women will be reassured. This information can fall into three categories: the biological, the psychological and the social. All too often, there has been an overemphasis on the biological aspects of menopause. We see the three areas as interconnected. In addition, the misinformation about women's biology has then been incorrectly attached to misinformation about psychology and women's social lives as well. The changes we describe will use the biopsychosocial model. This comprehensive approach has been used to teach medical students for over forty years but is still sometimes neglected. It is hard to imagine a woman's life that is affected by biology alone, psychology alone, or social factors alone. The comprehensive approach is more accurate and more powerful.

The three areas are interconnected. Bill Moyers's recent public television series and book, *Healing and the Mind,* highlighted this comprehensive approach (Moyers, 1993). Visits to doctors often involve psychological issues. Menopause has medical and psychological components and they should be treated together. A woman does not need to be suffering from symptoms or an illness in order to benefit from seeing a physician. She does not need to have a diagnosable psychiatric disorder in order to benefit from seeing a psychologist, or other mental health professional. By viewing the biological and psychological factors together, and by learning how to modify them during menopause, a woman can take charge of her own health care.

We need to look at social issues as well. There is a hefty amount of prejudice against women, especially aging women, in many of the writings on menopause. We plan to correct that. This prejudice has led to an unfortunate negative attitude toward menopause. It is internalized by too many of us and can lead to unnecessary anxiety. A second result of social forces is the polarization of women into two camps. The hormone replacement therapy (HRT) camp essentially portrays menopausal women as deficient and needing to have their hormones replaced. Many of these writings also prescribe estrogen for symptoms that have been shown not to be related to a lack of estrogen. The other camp, the anti-estrogen camp, sees estrogen as an evil medication, promoted by some larger medical and economic forces that exploit women. We see both of these views as limited. The question of HRT is only one of many issues that we need to explore during menopause, but it is a critical one. There are arguments to be made on both sides of the HRT issue, but this is not a war; this is your *life.* So polarization is not the answer.

Our belief is that each woman needs to make her own decisions in a comfortable and anxiety-free environment. We want women to participate actively in their health care during each crucial stage of life. As women facing menopause today, we have a variety of choices, and we want to help you make these choices.

The choices you make should be based on the information we provide, as well as your own individual symptoms, values and common sense. We believe that the best way for you to make these decisions is to be an active reader. Take the material provided here and apply it to your own life. We have found that the best way to learn is through this interaction. We have provided self-assessments and guided questionnaires that can help you assess your own needs during the menopausal years. By participating in these exercises, you can begin to make some tentative choices about your health care.

In each chapter, we also want to empower you to be able to communicate better with your health care professional. Each chapter will provide new communication strategies for interacting with your health care provider in an assertive and clear fashion. You can take your new-found information, your tentative choices, and talk them over. Most women want and need to form a partnership with their physicians and health care professionals.

Through our teaching at the Brown University School of Medicine, we have learned that communication is key. We have learned that women in particular value this communication and want to maximize each visit with their physicians. Many menopausal women visit their doctors primarily because they do not know what to expect during the menopausal years, not because they are suffering from any symptom. We want to respond to this concern. We understand this concern as well, because all of us are patients, as well as doctors. We know how it feels to be concerned about our health and to need information. We know that you are reading this book not only to learn about your own menopause but to learn how to deal with doctors, and we plan to help you do just that.

One study on doctor-patient communication revealed that over half of patients' complaints were not elicited by physicians, so we can't count on physicians to help us bring up our most pressing concerns (Todd, 1989). We have to identify them ahead of time. These communication issues are unfortunate. The three of us spend much of our time as faculty working with physicians during their medical residency, in order to improve their communication skills. We supervise these young doctors to help them become better listeners and to help them identify with patients' concerns. But in this book, we use similar strategies, and provide you, the patient, with a way to communicate better with your doctor. We know that being a patient can make you feel powerless and anxious at times. The suggestions in each chapter can help you regain feelings of control and competence about your own health care decisions.

Dr. Sherrie Kaplan at the New England Medical Center found that although women ask questions more often than men, the average patient asks less than four questions during a fifteen-minute office visit. Dr. Kaplan suggests that we prepare for the office visit by thinking through our concerns (Stark, 1992). Yet the anxiety-provoking nature of these doctor-patient encounters makes it difficult to process complicated information. Numerous researchers have written about the "data overload" that you get during an appointment. It is most important then to go to your appointment with a specific list of information and questions that you would like addressed. There is nothing wrong with taking notes before your visit and using them if you need to during the visit in order to talk with your clinician. In fact, many women use the list just as a "prompt" immediately before the appointment. Another way of coping with this data overload is to bring a friend or family member with you to the visit as some of our patients do. This is completely appropriate and quite common, especially if you are concerned about a specific problem that causes you significant anxiety.

As patients, we can try to approach the encounter with as much clarity as possible. Dr. Howard Beckman of Wayne State University studied over seventy patients and found that the beginning of the visit was a key time. When the doctor asked the patient, "What can I do for you?" Beckman's research found that the patient was interrupted on the average only eighteen seconds into the interview! (Beckman, 1984). No wonder patients might ask only four questions. We are amazed that they can manage to question that much after having been interrupted so early in the conversation. From this research we can learn two things: First, we should make our most important concerns known immediately. Second, we might need to be assertive in order to avoid being interrupted. It is a good idea, however, to try to be as succinct and clear as possible by thinking through your concerns ahead of time. Health care professionals, too, are under pressure. As health care providers we know that often we cannot share with patients the reasons for our pressure. The patient before you may have been twenty minutes late. Early in the day there may have been an emergency. This does not excuse clinicians who are routinely late, or excuse at all those who might be rude. But it is important to remember that health care professionals do have stresses outside of the examining room.

We know that as women you are aware of some of these issues. Patients are often concerned about their doctor's feelings. As women we've been taught our whole lives to be worried about the other person's feelings. Yet, if we do so in the doctor-patient interaction, we are often likely to become disappointed and perhaps resentful because our needs have not been met. Physicians have their own issues and may well be doing their best in communicating with us, but may not be answering our specific questions, or meeting our needs of that particular visit. In our residency training program, we focus on teaching physicians to be sensitive and to try to address the patient's agenda directly. However, many physicians have not been trained in this way and have a wide range of communication styles. Many are skilled interviewers and kind listeners; others can be abrupt and dismissive.

If the problem is embarrassing, it is important to address it anyway. We all feel vulnerable during the doctor-patient interaction, and when we are sick, it is extremely difficult to be "assertive." But it is possible to try and be clear. For example, an overweight woman might be afraid to talk to her doctor about chest pain, fearing that she will get a lecture about her weight. Nonetheless, that symptom is important and the doctor really does want to know about it.

It is also important to remember that you and your physician are only two members of the health care team. You may not be seeing a physician as your primary care provider but may be seeing a physician's assistant or a nurse practitioner. There is almost always a nurse or physician's assistant in the physician's office and she or he can answer your questions if you need to call back to get clarification. Health maintenance organizations offer many educational programs about specific problems like menopause. Many group practices also have clinical psychologists and other mental health professionals. Pharmacists can answer your questions about medication.

Another emphasis in the book is communication with families, so each chapter also contains a section on how to communicate about specific issues with family members. Problems in communications are the most frequent complaints presented to marital and family psychotherapists. The typical dynamic experienced by women is that their husbands don't listen to them and do not share feelings. However, their husbands often respond by saying something like, "I don't understand. I talk to her more than anyone else and she is my best friend." A man may feel most in touch when he is giving advice, while what his wife really wants is for him to listen and be empathic. Menopause can exacerbate this dynamic because many women feel particularly vulnerable and in need of support. At the same time, men are often going through their own transitions and are confused by their wives' concerns.

Similar types of communications problems exist in other communications patterns, between a woman and her lover, her friends and her children. We do not make the erroneous assumption that many books make, addressing women as if everyone is white, heterosexual and married for the first time. The present American experience is much more diverse. We find that all women can feel more connected to their friends and families when they can clearly identify their needs. We make specific suggestions for how to talk to spouses, partners, family members and friends about menopausal symptoms and midlife issues.

Communicating with other women about menopause is another crucial support system. Self-help groups and other resources are available to women. Often, just by acknowledging that hot flashes are driving you crazy, you will feel better. You will know that it might be time to take a walk with a friend who is a good listener. Or, your concerns about sexuality might be a signal that you need to discuss them with your partner or spouse. One of the gifts we have received from our patients is the knowledge that as women we have tremendous strength in our ability to change. Perhaps because we focus on relationships and put concerns for others first, we usually manage to go through life and make successful choices. Our strengths as women have led us to share problem-solving techniques and feelings with one another. It is important to remember that as women, we have long been experts at providing information for our family and providing support for one another.

The last part of the communications section in each chapter deals with resources. You will be amazed at how many resources there are for menopausal women. Pamphlets and educational materials are published by numerous foundations and self-help groups and are usually easy to read and free of charge. Menopause newsletters can put you in touch with a network of women who are eager to share information and support.

While we are on the subject of resources, let's remember that we all have many internal resources, as well as resources that we share with other women. We cannot let women be denied the opportunity that men have—that is, to approach our middle years with dignity and optimism. We can learn from lives of other women. Each chapter of this book will tell you the stories of many women—women from our practice, women who are our friends and colleagues, and women in literature and biography. We will mention only two for now. Janet Reno was named Attorney General of the United States while we were writing this book. A prosecutor in Dade County, Florida, for many years, Reno has led an active and exciting life. Prior to her accepting the nomination as attorney general, she had taken care of her mother who was in failing health and whom Reno describes as her best friend. This remarkable woman speaks passionately about the needs of women and children in her new role as attorney general. When the major networks complained because of her lack of makeup, Reno responded, "Like I can't go on their T.V. network unless I look good?" (Perspectives, 1993). Finally, a woman has enough power to challenge unreasonable expectations and to speak up! Janet Reno is clearly thriving at the age of fifty-three.

Also remember Margaret Sanger, one of the founders and leaders of the birth control movement in the United States. She was tireless in her work. When she was in her fifties, she was smuggling European-made diaphragms into the United States. This came after a career that had already spanned twenty years, and after she had launched a radical newspaper called *The Women Rebel* (Conway, 1992).

Yes, our lives change during our menopausal years, but there is nothing wrong with change. Change can bring new freedom and new power. Our work as founders of one of the nation's first women's health practices has taught us to value the lives of midlife women. Their stories are sometimes difficult, always moving and, ultimately, profoundly optimistic in their demonstration of the strengths of the female experience. We have developed a point of view best expressed by Ursula LeGuin:

> "It seems a pity to have a built-in rite of passage and to dodge it, evade it and pretend nothing has changed. That is to dodge and evade one's womanhood, to pretend one's like a man. Men, once initiated, never get the second chance. They never change again. That's their loss, not ours. Why borrow poverty?" (LeGuin, 1976)

The Complete Book of Menopause

CHAPTER ONE

The Natural History of Menopause

MENOPAUSE. IF YOU ARE LIKE MOST AMERICAN WOMEN, THE WORD fills your heart with dread. You don't know what to expect. You are worried—worried about hot flashes and disabling symptoms, worried about your sex life and worried about the rest of your life. Most of all, you are confused about whether or not to take hormone replacement therapy. But here is the good news: The negative aspects of menopause have been overstated dramatically, while the positive aspects have been virtually ignored. As you read on, you will find that the more you learn about the real facts concerning menopause, the better you will feel. And you will realize that with our comprehensive medical-psychological approach, you will be able to make good decisions about your health and you will enjoy the next ten years and more.

The next *ten* years? This phrase may strike you as odd since many women see menopause as some single threshold that we cross over. You don't just wake up one morning and become menopausal. Menopause is a natural, normal, developmental phase of a woman's life. Menopause is *not* a disease. It is the third major biological change in a woman's life, the last of the naturally occurring transitions. It is also the transition for which we receive little preparation. First, at menarche, or the onset of the menstrual cycle, we were given a pink pamphlet. It had floral borders and was titled something like "What Every Girl Must Know." The pamphlet introduced us to our reproductive system by providing a diagram of the uterus and ovaries and explaining the menstrual cycle. Later in our lives, books on pregnancy and childbirth provided a tremendous amount of information regarding the changes of the second transition many women experience as mothers. Until recently, there has been little written about menopause, the third transition. By helping you understand the natural course of menopause, you will be able to know what to expect and more importantly, what you don't need to worry about.

For most women the menopausal years are composed of three parts over about ten years. Figure 1-1 shows you the phases of the menopausal years. The perimenopause usually begins in the mid-forties. Menstrual periods become irregular, often closer together. At this time, many women begin to have hot flashes. This phase usually lasts about four years. We believe that the perimenopausal period deserves more attention. The onset of hot flashes can be extremely disturbing to some women, especially before they realize that the transition has begun. Some of the research about menopause suggests that some women begin to have problems with mood swings during this period. Most women are greatly relieved when they find that they have begun the perimenopausal period and that there is nothing else wrong with them.

Menopause itself is actually defined as the permanent end of menstrual periods which occurs when the ovaries stop producing hormones. Only in retrospect can anyone be certain that menstrual periods have permanently ended, since they may become very infrequent before they completely stop. Menopause is a gradual, natural process. Even if a woman's periods do end suddenly, without any warning (and this happens to 10 percent of women), the process leading to this has been a gradual reduction of the hormones produced by the ovaries. Previously, physicians diagnosed menopause if a woman had had no menstrual periods for twelve months, was not pregnant and was of the appropriate age, typically between forty-eight to fifty-five years. The lack of menstruation does not precisely define the change in hormone levels, and for that reason it is important that hormonal levels be tested. More recently, physicians have considered the diagnosis of menopause after there have been no menstrual periods for only six months. The average age of menopause is fifty-one.

Women are considered postmenopausal after the menopausal transition has occurred. We find postmenopausal women to be ex-

FIGURE 1-1
THE MENOPAUSAL YEARS

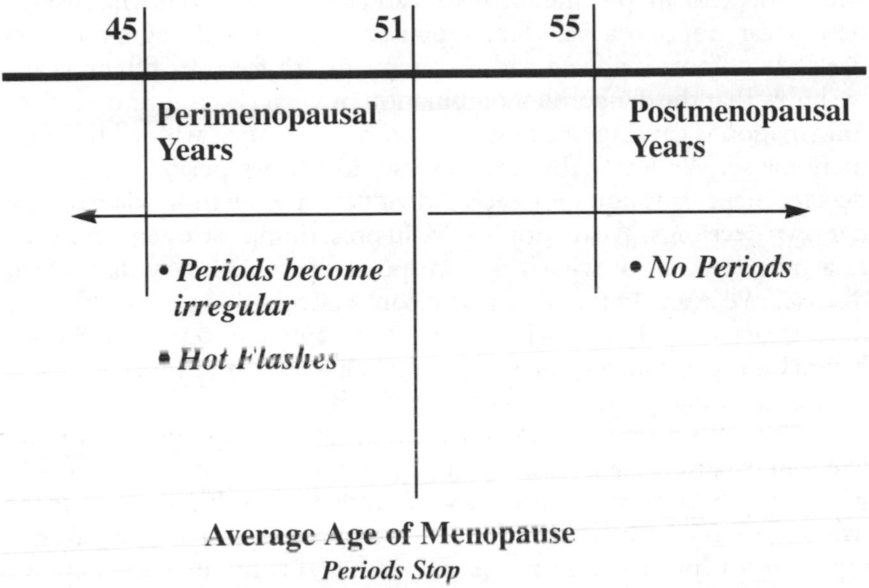

45	51	55
Perimenopausal Years		**Postmenopausal Years**
←		→
• *Periods become irregular*		• *No Periods*
• *Hot Flashes*		

Average Age of Menopause
Periods Stop

tremely generous in helping younger women understand menopause. When one of our wise postmenopausal friends heard that a younger woman expressed anxiety about menopause, she replied, "Menopause should be the worst thing that happens to us!" Here is another well-kept secret. Postmenopausal women are often like midlife men in one key way—they have more power! Many are free of family responsibilities for the first time in many years. Other women continue to cope with multiple family responsibilities but feel a new sense of energy during midlife. Whatever the situation, postmenopausal women can come into their own. We need only to think of Sandra Day O'Connor, Maya Angelou and Beverly Sills, just to name a few—not to mention Margaret Mead, who first coined the term "postmenopausal zest,"—to know that the postmenopausal years can be a time when we can be free at last.

These are the stages for women who experience menopause naturally. Hysterectomy and oophorectomy, or the removal of the uterus and the removal of the ovaries, brings on a sudden and dramatic change in hormone levels. Women who have had hysterectomies and oophorectomies, then, go through quite a different set of changes. Many articles about menopause confuse symptoms of natural menopause with those of oophorectomy. It is important to know that they are different. We discuss those differences in Chapter Nine, "Hysterectomy."

The contrast in attitudes between women who are premenopausal and those who are postmenopausal lead us to believe that what we see here is fear, not only a fear of menopause, but a fear of the aging process itself. As doctors involved with women's health for over fifteen years, we know that the dangerous combination of a fear of aging and a lack of information is causing needless anxiety. Most women will sail through menopause. We know that menopause, like other periods of human development, is unique for each individual. A woman needs to make her own decisions. We do not believe in prescribing estrogen wholesale as a miracle cure for what has been portrayed as a newly discovered disease. We want women to participate actively in their health care during each crucial stage of life. As women facing menopause today, we have a variety of choices, and we want to help you make those choices by providing unbiased and empowering information.

Although we can't tell you exactly what your menopause will be like, our experience has helped us understand what natural menopause will bring for most women. Since we founded a health care practice for women, we have treated hundreds of women using a medical-psychological team approach. Based on our work and combined research, we have come to understand the menopausal years. Our principal message to you is this: Do not expect major debilitating problems. It is going to be okay and you are going to be fine. It's just like our patients tell us: most women thrive during the menopausal years. The apprehension of this natural period in your life will most likely outweigh any real discomfort you will actually experience. So the tremendous fear and anxiety are unnecessary. The road to overcoming these fears and anxieties is to understand fully what menopause signifies. By doing so, you will dispel the many myths of menopause that have affected all of us. In fact, contrary to the stereotype, only 10 percent of all menopausal women find it to be a major disruption to their lives. Most everyone else finds it troubling at times, but certainly not a major problem. You may well have some symptoms, but they can be treated. Here is what will happen.

✦ WHAT WILL HAPPEN BIOLOGICALLY DURING MENOPAUSE?

The definitive study of the natural history of menopause has been conducted by epidemiologist Sonja McKinlay and sociologist William

McKinlay and their associates at the American Institute for Research. Their Massachusetts Women's Health Study followed 2,500 women ages forty-five to fifty-five for a ten-year period. Overall, they found that menopause was not a particularly problematic time for most women. One of their intriguing findings was that most women have neutral or negative feelings *before* menopause, but that feelings become more positive as women actually experience menopause (McKinlay and others, 1987). The first step toward developing a positive and more realistic attitude toward menopause is to understand our biology.

The change in our menstrual cycle occurs because of a decline in one of our female hormones, estrogen. Estrogen is produced by our ovaries. The ovaries gradually stop producing estrogen as our egg supply dwindles. The female baby begins life with approximately 400,000 eggs in her ovaries (they are *very* small). After the onset of menstruation, each month, approximately 1,000 eggs will try to develop but only one per month will be successful. Over a lifetime, about 400 eggs will be released to the tubes for possible fertilization. And sometime between the ages of forty-five and fifty-five, the eggs will be gone.

But the demise of these eggs is not a big deal. Unfortunately, all too often the medical profession, by continuing to use negative terminology about menopause, suggests that this biological change is, by necessity, a loss. A lecture at a major medical school included the sentence, "The ovary is the most precisely doomed organ in the human body." Menopausal women are accused of experiencing "ovarian failure." But rather than focusing on menopause as a negative, we can see it as a positive. Thus, we should not be talking about "ovarian failure" when we mean natural menopause. The ethicist Mary Mahowald has reviewed the overly negative vocabulary about menopause and points out that an organ is only doomed for a woman who has experienced herself primarily as a reproductive entity. If she has no interest in children in the first place, or if she has raised her children, then the lack of ovarian functioning should not be called ovarian failure but rather, "ovarian fulfillment," or perhaps "ovarian success" (Mahowald, 1992). It is important for all of us to counter this bleak outlook by expressing ourselves in more accurate and often humorous phrases.

✦ WHAT SYMPTOMS ARE COMMON?

We can certainly expect some hot flashes. Hot flashes begin before menopause, during the perimenopausal phase. Estimates vary, but anywhere between 30 percent to 80 percent of menopausal women will have a hot flash. This symptom is a sudden sensation of heat rising to the top of one's head and the upper part of the body. When the hot flash is over, a woman may begin to shiver. Most women who experience hot flashes are upset by the unpredictable and uncontrollable nature of them. The sweating and sudden temperature changes can also be disruptive to sleep patterns and some women visit their physicians for the related problem of insomnia.

One fact is clear: The hot flash is the hallmark of the menopausal experience. Interestingly, there are some cross-cultural differences in the experience of these symptoms. It is not clear that women in all cultures are plagued by the experience of hot flashes. Studies vary, but one compared Japanese and Canadian women. In this study, only 20 percent of Japanese women, in contrast to over 60 percent of Canadian women, reported hot flashes (Lock, 1991). These results could be explained by differences in diet and the use of naturally occurring estrogens like ginseng. It is also possible that Japanese women may be reticent about reporting such a symptom, or that Japanese women did not perceive the hot flash itself as negative. The same article suggested that many Japanese people believe that menopausal women should not be working outside of the home, so that they can take care of their aging parents. Some Japanese women, therefore, might believe they were self-indulgent even to discuss their hot flashes (Lock, 1991). In some cultures where older women are revered and have a special place in the society, menopausal symptoms are reported less often. So cultural differences are one of the many sociological factors that can affect symptoms at menopause.

The precise reason and physiological mechanism for hot flashes is unclear and we explore the possibilities in Chapter Two. Hot flashes may last for a period of months or up to a period of seven years. When they are severe and frequent they can be difficult. The most effective treatment for hot flashes is short-term hormone replacement therapy (HRT) described in great detail in chapters Two and Six. There are some other treatments as well. On the other hand, many women find hot flashes to be minimal, time-limited and thus are not an issue of great concern. If we were to wager on one symptom that you would have during menopause, it would be hot flashes.

A second common concern of menopausal women is vaginal dryness. Vaginal dryness is a gradual change that can be treated either with estrogen replacement therapy or with topical lubricants, and for most women is not a serious problem. It is a symptom that may occur suddenly in the case of surgical removal of the ovaries, but for those experiencing natural menopause it usually takes years to become noticeable. Vaginal dryness can be more of a problem to postmenopausal women who do not take hormone replacement therapy or use lubricants and who are not sexually active. Vaginal dryness can be uncomfortable, but it is not traumatic and should not be used as evidence of some dreaded "sexual decline." Some psychoanalytic authors have done women a tremendous disservice in not only emphasizing the problem of vaginal dryness but also in linking the biological changes of the reproductive system with psychological changes. The psychoanalyst Helene Deutsch and her views on the psychology of women have had devastating effects on midlife women. She connected the supposed physical decline of women in their forties and fifties to a lack of emotional warmth. Her words are frightening: ". . . everything she acquired during puberty is now lost piece by piece, and with the lapse of reproductive services, her beauty vanishes and usually the warm vital flow of feminine emotional life as well" (Deutsch, 1945, p. 461). There is no truth to this notion, but unfortunately, such prejudices remain throughout the medical care system and in American culture as well.

The last category of symptoms is called miscellaneous because there is a variety of symptoms that can occur in addition to hot flashes and changes in sexuality. We caution you here that although it is important to list some of these symptoms, you should not *expect* them to occur. The danger here is that any symptom can be connected to menopause when it may well be a random event or simply the result of the aging process. The fact is that many women go to physicians at the time of menopause rather than at earlier stages in their lives, and thus their symptoms, which may be long-standing, may be identified at this time. Some of the symptoms include headaches, mood changes, joint pain and fatigue. There are other changes in women that are associated with the aging process including hair changes, skin changes and a change in muscle tone. To some extent, these changes are affected by estrogen decline at menopause, but they are more often a result of the natural aging process. Yet what is important to remember is that this multiplicity of symptoms tends to be much less frequent and much less severe than either hot flashes or vaginal dryness. The most important consistent symptom is the hot flash. For this reason, one menopause newsletter is aptly named *Flash*.

✦ WHAT WILL HAPPEN PSYCHOLOGICALLY?

Psychological changes at menopause are usually based on our previous choices and our present relationships, and have little to do with hormones. Contrary to the popular stereotype of being "finished at forty or fifty," there is little evidence that midlife as defined as the forties or the fifties is necessarily a period of true crisis for men or women. In addition, many of the books on "life span" have assumed that women's development is just like men's. These theorists tend not to take into account that women make many specific choices that focus more on family issues and relationship issues. Given this family orientation, women may experience *more* freedom at the time of menopause, after their children have grown, rather than experiencing any sense of decline. In fact, studies of marriage reveal that the forties and fifties are the period of the second-highest level of satisfaction in marriages (the highest level is the prechildren era).

Some women, especially during the perimenopausal period, have sudden mood changes. We see this as some possible psychological vulnerability to the changes that women are beginning to experience. This fluctuation is similar to premenstrual syndrome (PMS). There are some anecdotal reports that suggest that women who have had difficulty with PMS also have difficulty with mood swings during menopause (Sherwin, 1993). However, mood swings do not constitute a serious clinical depression. The mood swings associated with perimenopause tend to be sudden but minor, and can be handled.

Depression, on the other hand, is a serious, psychological problem distinct from menopause that will often require psychological treatment. We discuss depression at length in Chapter Seven. There is no such thing as a menopausal depression, but the erroneous belief that hormonal changes cause depression persists. Many women believe that menopause causes some horrendous sudden depression. This may be a problem of definition, because of the mood swings associated with the perimenopause. True clinical depression is something else. It involves a more overwhelming and persistent feeling of sadness, combined with other symptoms such as weight loss, sleep disturbance, and difficulties in concentration. When we look at true clinical depression, there is no increased risk at the time of menopause. In fact, younger women are at greater risk for depression.

For the menopausal women who do become depressed, there is no evidence that changes in hormones cause the depression. Studies of women who have become depressed during their menopausal years have found a link with such social stressors as unhappy relationships and coping with aging parents. These women, as studied by the McKinlays, had multiple sources of worry. These worries and social factors, not differences in hormones, seemed to be directly related to the depression (McKinlay and others, 1987).

We do not underestimate the problem of depression in American women in today's society. Many women are depressed during their menopausal years, just as many women are depressed in any point in the life cycle. We outline treatments for depression in Chapter Seven, but you should not approach menopause with the view that the hormonal changes at that time cause clinical depression.

✦ WHAT WILL HAPPEN SEXUALLY?

Sexuality depends on the quality of your relationship, the stress in your life, your health and your attitudes toward sex in general. Obviously there is tremendous variability in these factors in the lives of menopausal women. Some women have been in sexual relationships with men for over thirty years when they reach menopause. Others are beginning to date again. Some are relating sexually to women, either for the first time, or in long-term relationships. So it is difficult to say what will happen to women sexually during menopause. There are a few reports of women who reported a decrease in their sexual interest, or their libido, during the menopausal years, but overall, this is not true for most women. There are some biological changes, though, during menopause that may impact on the sexual relationship.

The first issue is that vaginal dryness can cause discomfort during intercourse. This can be a definite problem sexually but can be treated with topical lubricants or hormone replacement therapy. However, some of the reports that we have read written by men, insisting that women be placed on estrogen because of this problem alone, strike us as being overly phallocentric in their concerns. We believe that vaginal dryness, with respect to sexuality, should not be categorized as the woman's problem, but that it should be seen in the context of a relationship. For example, many women are in long-term marriages to men and the men are having sexual changes as well. One male change is that the hormones are no longer sent out in pulses rising and falling in a daily rhythm, but become more consistent. The concentration of testosterone remains the same all day long rather than peaking early in the morning and subsiding later in the day. At the same time, men's sexual responses slow down and it takes longer for them to attain an erection and longer to reach climax. For some couples, this change can be positive, especially in the case when the man has had previous problems with premature ejaculation.

Thus, rather than identifying women as suffering from menopausal deficiency, it is more important to view men and women alike within the context of aging. Adaptation to these changes in sexuality can often be associated with very positive changes in a relationship. Some of the biological changes in menopause can actually force couples to communicate. An informal study of lesbian women also suggests that the ability to share feelings about sexuality, and the ability to communicate, may be more important than any biological changes.

One woman told us that she did not have time to worry about sexuality at menopause because she had just fallen in love with a younger man and had a great sex life. Isabel Allende tells us, "My husband and I got together very late in our lives and we discovered a passionate love affair. There is passion for older women in midlife. Absolutely!" (Rountree, 1993, p. 157).

So, the reports of the death of the libido at menopause have been greatly exaggerated. This is not a common symptom, but even for women who do have a decrease in sexual interest, there are many treatment options. We discuss them in Chapter Three.

It is true that hormone replacement therapy and/or topical lubricants will treat the problem of vaginal dryness that occurs during menopause. Other studies suggest the "use it or lose it" phenomenon. That is to say that continued sexual functioning can, in and of itself, help the sexual adjustment during menopause. Some women, when faced with some minor sexual problems, withdraw from sexuality and this can be a serious problem. In contrast, by continuing to remain sexually active, not surprisingly, sexual adjustment can be positive.

By now you are probably worried about what you can do about all this. The answer is, in short, a lot! The menopausal years provide us with many choices and opportunities to change and improve our health.

Although estrogen has been promoted as the cure to the "menopausal disease," it is only one option for treating some of the symptoms of menopause. This book will help you decide whether or not you want to proceed with hormone replacement therapy. Too many books on menopause emphasize the issue of hormone replacement therapy alone, as if that alone will keep us young and prevent osteoporosis, coronary artery disease and hot flashes. Indeed, as described in Chapter Six, hormone replacement therapy can be beneficial for many women, but it is only one of many issues that should engage us. Equally important are our attitudes toward menopause and life changes, our overall health and our health care.

✦ MAINTAIN A POSITIVE ATTITUDE

There are many choices and challenges that we face in the menopausal years. Overall, the most important coping strategy is to maintain a positive attitude. By the time we are menopausal, we have been inundated with negative stereotypes from many sources. We all understand why any woman may come to menopause with a negative attitude. Until recently, we've seen little in the popular culture about menopause. Older women are virtually absent from television news programs and other types of entertainment. In the popular media, women are rarely seen in advertisements after the age of thirty-five, with the exception of advertisements for hair coloring products, diet programs, support bras, laxatives, denture cleaners, sleep preparations, and a sundry of other problem solving products. Interestingly, older women, such as in the popular television series *Murder She Wrote* with Angela Lansbury and the *Golden Girls,* have gained attention in the past few years, but middle-aged women in their late forties and fifties continue to be absent. This tells us something about our fears about this transitional period.

In the 1990s, menopause has become a hot topic on television. We did suffer through Edith Bunker's menopause in the 1970s, only to see her become "even more crazy" in dealing with her husband's verbal abuse. By the 1990s Julia Sugarbaker was allowed to go through menopause with humor on the television program *Designing Women.* Yet the negativism remains. In the television program *Sisters,* Teddy, a fashion designer in her late thirties, is distraught by the way she is being unjustly criticized by an older critic. Her response to this is to call a press conference where she sympathizes with the woman for having "such a difficult menopause." Now that menopause is in the public domain, it unfortunately serves as the brunt for hostility that is especially troubling when it is between women.

Even two recent books about menopause have had negative undercurrents. Gail Sheehy's book *The Silent Passage* brought the subject of menopause out into the open. But Sheehy overestimates the power of estrogen. "Within days the blue-meanie moods lifted, I was able to write for twelve hours straight on deadline . . . I was staggered by the potency of the female hormone" (Sheehy, 1992 p. 19). In addition, Sheehy's description of a group of women in Beverly Hills is strikingly lacking in empathy and by its detailed description of each woman physically, only emphasizes the myth that as women we must define ourselves either through our reproductive organs or through physical youth and beauty. She writes, "Surely what they all wanted to hear from me and Doctor Allen was that some magic regimen—yoga and yogurt, or yams and ginseng and green leafy vegetables—would allow them to remain as middle-aged women exactly as they had been: youthful wives, sexually appealing and responsive lovers, efficient career builders. They were not ready to consider a new self-definition" (Sheehy, 1991 p. 48). This "I am more self-aware than you are" approach, only feeds into our fear of aging rather than casts it aside. Although *The Silent Passage* ends with exhortations for a new life and growth, the overall tone of the book up until that chapter is so strikingly negative that it is hard for the reader to recover. When we recently discussed this book with one of our patients, we pointed out that the last chapter is positive and she replied, "Are you kidding? I quit reading long before then."

In Germaine Greer's *The Change*, the author contends that sexuality will probably end for most women and that our best bet is to retire to our herb garden, read books and become "crones" (Greer, 1992, p. 362). There are many problems with this analysis. The first is that Greer assumes that menopause must be a crisis. This is not the case, as documented by numerous longitudinal studies of women. The second problem is that Greer, although provocative and entertaining, has always been overly fixated on sexuality and has paid less attention to other aspects of women's development (Greer, 1970).

Although Greer is correct in noting that estrogen has a strong placebo factor, it has been shown to be more effective for stopping hot flashes than anything else. Since hot flashes are the most prevalent and the most troubling symptoms to many women, this is an important consideration, and Greer is doing us a disservice by overestimating the risks of hormone replacement therapy while also misjudging the use of natural substances. Greer is also in danger of becoming the Martha Stewart of menopause when she suggests that we should grow, collect *and* prepare our own herbs since, "Most dried herbs sold in commerce are not only old and valueless but can be contaminated" (Greer, 1992, p. 231).

So is it any wonder that we approach menopause with such negative beliefs? We have been taught that our ovaries are shrinking, our eggs are dying, we are going to become psychotically depressed and that our only hope is to take estrogen or become a crone and, let's face it, we *are* getting old! It does not matter that most of this is nonsense and that our alternative to becoming old is to die young. Given this choice, we should approach menopause with a sense of humor and with a commitment to maintain our health. Perhaps rather than bemoaning our fate, we should continue to enjoy life.

One way to not only enjoy the menopausal years but to rejoice in them is to read other women's stories. If we do so, we will learn that each of us is unique and that menopause may well be easier than other stages of life! Three books that have helped us listen to women are *Women of the Fourteenth Moon,* edited by Dena Taylor and Amber Coverdale Sumrall (Taylor and Sumrall, 1991), *Written By Herself,* edited by Jill Ker Conway (Conway, 1992) and *On Women Turning Fifty,* by Cathleen Rountree (Rountree, 1993). We learn, for example, from Cathleen Rountree's interview with the lawyer Gloria Allred who says, "I like being in my fifties. I don't think it's anything to be ashamed of. We should get medals for having survived what women have to go through to reach the age of fifty and the obstacles they face. It's a real test of survival" (Rountree, 1993, p. 63).

Changing our beliefs about menopause is critically important, for our physical, as well as our psychological well-being. A study by Dr. Myra Hunter in Great Britain reveals that a woman's belief in the negative stereotypes about menopause can be linked to depression (Hunter, 1990). Other studies have also documented this correlation: Women who fear menopause and have negative beliefs about it may well do worse than women who have an optimistic attitude. So it is our attitude and our outlook toward midlife and not our hormones that can lead us to sadness, depression and preoccupation with physical symptoms.

✦ PAY ATTENTION TO HEALTH, NOT ILLNESS

Menopause is a time when we need to pay attention to our overall health. For many women, menopause may be the first stage of life when there is enough leisure time to even consider sports and physical activity as part of a regular routine. For others, the beginning rumblings of our body, such as the beginnings of arthritis or a lack of energy, pinpoint that it is now time to pay attention. Exercise is a key factor in the prevention of osteoporosis and heart disease and in creating a feeling of general well-being. In fact, there is a strong interaction between physical and psychological health. People who are in good physical health are reporting the fewest psychological symptoms. A study of the readers of the journal *Melpomene: A Journal for Women's Health Research* revealed that these women found exercise to be an important source of satisfaction. In contrast to the average American woman, only 15 percent of these women said they were on a special diet, 9 percent in order to lose weight and 5.5 percent for other health reasons. This is in contrast to somewhere between at least 40 and 50 percent of the more general population of American women. The Melpomene women, to a large degree used physical activity as well as talking and individual time for themselves as a way to cope with stress (Lutter, 1992).

Our chapter on healthy bodies (Chapter Ten) emphasizes the need to pay attention to nutrition, exercise and to avoid substance abuse. We have no interest in becoming the "health police," to overburden you with too many prescriptions for a variety of health maintenance and exercise regimens. On the other hand, if you can find a specific physical activity that you enjoy, this can probably be one of the most important health decisions of your life.

Another way to focus on health is to accept that we do change as we grow older. Another story from *Women Turning Fifty* can help us here. Dolores Huerta is one of the founders of the United Farm Workers and has led an amazing life. As a young mother, she took her children with her when she worked with migrant farm workers. Now that Huerta is older she says, "I know that I will have to slow down some day, because I've seen it happen to other people. When I do reach that point, I'll be able to read books and do a different kind of activity" (Rountree, 1993, p. 133). She's not slowing down yet, though. When she was in her fifties, Dolores Huerta was beaten unconscious in a demonstration against George Bush in San Francisco. She survived.

✦ TAKE CHARGE OF YOUR HEALTH CARE

We have learned a lot from our menopausal patients. We have learned that women want information. They want a physician who will listen to them. They want access to other health care professionals as well. They want to be actively involved in choices regarding their own health. We will help you create your own Women's Health team in the last chapter of this book. For now, there are some general communications strategies that you can use to take charge of your health.

The typical physician-patient interaction puts the patient at a terrible disadvantage in communication. Many courses on effective communication emphasize nonverbal aspects including: eye contact, posture, gestures, dress, voice and natural expression. Now consider the typical doctor-patient interaction. In many cases a woman is seeing her male primary care physician. All too often she may be sitting at the edge of an examining table wearing a hospital johnny, feeling either too cold or too hot and is anxiously awaiting information about her health. The physician may be standing, fully clothed, looking down at the patient and is acting hurried. Even the best of communicators would find this situation untenable. The power dynamics are such that the woman patient is at an incredible disadvantage. The problems in doctor-patient, male-female communication can become so difficult that one study was aptly titled, "Intimate Adversaries" (Todd, 1989).

What to do? As a patient you have several choices. We suggest that you make an appointment specifically to talk to your physician. Many primary care physicians now schedule time with the patient (fully clothed!) for a consultation in the office. If this is not the normal procedure in the practice you go to, you have the opportunity and right to schedule such a visit. Another possibility is to specifically ask the physician to sit down after the physical exam is over. You can state that you would like to discuss some concerns and need a few minutes of his or her time. Not many physicians would say no to this request.

Remember the other members of the health care team—nurse practitioners, mental health professionals, physician assistants and pharmacists. All too often a woman is given a prescription being told, "take this for your blood pressure." One of the most important problems as we get older is that medications interact with one another, and can cause unexpected side effects. So you have the right to know the precise details of a medication plan, or regimen. Your physician should give you these details. If for some reason that does not happen, don't forget your pharmacist. Most pharmacists are very comfortable and eager to discuss the issues of medication with you. Some of the questions you might want to ask include: What will this medication treat? How should I take it? How many times a day? With food, or on an empty stomach? With water, or is water not important? If I decide to stop the medication, can I stop suddenly, or should I taper off? What will happen if I stop the medication? Are there other medications that I should not take while taking this one? Are there foods and beverages that I should avoid? Can I be exposed to the sun while taking this medication?

Studies have shown that over 50 percent of prescriptions filled each year are not always taken properly. Another study found that 50 percent of people on medications for a long period of time stopped taking their medication before they should have. Finally, 20 percent of prescriptions are never even filled (Katz, 1992). It is important then to know why and how to take the medication. If you have any reservations, it is much better to discuss them with your doctor, nurse or pharmacist than to become quiet and not let the physician know of your concerns.

By communicating clearly, setting your priorities for each appointment, and asking questions, you can take charge of your health care. You *can* take the power. In fact, many women come to our practice because they "just couldn't take it anymore," and were fed up with the previous health care system. Creating a new health care team with a new attitude can help you through this developmental period and can be one of your strongest support systems.

✦ LEARNING FROM THE EXPERIENCE OF WOMEN

So you want to know what your menopause will be like. What *can* you expect? We wish we could tell you exactly what your menopause would be like, because we know that you feel anxiety and that you would feel better if you could prepare. However, menopause is much more variable than other women's transitions like menarche or pregnancy. Each woman brings her own genetic background, her psychological issues and her social context to menopause. Her overall physical health is another issue. If you are like most women, you will be just fine, and you will experience a few hot flashes. You may have some other symptoms but the changes will be gradual, not dramatic and can be treated. To help you appreciate the variety in the menopausal experience, here are the short stories of four women who represent some of the possibilities during menopause.

• Allison is a forty-nine-year-old divorced woman who has returned to Brown University in the Resumed Undergraduate Education program. We have seen her on our way to meetings on campus, sitting on the Green, wearing a baseball cap, a comfortable sweatshirt and blue jeans, running shoes and obviously enjoying her studies in American History. She and her husband have been divorced for ten years, and her two children are grown and doing well.

Allison came to us originally because she was concerned about her blood pressure, which was at one time 160 over 116. She had had very few hot flashes and they were fleeting and not debilitating. Allison had not had a period in about six months. Allison was slightly overweight and there was no history of osteoporosis in her family. She did not smoke or drink. She was concerned about hormone replacement therapy because there was a family history of breast cancer in her mother and her aunt. Although Allison was doing quite well overall, she was terrified that menopause would cause her health to deteriorate. She came to us with a high level of anxiety.

We met with Allison in order to discuss her concerns. We reassured her that menopause, in and of itself, would not make her health deteriorate. Allison had believed many of the myths that we have discussed previously, and now experienced a great feeling of relief. We did share our concerns with Allison about her blood pressure. She was surprised to learn that it is heart disease that is the most significant cause of death for women over the age of fifty. Allison, upon hearing this news, became highly motivated to lower her blood pressure, and reduce any other risk factors for heart disease. She worked with our nutritionist to lower her fat intake and began a walking program. She was a woman who had never engaged in any physical activity and had little interest in aerobics or any activity that was strenuous. But she learned to enjoy walking and we now see Allison walking on a local boulevard two miles a day, three or four times a week.

Allison also appreciated the opportunity to think through the issues about hormone replacement therapy that we detail in Chapter Six. After thinking things over, and given her family history, she decided not to take hormone replacement therapy. Allison returns to see us now on a yearly basis, and is approaching her menopausal years with a new sense of optimism and commitment to her health.

• Gladys is an African-American woman who lives with her husband, three dogs and several cats. She and her husband are both retired from jobs in accounting firms. They had no children and are devoted to one another. Although they are not wealthy, they had saved quite a bit of money and enjoy traveling. Gladys, at age fifty, had serious problems with hot flashes. Her sleep was becoming disrupted, and she was feeling fatigued and out of sorts, something extremely unusual for her. Her husband came with her to her appointment and, after discussing the issues of hormone replacement therapy, Gladys decided to begin treatment. Her hot flashes stopped almost immediately and she was greatly relieved. Gladys is an example of a woman who benefited tremendously from hormone replacement therapy.

• Sarah is a forty-nine-year-old lesbian woman who is an advertising executive. She came to see us because she has begun to wake up sweating at night. Sarah has a history of panic attacks and is concerned that the stress of her high-powered job is affecting her mental health. We have seen Sarah for several medical and psychological sessions and have ascertained that she is generally in good health. But Sarah is a good example of someone who needs to work on problematic behaviors in order to preserve her health. Sarah smokes two packs of cigarettes a day. She functions well at work, and is content in her relationship of ten years. Her FSH (follicle-stimulating hormone) level is 42 MIU/ ml, indicating that Sarah may be entering menopause. We explained to her that smokers tend to have earlier menopause and that nicotine does not help at all with anxiety. Although Sarah uses smoking to cope with stress, she has agreed to consider a smoking-cessation program. We've worked with her to set a quit date and to explore a stress management program. Sarah does not wish to consider HRT at this time.

• June came to see us originally because of her concern for her twenty-one-year-old daughter. Her daughter had been a victim of date rape and was having terrible difficulty going back to college. We saw her daughter for a few sessions of psychotherapy and referred her to a psychotherapist located near her college. After her daughter returned to college, June talked more with us about her health and her concerns. Although June has been troubled by hot flashes, she has become increasingly depressed at the same time. Not only is she concerned about her younger daughter, but her older daughter is having difficulty in her marriage. June exemplifies some women who do become depressed during menopause. Although her hot flashes were one issue, another issue was June's multiple sources of worry. She was worried about both of her daughters, her husband's response to his unemployment and financial worries. We worked with June for several months, focusing on these issues. First, we taught her relaxation exercises to help deal with the hot flashes. In addition, she learned to dress in layers of clothing and to carry a fan with her. In order to help June develop more social support, we encouraged her to reach out to a neighbor who had been interested in establishing a deeper friendship with her. June and her neighbor now "walk and talk" every morning and have developed a close friendship. We helped her husband find career counseling, but he continued to have difficulty securing employment. June still has many difficulties but is coping better now through the techniques she has learned and through the social support she now enjoys.

These four women, from different lifestyles and backgrounds, all have some things in common. First, they all were eager to discuss the issue of menopause and to get as much information as possible. Each of them wanted to make the decision about hormone replacement therapy for herself. All of them benefited from relationships that they found supportive and felt great relief in talking about their problems with a friend or family member. These women viewed menopause not as a crisis but as a new phase in their lives. You will hear the stories of other women's lives as we go through each chapter.

We cannot forget Rae, who comes to see us for health care on an annual basis. She is enjoying menopause just as she has enjoyed other stages of her life. She loves working as a newspaper editor, she has a wide network of friends, and she is active in local politics. When we specifically ask her about menopause she looks puzzled, then smiles and responds, "No periods, remember?" Rae is having a great time. She reminds us that menopause is just part of life.

You will be able to think through the issues for maintaining your health as you read through each chapter of this book. But we have to remember to look at the big picture: as women, we have coped through earlier stages of life and we will cope and thrive during menopause as well. You have already met some of the women from our practice, and you know many menopausal women who are thriving. The fact is that we can rejoice in our menopausal years, enjoy life to its fullest and reach new heights. Our philosophy is that if we provide women with a comfortable health care environment, and with a maximum of information, women can use their resources to make important decisions. We can take charge of our health care in order to get relief from any menopausal symptoms. We can all use our internal and external resources to maintain our health and prevent health problems.

So now you know. Menopause brings a certain number of changes and in some cases, difficult symptoms. None of them are debilitating and most of them are not serious, but they can trouble you. As you read on, you will learn about each category of symptoms, and other issues that should concern us at midlife. You will learn that midlife brings with it a set of choices and that each of us can deal with these choices with help from our physicians, family and friends. Ultimately, we have as much control over menopause as we do over any other phase of our lives, and maybe even more. Read on.

CHAPTER TWO

Hot Flash!

DEATH, TAXES, AND NOW HOT FLASHES? WHILE IT IS TRUE THAT most menopausal women will experience hot flashes, we can be reassured that they are neither as inevitable as death, nor as bad as taxes. The only guaranteed consequence of menopause is the usually welcomed end of menstrual periods. Hot flashes are the second most predictable consequence of menopause but get more press because they are much more newsworthy than the last period. In fact, hot flashes are so common in the menopausal years that some have called them the calling card of menopause.

What is truly remarkable about menopausal hot flashes is the tremendous woman-to-woman variation. While Ethel, who is now ten years postmenopausal, concedes that she had years of hot flashes, she scoffs at their significance in her day-to-day existence. On the other hand, Victoria has been having hot flashes now for six years with only recent relief after doubling the dose of her estrogen patch. Pam was in the enviable position of experiencing not one hot flash in the eight years since she stopped menstruating, even without hormone replacement therapy.

We learn from these varied experiences that there is, in fact, no consistent pattern to menopausal hot flashes or any woman's reaction to them. One woman's "symptom" is a passing "sensation" to another. Unfortunately, this variability in the frequency and experience of hot flashes has created yet another opportunity to blame the victim. Women who do have debilitating hot flashes are often chided by their physician or family members for their poor tolerance, exaggeration of symptoms and inability to cope. Compounding the problem of individual variability in experience of hot flashes is the scientific community's poor understanding of them.

Not unlike premenstrual syndrome, hot flashes are poorly understood and are often discounted as yet another "female problem." Unlike premenstrual syndrome, however, there is a highly effective treatment which many physicians eagerly prescribe. While hormone treatment may be appropriate for many women, for many others it is unnecessary. What women really need is adequate information to make an informed decision about hormone replacement therapy and alternative methods of treatment rather than a prescription completed hastily as if to write off the entire problem. This chapter will give you the facts about hot flashes, including the lingo used to describe them, the likelihood that any woman will experience them, the consequences, the proposed causes and available treatments.

Despite the fact that hot flashes are so common, many women continue to be embarrassed by them. We prefer the approach of one of our patients, Kai, who is a professor at a small college. She dealt with her hot flashes with humor. When she began to sweat and turn red during a lecture she'd say to her students, "Let's take a break." She would then remove one of her carefully planned layers of clothing and her students would joke with her, calling these episodes "Flash Alerts."

✦ FLASHES, FLUSHES AND NIGHT SWEATS

The medical terminology that describes hot flashes is confusing, since the physicians who initially wrote about hot flashes chose to divide them into the subjective feelings of the patient, versus the objective measurable physiological changes. No other medical condition is so strictly divided into its subjective and objective aspects. Logically, the entire event could be designated as a *hot flash* and it is obscure why it is not. The experience of a heart attack is not divided into the subjective pain versus the objective electrocardiogram changes. Since you're reading this chapter, you might want to know how the medical profession describes hot flashes.

Hot *flash* refers to the subjective experience that precedes any measurable physiologic changes. Although there is considerable variability in the experience, most women first notice an intense feeling of warmth throughout the upper body. Some women additionally note an aura and state that they "just don't feel normal" prior to the onset of the actual warmth. These feelings may be accompanied by rapid or irregular heartbeats, headache, weakness, faintness, anxiety or dizziness. Most often, the entire episode ends with significant sweating and a cold clammy, chilled feeling.

In contrast, the hot *flush* constitutes the objective changes that occur during the episodes. In most cases, the hot flash precedes the hot flush. During the flush, there is visible redness of the upper chest, neck, face, followed by perspiration in the same areas. There is a measurable increase in skin temperature, blood flow and heart rate. Finger temperature increases as much as 6 degrees Centigrade during an episode. The skin temperature drops at sites where sweating occurs. (That is the whole point of sweating, after all.)

Now that you are familiar with the lingo, you may appreciate a story retold in *Women of the Fourteenth Moon*. It seems that a male gynecologist corrected a woman's use of the term "hot flash" saying, "No, dear, they are called hot flushes" to which she replied, "Well, dear, when *you* get one you can call it anything you want" (Parke, 1991, p. 7). You may want to use this line if you find yourself in a similar situation, then change doctors.

Night sweats are the nocturnal form of hot flashes. Most women who experience night sweats complain about them more bitterly than daytime flashes. Hot flashes are more frequent at night and may awaken women from sleep. This disturbance of sleep can, in turn, cause severe daytime fatigue, irritability, inability to concentrate and impaired memory. In 1981, Dr. Erlik and associates demonstrated that nighttime hot flushes, measured by increased skin temperture, are clearly associated with episodes of waking. The authors conclude that "the occurrence of waking episodes with hot flushes contributes to the insomnia seen in older women. This chronic sleep disturbance could alter psychological function." They add that estrogen probably improves mood and cognitive functions by eliminating night flushes (Erlik and others, 1981, p. 1744). We know that many women who have hot flashes at night complain of sleep disruption. They may awaken drenched in perspiration and be forced to get out of bed to change their clothes.

In their study of menopausal hot flushes and waking episodes, the same researchers found that women were awakened before any changes in skin temperature occurred (Erlik and others, 1981). These findings suggest that the subjective hot flash, rather than the discomfort associated with flushing and sweating, causes the sleep disruption. Many women can sleep through the hot flash experience, especially when they are in a cold room. This seems logical enough.

Vasomotor symptoms refer to the whole array of subjective and objective events that constitute hot flash, flush and night sweats. These refer to changes that occur in the circulation, including increased blood flow, temperature and heart rate.

✦ THE NUMBERS

Although almost 75 percent of menopausal women in the United States experience hot flashes, only 10 to 15 percent of women have symptoms that are severe enough to cause them to consult a physician (Kronenberg, 1993). Interestingly, there is tremendous cultural variation in the report of hot flashes among women, ranging from 25 to 85 percent. Japanese women report hot flashes much less frequently than women from Western cultures (Lock, 1991). Many now feel that the Japanese diet, high in naturally occurring plant estrogens, may account for these differences.

The occurrence of hot flashes is highest during the first two years after menopause and lessens with increasing years from the last menstrual period. Of the women who experience hot flashes, 85 percent will have them for more than one year and 20 to 50 percent for up to five years. Women who have surgical menopause (oophorectomy) often have frequent and severe hot flashes soon after their ovaries are removed (Kronenberg, 1990).

Hot flashes are not limited to perimenopausal or postmenopausal women. Guess what? Men can have hot flashes too. According to Drs. Isaac Schiff and Brian Walsh, hot flashes are a result of the sudden withdrawal of estrogen (Schiff and Walsh, 1989). Men often have hot flashes when they experience a sudden withdrawal of the male sex hormone, testosterone. One study found that 73 percent of men have hot flashes after the removal of their testicles to treat prostate cancer. Also, men who have other types of testicular insufficiency have also reported hot flashes. As many as two-thirds of premenopausal women may also experience hot flashes (Kronenberg, 1990). Many women have their first hot flashes after childbirth, presumably related again to the sudden drop in estrogen levels. When hot flashes occur before the end of menstrual periods, they signify that estrogen levels produced by the ovaries are reduced, but not enough to stop menstruation. Women who experience hot flashes while still menstruating need to have other causes of these symptoms, like hyperthyroidism, evaluated. Your health care professional can order a blood sample of hormone levels in order to diagnose menopause.

The good news is that hot flashes improve with time. Most women will be completely hot-flash free within five years of the last menstrual period. However, for some they can last for five years or more. There is little to predict which women will experience prolonged hot flashes. We do know that women who have surgical menopause when both ovaries are removed may experience more severe hot flashes for a longer period of time. So far, there has been no clear relationship established between the occurrence of hot flashes and a woman's menstrual history, including the age of her first period, the age of menopause or the number of pregnancies. Neither do a woman's employment status, social class, age, marital status nor workload predict hot flashes (Kronenberg, 1993). Even today, prejudices flourish, with hot flashes and other menopausal symptoms being seen as the self-indulgence of middle- or upper-class women. Women who experience hot flashes tend to weigh less than women who do not (Kronenberg, 1990). Since estrogen is stored in fat, women who have a higher percentage of body fat are likely to have a less dramatic decline in their estrogen levels at menopause. At last, the corpulent get revenge on the emaciated!

◆ ANATOMY OF A HOT FLASH

Hot flashes can occur any time during the day but seem to be most frequent from six A.M. to eight A.M. and six P.M. to ten P.M. This may be good news for the women who work outside their homes from nine A.M. to five P.M. and fear that hot flashes will interfere with their work (Doress and others, 1987). The frequency of hot flashes varies considerably from woman to woman, from day to day, from year to year. It appears that almost half of women in the forty- to sixty-year-age group report hot flashes on a daily basis. Far fewer report multiple hot flashes in a day, or as few as one hot flash per week (Kronenberg, 1990).

Researchers have tried to identify the factors that precipitate hot flashes. Stress usually leads the list of possible triggers of hot flashes, but this is still controversial (Kronenberg, 1993). One study was completed to specifically answer the question, "Does stress actually trigger

TABLE 2-1
If you have never had a hot flash, this is what it is like:

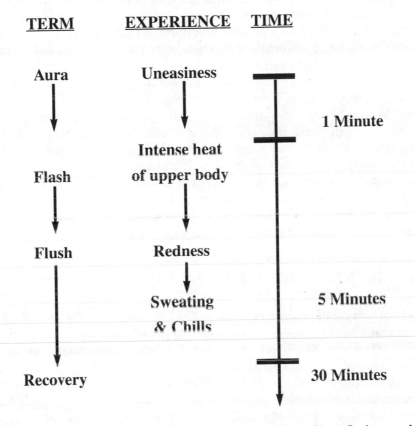

TERM	EXPERIENCE	TIME
Aura	Uneasiness	
		1 Minute
Flash	Intense heat of upper body	
Flush	Redness	
	Sweating & Chills	5 Minutes
Recovery		30 Minutes

hot flashes or does stress make women more aware of hot flashes and, therefore, more likely to report them?" The authors found that stress does not make women report more hot flashes but probably does cause a specific physiologic change that triggers them (Swartzman and others, 1990). Warm weather also triggers hot flashes and worsens both their intensity and frequency. Ethel recalls that she really didn't have time for hot flashes while caring for her failing father-in-law, but she did acknowledge fairly predictable hot flashes in the late afternoons of one summer. She recalls that it was "no big deal" and would get in her car, roll the windows down and go for a ride when she felt an impending flash. Ethel's story emphasizes that anything that can raise the normal body temperature can trigger hot flashes, including hot weather, hot drinks, rooms, beds, foods and alcohol.

The typical hot flash may begin with an aura—an initial sensation of uneasiness. Some women also report palpitations, headaches or dizziness. Many women are relieved when they learn that this experience is a prelude to a hot flash, not an anxiety attack. The aura is followed by a sensation of heat across the upper chest, neck, face and head. This sensation usually precedes the flush by less than a minute. The flush is heralded by redness in the same distribution that lasts for several minutes. Sweating, accompanied by chills, often follows. The total duration of a typical hot flash and flush is five minutes. Although dramatic flashes and flushes last only five minutes, it may take a woman approximately thirty minutes to return to normal (Budoff, 1983).

While there is a fair amount of uniformity in the experience of an individual hot flash and flush, there is very little consistency in the frequency, intensity and duration of hot flashes for women. Our experience with our patients has shown us the variety of women's experiences. Whereas Sue is completely thrown by her night sweats, Jenna uses them as a time to get up, stretch for a while and then return to bed. One difference between these women is that Jenna can make her own hours and Sue has an eight-thirty to five job.

◆ THE MYSTERY OF HOT FLASHES

It is quite remarkable that as late as 1978 investigators wrote, "Rather surprisingly, the flush has received very little scientific investigation. The rationale for estrogen treatment has been questioned with some justification" (Sturdee and others, 1978, p. 79). Alas, the specific biochemical cause of hot flashes and flushes remains elusive even now. Certainly the slow start to investigate the basis of hot flashes has contributed to this problem, and we have made relatively little progress even with the intensified study in the 1980s.

It was initially assumed that a lack of estrogen was solely responsible for hot flashes. Yet women who have had no estrogen production from birth do *not* suffer from hot flashes. It has become clear that it is the relative drop in estrogen levels that causes hot flashes. As with other substances that cause symptoms, when they are withdrawn, the body becomes accustomed to the presence of estrogen and its disappearance causes a disequilibrium.

More specifically, the levels of female hormones are regulated very carefully by the feedback loop between the blood and two sensing areas of the brain known as the pituitary gland and hypothalamus. Both areas respond to low levels of estrogen by increasing the hormones that they produce. The pituitary gland produces luteinizing hormone (LH) and follicle-stimulating hormones (FSH), which are the hormones typically measured to diagnose menopause. The hypothalamus produces gonadotropin-releasing hormone (GRH), which acts on the pituitary gland to produce FSH and LH in response to low estrogen levels. Initially, researchers believed that the elevated levels of FSH and LH were the sole cause of menopausal hot flashes, but this turns out to be untrue.

Although scientists have explored a number of theories, currently the most promising explanation for menopausal hot flashes lies in the hypothalamus. Although we don't know the exact biochemical cause of hot flashes, it does seem that it is related to the hypothalamus' role as the body's temperature regulation center. The hormone (GRH) produced in the hypothalamus in response to lowered estrogen levels seems not to be the sole cause of hot flashes, but is likely to be a major player in the reaction.

We do know that the substances responsible for revving up the body's nervous system increase during hot flashes. Specifically epinephrine (adrenaline) rises during hot flashes and may be responsible for the increased heart rate, increased blood flow through the circulation and increased temperature. It may also explain the subjective feelings of anxiety or dread that many women experience preceding and during hot flashes. It is unclear what causes the surge of adrenaline during a hot flash, but it may be a response to an event in the hypothalamus. Although estrogen withdrawal and the body's reaction to it are the underlying causes of hot flashes, the specific symptoms and physiologic changes observed are likely to be caused by the effects of epinephrine on the nervous system. This becomes important when treatment options are considered. Although estrogen replacement is the most logical choice for treatment, there may be alternative approaches that prevent or lessen the severity of hot flashes by other means.

✦ THERAPY FOR HOT FLASHES

As with any treatment decision, the first step is to evaluate the severity of the symptoms you are experiencing. We have included a hot flash diary for you to review and complete. By filling it out, you can get a true picture of how much hot flashes are interfering with your life. Also, you may be able to pinpoint some triggers such as stress or caffeine. This will help you develop a plan for preventing hot flashes that can be monitored by continuing the diary. In addition, you can use this diary to assess your response to any specific treatment that you are trying.

HORMONES

Estrogen withdrawal, unquestionably, sets off the cascade of events that lead to hot flashes. Estrogen is a highly successful treatment for hot flashes. Estrogen is over 90 percent effective in relieving hot flashes; an impressive statistic for any therapy. If you have no major reason to avoid estrogen, then remember that estrogen is truly the "flash blaster." In many cases, hot flashes can be treated with as little as .3 milligram (mg) of conjugated estrogen but may require up to 1.25 mg per day. We discuss the dosages of estrogen in detail in Chapter Six. The estrogen patches are equally successful in treatment at doses of .05 mg to .1 mg (Ravnikar, 1990). Symptom relief with estrogen is not immediate, however, and it may take up to four weeks of therapy to assess effectiveness. This is important to remember when your doctor suggests an increased dose of estrogen before the completion of a full four-week trial on the lower dose.

If an adequate trial of estrogen therapy at the higher dose fails to eliminate hot flashes, then there are several other possible causes. Common conditions that can mimic menopausal hot flashes include hyperthyroidism, alcoholism and diabetes. Carcinoid syndrome, a rare condition of an excess of the chemical serotonin, can also cause episodic flushing.

Because most women's hot flashes dissipate after three to five years from the last menstrual period, treatment with estrogen may be time-limited if it was started only for hot flashes. If, on the other hand, hormone replacement therapy is also being used to prevent the long-term consequences of menopause like vaginal dryness, osteoporosis and coronary artery disease, then therapy may be continued for many years. Women who have successfully been treated with hormone replacement therapy and wish to discontinue this therapy may choose to try a period off hormone replacement therapy on a yearly basis. Beware that if estrogen is stopped abruptly, hot flashes will return, and probably in a big way! If, however, the estrogen is tapered over weeks to months, then the body has an opportunity to reequilibrate, and it is possible that hot flashes will not recur once the medication is stopped completely. An older regimen of hormone replacement therapy involved daily estrogen doses for three out of four weeks of any month. Many women experienced hot flashes during the one week off estrogen, thereby demonstrating the importance of tapering the dose of estrogen rather than abruptly stopping it.

Table 2-2

HOT FLASH DIARY

Date	Day	Time	Food	Stress	Flash	Severity (1–5)	Notes
2/1	MONDAY	6:00 A.M.			√	4	Awakened from sleep
		7:00 A.M.	Muffin Coffee		√	5	On way to work
		Noon	Tuna Sandwich Diet Coke Brownie				
		1:30 P.M.			√	3	Sitting at desk
		3:00 P.M.		Argument with co-worker			

- After two full weeks, count the number of hot flashes per day and average.
- After two full weeks, average the severity of hot flashes experienced.
- Look for any patterns in flashes—food, caffeine, stress, days of week, times of day.

Alternative forms of hormone therapy have been investigated because so many women are unable to take estrogen and many women prefer not to take it. The use of the other major female hormone, progesterone, has been investigated thoroughly. Hot flashes can be reduced by 70 to 90 percent with medroxyprogesterone alone (Schiff and others, 1980). It is intriguing that women who were treated with placebo consistently showed a rather significant decrease in hot flashes (as much as 25 percent in women receiving placebo alone) (Albrecht and others, 1980; Bullock and others, 1975). There is no clear explanation for this response to a supposedly ineffective substance. Perhaps the expectation of a response to treatment increases a brain substance that can by itself decrease the frequency of hot flashes. This is not evidence that women who respond to placebo are exaggerating their symptoms. This phenomenon of placebo response is seen to some extent in all treatment studies of females and males. What it does mean is that any therapeutic response must be compared to response that is seen with placebo alone. If, for example, a therapy is touted as effective but only reduces hot flash frequency by 25 percent, then it is not better than placebo. Medroxyprogesterone is not without side effects but it may be an alternative therapy for women who are not candidates for estrogen therapy but have severe frequent hot flashes for which they desire treatment.

NONHORMONAL DRUG THERAPY

A number of nonhormonal drugs have also been used in the treatment of hot flashes with variable success. Many of the drugs found to be effective in treating hot flashes were developed to treat high blood pressure. Their success with hot flashes probably relates to their effects in the circulatory system.

The most promising medication to date has been the blood pressure medicine Clonidine. Clonidine has also been used in the treatment of nicotine, alcohol and heroin withdrawal. This is not to imply that hot flashes are analogous to heroin withdrawal! Clonidine acts in all these situations to modify the overdrive of the circulatory system. It has no effect on hormones and does not treat the other symptoms or consequences of menopause. In one study, Clonidine doses lower than those used for high blood pressure reduced the number of hot flashes and their severity significantly when compared to placebo (Clayden and others, 1974). A similar medication, Lofexidine, can also decrease the number of hot flashes (Jones and others, 1985). The beta-blockers, another class of blood pressure medication, have had some promise as well. Sotalol has been found to decrease hot flashes by 62 percent

(Young and others, 1990). For many of these medications, there may be side effects related to lowering blood pressure. Some women may experience light-headedness and fatigue when begun on any of these drugs, depending on the dose.

Another class of drugs has been somewhat successful in the treatment of hot flashes. Veralipride is a medication that acts on yet another substance produced in the brain called serotonin. Total elimination of hot flashes has been found in 60 to 80 percent of women. After the medication was stopped, hot flashes were eliminated for three months, but returned in six months. The medication is also associated with breast tenderness and some production of milk by the breast that disappears rapidly after the medication is discontinued (Young and others, 1990).

While many of these medications hold promise in decreasing the frequency and severity of hot flashes, none of them are as effective as hormone therapy. Additionally, none of them treat the other symptoms of menopause or prevent the long-term consequences. For women who cannot take or choose not to take hormones, these may be reasonable alternatives when hot flashes cannot be managed otherwise.

NONPRESCRIPTION REMEDIES FOR HOT FLASHES

There have been a number of substances that have been suggested as effective in treating hot flashes. Most of these have not been studied rigorously. In the case of hot flashes, this is particularly important since the response to placebo is so high. As is true with prescription drugs, a woman needs to consider the potential side effects, complications and financial cost compared to its benefits in treating the symptom. We wish there were more studies about the effectiveness of nonmedical approaches to hot flashes. The truth is, though, that as little as women's health has been studied, nonmedical treatments of symptoms have been studied even less. We are delighted that the National Institute of Health finally established the Office of Alternative Medicine, because that means that new research will be forthcoming. But here is some of what we do know:

Vitamin E appears in many lists of treatment for hot flashes, but much of the information we have about it is anecdotal at best. Vitamin E occurs in a number of food substances, including wheat and rice germ, legumes, corn, almonds and egg yolks. It can also be taken as a vitamin supplement beginning at 100 international units a day and increasing to 400 international units a day. Although vitamin E is a relatively safe vitamin, if you have heart disease, hypertension or diabetes, you should consult your physician before starting to take it (Dukes, 1992). Vitamin E is a vitamin that can be stored in the body's fat and it is important that doses be kept at no more than 400 international units per day to avoid toxic effects. For some women, vitamin E may completely relieve hot flashes. Up to two-thirds of women may experience relief from hot flashes with daily vitamin E.

Vitamin B complex is important for the normal functioning of the nervous system and some women have reported help with hot flashes and the daytime consequences of night sweats.

Ginseng is an herbal source of estrogen and is available as a tea. Although ginseng is available in health food stores it is, nonetheless, a form of hormone therapy. It can be effective in treating hot flashes as well as the other symptoms of menopause but it carries the same risks as estrogen replacement therapy. The dose of estrogen taken is very difficult to estimate and, therefore the effects are difficult to predict. It is also very expensive.

Many other *herbs* have been used in the treatment of menopause and are highly recommended by many women, including Germaine Greer. Again, there have not been many studies of most of these substances and some, including black cohosh, contain estrogen. Most of the herbs used in the treatment of hot flashes and menopausal symptoms are available in a dried form for tea but may also be available in capsules and as powder. It is important that herbal therapy be used cautiously and based on a clear understanding of the active substance. Herbs that contain estrogen carry the same potential for complications as hormone replacement therapy and need to be considered in the same context. Some women have used these "natural" substances and have experienced unpredictable bleeding, so, even "natural" products may have very significant side effects. Some of the herbs used in the treatment of menopausal symptoms include dong quai, damiana, cramp bark, golden seal, licorice root, oil of primrose, red raspberry leaves, sarsaparilla and spearmint.

We do not want to leave you with the impression that we are against the use of herbs and alternative treatments. The problem is that there has not been enough research to evaluate their effectiveness. In general, we feel that if they are safe and work for you, by all means, try them.

OTHER STRATEGIES TO DEAL WITH HOT FLASHES

A number of other techniques have been used in the management of hot flashes. Relaxation techniques, biofeedback, visualization, hypnosis, meditation and massage have all been used with some success. Because each woman's experience with hot flashes is so different, it is impossible to predict her response to the many forms of treatment. You may want to try some of these methods. All of these behavioral treatments are essentially educational. They involve skills that require practice. As you practice these and become comfortable with them, they can be easily and quickly used to deal with any stress, including hot flashes.

Paced respirations or controlled breathing has been shown to be more effective than either relaxation or biofeedback in dealing with hot flashes. The same principles apply here as they did to labor or childbirth. You need to focus consistent breathing in order to relax, rather than "fight" the flash. Relaxation techniques may be particularly effective in women who do experience more hot flashes when stressed. When increased stress is recognized, relaxation techniques may actually be used to avert hot flashes. When hot flashes begin, many women also find relaxation techniques helpful to lessen the severity of the attack and avoid the escalation that can occur during the episode.

Amy, a sales representative for a computer software company, found paced respirations and relaxation techniques very effective. She was having relatively infrequent hot flashes but they occurred at the most inopportune times. It seemed that anytime she was about to give a major presentation, she would experience a flash. This is completely understandable, since stress can increase the occurrence of hot flashes. Amy did not want to take HRT. She was able to learn relaxation techniques and practiced them before major presentations in order to decrease her anxiety and thereby avoid her dreaded hot-flash trigger.

Biofeedback would seem to be an ideal technique since it capitalizes on an individual's ability to monitor and alter involuntary functions. Because subjective symptoms of hot flashes are so dramatic this would seem to be a perfect opportunity to alter the body's response. Biofeedback teaches the techniques of changing muscle tension, lowering blood pressure and heart rate, as well as temperature. Specifically in the case of hot flashes, the woman is instructed to think of increased blood flow in her hands that may allow a diversion of blood from the head and upper chest to the extremities.

Visualization is another mind-body technique. It builds on relaxation techniques. During the hot flash, the woman is instructed to imagine herself in cold water or snow that will allow the mental removal of the sensation of heat from the body. Similarly, self-hypnosis creates a mental and physical state of relaxation. While in this state, a woman can suggest methods of dealing with symptoms such as hot flashes by establishing a detailed image that can be called upon during subsequent episodes. In the case of a hot flash, this image may be one of cooling and can be called up during each episode. Meditation has been shown to lower heart rate and blood pressure and may ease the discomfort associated with the hot flashes in this way.

One study found that acupuncture reduced the frequency of hot flashes. This is an area that needs more attention.

HOT FLASH PREVENTION

A number of substances can precipitate hot flashes. Included among the lists are hot drinks, hot rooms, hot beds, hot foods, alcohol, and stress. If these substances do trigger hot flashes even if only in some women, avoidance is a logical first step if hot flashes are bothersome. Some of the behavioral techniques outlined above may have a role in prevention if stress is a major contributor to the episode.

Nutrition may play a role in prevention as well. We know that women who are underweight are likely to experience more severe symptoms of menopause because of the relative lack of estrogen stored in their body fat. For this reason, it is advisable that women not be significantly underweight. A diet supplemented with plant estrogens, that is soy flower and linseed, may benefit women with hot flashes as well. This could, in part, explain the lower occurrence of hot flashes among Asian women who consume a large proportion of their calories from foods high in plant estrogens. If caffeine, alcohol, sugar and spicy foods are possible triggers of hot flashes, then they should be avoided. The most sensible dietary approach is to eat a balanced variety of foods that are nutritious and to avoid any foods that may precipitate hot flashes.

Exercise has a significant beneficial effect on menopausal symptoms as it does with premenstrual symptoms. Regular exercise probably decreases FSH and LH and in this way decreases some of the symptoms of menopause. Exercise increases the natural endorphins, or opiate-like substances produced by the brain, and these may have a beneficial effect on menopausal symptoms and stress as well. If you are going to start an exercise program, you should check with your doctor and you may want to also consult an exercise physiologist in order to achieve aerobic effects. (See Chapter Ten, "Promoting a Healthy Lifestyle.") It is best to exercise three to four times per week. Yoga may be used also or as additional exercise and may achieve the same beneficial effects.

✦ COMMUNICATION

COMMUNICATING WITH YOUR
HEALTH CARE PROFESSIONAL

We have found that hot flashes are often the symptoms that bring menopausal patients to our practice. Therefore, hot flashes often begin the conversation with your health care professional. This interaction is a critical part of your health care. In each chapter, we will be reviewing different communication strategies specific to the topic covered. Remember, in general, you should expect this communication to be part of your office visit. Do not be afraid to ask questions. You should ask follow-up questions if you don't understand the answers. It is our hope that by the end of this book, you will have an ample repertoire of communication strategies.

To begin your conversation regarding hot flashes, you may wish to review, with your health care professional, your hot-flash diary. Make a special effort to communicate to your health care professional the disruptiveness of your hot flashes. Even if your hot flashes are infrequent but debilitating, you might consider some form of treatment. Together, you may identify specific triggers and try some prevention strategies before considering other treatment. Clearly communicate what types of treatment you would and would not consider. You may wish to review the treatments presented in this chapter and rate them as *yes, no,* and *possibly.* This designation will help you plan a strategy of treatment. It may be that if all else fails, you would be willing to try HRT, but that you'd rather use prevention and behavioral techniques first.

If you do decide to try medication, remember that you have not failed. Many of us learned this lesson anticipating our pregnancies and deliveries. After all, this is not a competition to see who can tolerate the most pain and suffering. Even if you are one of those die-hard natural childbirth types, remember that hot flashes can give you as many sleepless nights as newborns, without the irresistibly cute faces to greet you. If you are feeling pressured by others in either direction, toward or away from treatment, express your concerns about this with them. This includes your doctor. Many physicians have strong opinions about hormone replacement therapy. Most of them (but not all) are pro-HRT. You need to be clear that you value your physician's advice but that the decision must ultimately be your own. Do not be discouraged if your physician only recommends hormone replacement therapy for your hot flashes. Persevere and ask follow-up questions such as: Can you recommend any other forms of treatment? We have found that these follow-up questions are as important as the initial questions for women to ask. The issue of hot flashes is just one part of the HRT decision, but a crucial part since HRT can be so effective. You will weigh other factors as we progress through this book.

COMMUNICATING WITH FRIENDS AND FAMILY

Family and friends can be very helpful if you share your symptoms and decision making with them. They may be in a good position to help you assess how hot flashes have affected you and your interactions with others. They may also be willing to help with solutions. Amy's family was willing to keep the temperature lower in their house after they realized that the hot rooms triggered her hot flashes in the evening and during the night. Amy's husband and children layered on extra clothing to help keep her hot flash–free.

To summarize, hot flashes are very common among menopausal women but are not usually severe enough to warrant medical treatment. It is important for each woman to assess how bothersome they are in order to make decisions about treatment. Severity is not just frequency. Hot flashes may be relatively infrequent but very disruptive. Remember that hot flashes do not last forever nor do the treatments. For many women, controlling hot flashes, rather than being controlled by them, is critical to improvement. This philosophy of taking charge of your health is at the core of the women's health movement.

Our patient Kai ran into a perimenopausal friend, Donna, who was just beginning to experience her first flashes. Kai shared her humorous approach to hot flashes with Donna who responded, "That's great! But haven't you heard? They're called power surges now!"

RESOURCES

Women's best resources for dealing with hot flashes are other women. Newsletters about menopause are multiplying like rabbits! Here are three:

A Friend Indeed
Box 515, Place du Parc Station
Montreal, Canada H2W 2P1

Published by Janine O'Leary Cobb, "A Friend Indeed" is the grandmother of them all. It is especially intriguing because it contains *both comments from Canadian and American women. It provides information on recent research, a forum to exchange experiences and support for the woman approaching or experiencing menopause. It reviews almost all of the books that deal with the various aspects of menopause. It comes out ten times a year and a subscription is $30.*

Hot Flash: Newsletter for Midlife and Older Women
Dr. Jane Porcini
National Action Forum for Mid-life and Older Women
Box 816
Stony Brook, NY 11790-0609
(212) 725-8627

This quarterly newsletter gives information on political and social issues related to the physiology and psychology of menopause, and resources. $25 a year with a membership.

Menopause News
2074 Union St.
San Francisco, CA 94123
(415) 567-2368

"Menopause News" is published six times a year by Judith S. Askew. It provides medical and psychological information, publishes letters and reviews books and videotapes. The cost is $24 a year.

If all else fails . . . consider a portable fan. One of our favorites is called the "Tiny Tornado," available from the Solutions Catalogue (P.O. Box 6878, Portland, Oregon, 97228).

CHAPTER THREE

Sexuality

"WHY DO WOMEN FAKE ORGASMS? . . . BECAUSE MEN FAKE FOREPLAY!"
This is one of the best jokes of Miriam, our fifty-five-year-old patient
who regales us with funny stories whenever we see her. Miriam went
through menopause four years prior to our meeting her. She comes to
see us every year for her annual physical, Pap smear, to have her blood
pressure checked and to schedule her mammogram. Over the years we
have enjoyed our relationship with Miriam and she has taken advantage of the abundance of information and resources available through
our practice. Most recently, we provided a referral for infertility evaluation because her thirty-two-year-old daughter and husband had not
been able to conceive.

Miriam worked as a secretary full-time, but recently reduced her
hours to part-time. She is bright, engaging and articulate. Her husband Tom is a journalist, a quiet and wryly humorous man. He and
Miriam have been married for thirty-three years and have three children, who are now in their late twenties and early thirties. When asked
about her own sex life Miriam replied, "Now that's foreplay! We take
longer than we used to and I love it." Miriam was eager to share her
story with other women. Miriam and Tom have always communicated

well, partially because they have so much in common. They are both active in their church and enjoy hiking, camping and other outdoor activities. She told us that she and Tom have always enjoyed sex but that their patterns had changed with time. Originally slaves to the missionary position, Miriam read Masters and Johnson in the early seventies, and she and Tom began to be more sexually adventurous, exploring different positions and incorporating more romance into their lovemaking. Now that they were in their fifties, they had intercourse somewhat less often, but still enjoyed themselves and were both orgasmic. Miriam often was on top during sexual intercourse. This helped when she had some problems with vaginal dryness, in that she could control the pace and the positions during intercourse. She added that, "Tom just turned sixty and his back hurts now and then, so this position is great for both of us." When we commented on the couple's ability to communicate well about sex, she retorted, "After three children and thirty-three years of marriage, if we can't talk about sex, what's it all about?"

Miriam is an especially open and humorous woman, but her story is not all that unusual. Most menopausal women enjoy their sexuality and adjust quite well to the biological changes associated with menopause. This may surprise you, if you've believed the stereotypes of frustrated, sex-starved menopausal women. There is a long history of viewing older women primarily as asexual. Other popular myths have portrayed older women as sexually depraved and voracious. We see little about well-adjusted, mature women. Even as recently as 1992, Germaine Greer was exhorting menopausal women to give up sex and men and retire to their gardens, because she believes that sexuality is a useless endeavor (Greer, 1992). These antiquated myths and this unsound advice do a disservice to the millions of sexually active menopausal couples.

❧ SEXUAL ADJUSTMENT: PSYCHOLOGICAL ISSUES

Entirely too much of what we have read and seen about menopause has focused exclusively on the female biological changes. This is problematic for two reasons. First, biology is *not* our destiny, especially with regard to sex. Second, sex occurs in the context of a relationship and therefore, partners bring issues to the sexual encounter as well. So if you are in a hurry to get to the biological changes, you can skip ahead a few pages. Otherwise, settle back and read on—we have some unlearning to do!

The brain is the most important of all the sexual organs, when we are younger, and as we age. Most sex therapists find that concern and worry about sex are usually more problematic than any physical or sexual changes themselves. It is almost impossible to enjoy sex if you are worried or anxious about it. Whatever the biological problem, when it comes to sex, your attitude will be the most important determinant of how well you cope.

Women who have enjoyed healthy sex earlier in their lives are exceptionally able to maintain their sexuality at midlife. (So, if you're reading this when you're perimenopausal and not enjoying sex, get going!) This is probably true because these women have seen sex as an integral, enjoyable part of life and have learned to value communication with their partners about sex. Couples who are affectionate physically tend to feel connected sexually as well. This connection leads to a well-established pattern of sexuality and can be easy to maintain, despite any biological changes associated with menopause. If sex has never been enjoyable for a woman, the additional stresses of menopause may be more difficult to overcome. One author has suggested that some menopausal women use "the change" as an excuse for avoiding sex that has never been fulfilling throughout the marriage (Hallstrom, 1977). In our experience, it is not that women in this situation purposefully lie to their husbands, but that menopausal symptoms may be "the last straw" in a marriage that has a marginal sexual adjustment. If you add vaginal dryness and the possibility of painful intercourse to a sexual relationship that has not been fulfilling, you can see how that relationship could deteriorate. Yet, even for these women, if menopause becomes the time when they finally address the sexual problems with their partners, they can learn to communicate directly and openly with their partners. Then the next phase of their sexual life can be vastly improved.

This brings us to the "use it or lose it" phenomenon. Good sex at menopause breeds more good sex (without breeding babies!). An intriguing study conducted by Drs. Gloria Bachmann and Susan Leiblum found that postmenopausal women who are more sexually active have fewer problems with lubricating and vaginal changes than other women. They reported higher levels of sexual desire, greater sexual satisfaction and more comfort expressing sexual preferences (Bachmann and Leiblum, 1991)—proof again that it is the interpersonal, not just the hormonal changes associated with menopause that determine adjustment. We emphasize the interpersonal aspects of your life because you can have a lot of control over the them. We don't want you to see menopause as a menacing hormonal event that happens *to you*. Rather, the entire menopausal transition is just another phase of life that you have the power and resources to deal with.

Sexuality is also part of a woman's more general physical sense of self. Women who are physically active feel better overall, and therefore can be more active sexually. The nature of physical activity doesn't need to be strenuous or intensive. You do not need to go to the gym on a daily basis to maintain a feeling of physical activity. But getting some movement into your life will preserve your health and maintain your activity level. Walking, swimming, dancing, gardening or any movement that you enjoy can be a regular pleasure in your life. We discuss this more in our chapters on stress and promoting a healthy lifestyle, because feeling physically fit can improve our sense of self-worth. Since all of us have internalized negative attitudes toward aging, it is important to feel good about ourselves physically. Any effort we take to improve our lifestyle in the area of physical activity relates directly to feeling better psychologically at midlife. It is also clear that in addition to releasing tension, exercise and physical activity can increase sexual energy.

Sexuality is only one part of the general area of sensuality. Sex does not just mean intercourse, but can involve a deep emotional attachment and a wide variety of sensual and enjoyable activities. For some couples, if the man has truly been faking foreplay, as Miriam jokes, then the woman may become resentful. One of the most common problems in long-term relationships is that the partners lapse into routinized, predictable, nonromantic sex. Each member of the couple can foresee exactly what will happen next. We have actually had some women tell us that they work on their grocery lists in their mind during these boring sexual encounters. In the case where a menopausal woman has been with her partner for many years, it may be difficult for the couple to find themselves sexually attracted to one another if there has been little intimacy or physical affection.

However, many couples use their time at midlife to rekindle their relationships. With the children out of the house (or at least out of diapers), or with the extra time gained from reduced work pressures, couples can turn to one another and start again. This involves a renewed commitment from each member of the couple, but many couples find that midlife can be an extremely happy period where sex is just one of many activities they share together. Other couples like Miriam and Tom have always worked together well and also see that sex can change over a lifetime. They can remain intimate and are not limited by some specific sexual routine. We have found that couples who are maintaining a physically active and intimate relationship are the same couples who continue to value their sexual intimacy and self-expression. These fortunate couples who value communication continue to share their feelings about sex, as well as other aspects of their lives.

✦ BEWARE OF STEREOTYPES

We need to look at some of the social stereotypes of sexuality and menopause. Do not believe them! The most destructive myth of "finished at fifty" is just a new spin on "finished at forty." Both medical materials and popular press articles have overplayed sexual problems at menopause. This exaggeration was not always the case. An analysis of articles appearing in the popular media found that prior to 1950, menopause was seen as both positive and negative. Often it was portrayed as a serene period in women's lives. But by 1960, the view that menopause meant a loss of sexuality and youth grew substantially. Interestingly, prior to 1960, HRT was recommended for severe symptoms only, but after that date it was being promoted as a cure for a wide variety of mild and cosmetic as well as severe symptoms (Bell, 1990). Of course, the 1960s were the height of Robert Wilson's *Feminine Forever* propaganda. This book claimed estrogen to be a treatment for every older woman's symptoms and neglected to mention the author's ties to pharmaceutical companies (Wilson, 1966). The promises of this book were seen in a different light once the increased risk of uterine cancer was later linked to unopposed estrogen.

An additional stereotype of the menopausal women was provided by the infiltration of orthodox psychoanalytic theory into the popular culture. Freud's original theories, after all, really did women a tremendous disservice. Much of Freudian or psychoanalytic theory focuses only on the reproductive aspects of a woman's life. Thus, menopause was seen as the end of the road for women. Helene Deutsch, one of Freud's students, was a notable psychoanalyst but did terrible damage to women's views of midlife. Her comments on sexual changes can be summed up in one word—"horrifying." Her words were, "Everything she acquired during puberty is now lost piece by piece." If one were to point out that most menopausal women were quite active and happy, Dr. Deutsch had this response, "She herself has the feeling of heightened vitality. . . . She becomes enthusiastic about abstract ideas, changes her attitude toward her family, leaves her home from the same motives as in her adolescence . . . narcissistic self-delusion makes her painted face appear youthful to her in the mirror" (Deutsch, 1945, p. 462). So Dr. Deutsch promulgated three myths. First, we lose all of our sexuality. Second, we lose our psychology of being female as well. Finally, to add insult to injury, any sign of vitality at midlife is seen only as a form of narcissism. Unfortunately, the views of Dr. Deutsch and other psychoanalysts have permeated society for a long time, despite the fact that they were never supported by any data. Combine them with the mass media emphasis on youth, and the prescribed form of female beauty, and it is no wonder that a woman over fifty is bound to be worried about her appeal.

American women see middle age as an unattractive physical stage of life for women. But not so for men. Although we can hope that times have changed, evidence proves much the contrary. The Disney company, for example, continues to elaborate their portrayal of sex-starved, unsightly and even monstrous female villains that helps to shape the way society views the sensual nature of middle-aged women. Powerful images of women at midlife struggling to repossess their youth are prominent throughout folklore—from the old Russian tale of the "Baba Yaga," where a middle-aged homely witch attempts to destroy and consume youthful innocence by breakfasting on the lovely heroine; to Ursula the Sea Witch in Disney's recent movie *The Little Mermaid*. Ursula, through trickery and sorcery, steals the sweet, cherished voice and youthful appearance of the heroine, Ariel, to seduce her handsome prince. Ursula takes her place following earlier Disney villainesses envious of youth and beauty including the Wicked Step-mother in *Cinderella*, the Evil Queen in *Snow White* and Maleficent in *Sleeping Beauty*. These films, already etched in the memories of today's menopausal women, are now made readily available on videocassette and are greatly contributing to how children view aging women. We should not be surprised when they grow up thinking that older women are witches, hags and just plain nasty.

We are making some progress in the war against the stereotypical aging female as women gain power in all areas—business, arts and entertainment, industry and even the medical profession. But these stereotypes do remain. It is only recently that we are beginning to have role models of women who are over the age of fifty and are still active in all areas of life. From women like Joanne Woodward to Rita Moreno to Tina Turner, things are changing. We are slowly but surely shedding old stereotypes and accepting women as competent, powerful and yes, even sexual role models.

Hasn't sexuality for women always been about relationships? As women, we know this, even though advertising has tried its best to convince us otherwise by emphasizing physical attractiveness alone. There is no reason to assume that the relationships themselves will deteriorate at menopause. In fact, sex and relationships often improve with age. Women who go to marital therapy, for example, usually complain about the lack of intimacy with their husbands. Many midlife men though, are reevaluating their lives and taking more time to develop relationships. Therefore, midlife becomes a developmental period when men and women often have time to improve their long-standing relationships. Many midlife women who are lesbian have a heightened sense of sharing because they go through the menopausal experience together. We have also found that lesbian women are not as burdened by the socially restrictive view of sexuality as young and physically attractive in a prescribed way. Many lesbians have been able to escape the stereotypes of midlife women by recognizing and battling them together. It is clear that sexuality, when seen in the context of a relationship, does not need to change in a negative way at the time of menopause.

Two of our recent cases make this clear. Both of them experienced sexual reawakenings in their late forties and early fifties. Maria is a forty-nine-year-old lesbian woman who works as a computer programmer. She came to see us originally for numerous complaints, including concerns about her adjustment to perimenopause. She was able to work with many issues in individual therapy. However, she also wanted to talk about her sexual adjustment. Maria had been in psychotherapy ten years previously for an extended period of time. At that time, she experienced the loss of her grandmother, "my role model for female strength," and her sister, who died of cancer in her twenties. She knew that she was lesbian from an early age, but never felt comfortable acting on this feeling. During her earlier psychotherapy, she worked on issues of how it felt to be a gay adolescent in a traditional family in conservative Boston. Maria is a strong and courageous woman who also has a deep commitment to psychotherapy as a process. In individual therapy and in group therapy she was able to work through many issues, including her sexuality and sexual orientation. Over the past ten years, Maria had been involved with several women but never felt that she was in an intimate relationship or one that felt right to her.

Maria describes herself as a "late bloomer," and so she knew that she needed more work in order to develop an intimate relationship. In her second phase of psychotherapy, she felt like she was coming together psychologically and sexually. Previously Maria was involved in relationships that were limited by their very nature: either women who were involved with someone else, or were unavailable psychologically. As she continued to work in psychotherapy, however, Maria realized that by allowing herself to become involved in an intimate relationship with another woman, she would take the final step toward accepting her sexuality and improving her life. Over time, Maria became involved with Liz, another woman who worked in the same company. They developed an intense and close relationship based on equality and commitment. Maria shared her previous feelings of loneliness and isolation while Liz talked about years in an unhappy marriage.

Together, they worked on similar concerns and were able to support and help one another. They have an active sexual life, and Maria felt that her sexuality had finally begun to flourish in midlife. She and Liz spend time traveling, enjoy hot tubs and women's folk music, and feel relaxed in their new-found sexual life together. Maria and Liz now share their home with one of Liz's daughters who is in college. Maria and Liz tend to their garden, work on joint political projects and are quite contented.

When Maria began to have hot flashes, she asked Liz about it, since Liz was fifty-three. Liz told her that her own hot flashes had not been severe, but that she had been troubled by a few months of night sweats. Maria is keeping track of her hot flashes with her hot-flash diary, and how much they interfere with her life, while considering the information about estrogen, osteoporosis and heart-disease prevention before making her decision.

Many lesbian women who come from extremely traditional backgrounds find that midlife can be a time of integration. Freed from the pressures of needing their parents' approval and often secure in their careers, they can become completely comfortable with their sexuality. For these women, midlife can be a time of deep sexual satisfaction. Positive sexuality for Maria and Liz came to them late in life. Other lesbian couples who have been together for many years may have problems similar to those of some heterosexual couples. Janet and Bob present a frequent pattern. Janet, one of our fifty-six-year-old patients, came to us with the most common sexual complaints of midlife heterosexual couples. As she described a typical day of established routine, we began to see how her sexual problems had become serious.

Janet awoke on a Friday morning at 7:30 a.m., just as she did every week-day morning. On weekends, she and her husband of twenty-five years, Bob, allowed themselves to sleep until 9:00, but no later, as their cocker spaniel, Bessy, demanded that their schedule be pushed no further. At 7:30, Janet was the first in the family to rise. She made her way to the kitchen, awakening her sixteen-year-old son along the way, and then pushed the button on the automatic coffeemaker (which she prepared religiously the night before). After fixing her family breakfast, she waved them off with the customary exchanges, "Have a good day." Janet was then left standing alone in her bathrobe to begin her typical Friday chores. Bathroom cleaning and laundry were at the top of the list. Later in the day, she found a spare moment for a walk to the park with her neighbor Julie, a chance to chat with her friend and walk Bessy at the same time. At 2:00 p.m., she did her usual Friday marketing for the weekend meals. At 3:30 p.m., she picked up her son from a friend's house across town and then wrote a letter to her daughter at college. By the time Bob arrived home, she had dinner on the table. After eating, Janet's son left almost immediately for a date.

Left alone, she and Bob did what they did almost every other night. Bob helped clear the dishes and then Janet washed them while they both watched *Wheel of Fortune*. After cleaning up, they sat together on the couch while Bob flipped through the channels to see what movie or television show they would choose for the evening. Janet found her mind wandering that night, watching her husband watch the television and wondering why it was she could not bring herself to reach out and touch him. When she thought of asking him to make love, she was discomforted by the question and forecasted the same predictable preparations for sex. She would go to the bedroom first. He would follow five minutes later when he knew that she had undressed and washed, and then they would both lie on the bed. He would kiss her gently, only a few times, and then he would touch her to see if she was lubricated. If all went well, Bob would reach climax in five minutes, tell her that he loved her, and then they would both return to witness the outcome of the sitcom that had been interrupted.

On that particular Friday night, Janet did not ask Bob to make love to her. She was frustrated by the fact that they were not able to spend a longer time loving each other and she felt there was little hope of ever changing their dull sex life. What Janet did not know as she sat on the couch with her husband was that Bob, too, was feeling a need for greater companionship and heightened sexual experience. Because of their well-established lack of communication, they had no idea that what they shared most was a deeply felt need for one another.

Although this pattern had existed for most of their marriage, as Janet reached her postmenopausal years she began to blame herself. She felt that because she was lubricating less and had been experiencing some pain during intercourse, that it was her fault that she had no desire for her husband. This self-blame is what lead her to visit our practice, and prompted her decision to change a marriage lacking in communication and sensuality. We referred Janet and Bob for sex therapy. Although Bob was nervous, he was anxious to cooperate. During sex therapy, they uncovered that Janet and Bob had enjoyed intercourse when they were first married. But, neither of them had talked much about individual sexual needs. Janet had always deferred to Bob sexually, but she was unclear which parts of the sexual experience he enjoyed most. This lack of communication had not allowed their sexual experiences any room for growth or exploration.

During therapy, it was also discovered that they had avoided experimentation with foreplay and had a relationship that otherwise did not include a lot of affection or sensuality. Even though Janet and Bob had been uneasy about accepting the referral to sex therapy, they were quickly amazed at how they were able to learn new communication patterns and sexual skills. After a relatively short period of sex therapy, Janet and Bob were able to articulate their needs and listen well. They discovered a whole new experience involving the nonintercourse parts of the sexual encounter. In addition, Janet and Bob felt comfortable using a lubricant like Astroglide when necessary. In their fifties, they are finally enjoying sex as equal partners. Now a typical Friday night is far from typical. They make a point of getting out of the house, seeing a movie, or sampling different restaurants. Even if it is only for a long walk (holding hands!), they have shared something by relaxing with each other. These days, when Janet and Bob awaken on a Saturday morning, it is their son who takes Bessy for her morning stroll through the park. There's no need for them to rush.

The stories of Maria and Janet illustrate only two of the many women we have seen who indeed experienced some biological changes at the time of menopause. But like all women, their lives were affected by psychological and sociological factors as well. Sexuality is a complex and delicate issue, and improving your sexuality at midlife can involve numerous biological, psychological and social changes.

◆ THE BIOLOGY OF SEX AT MENOPAUSE

Fear not! This is not meant to be affirmation of all of your worst fears about menopause. If we are completely honest, our greatest dread is that at the time of menopause our sexual organs will, at best, dry up and, at worst, fall out. Thankfully, this is far from the truth. There are several biological changes that are associated with menopause. However, most of them do not occur until five years after the final menstrual period. In addition, we know that women's lives are extremely variable, so that not every woman will have difficulty with these changes. Some of the changes that do occur in menopause are difficult to separate completely from changes that would occur with aging alone.

Whatever the cause, the specific biologic changes that are experienced can be divided into two large categories: those that relate to anatomy and those that relate to physiology. In other words, there are changes that occur in the actual sexual organs as well as changes in the sexual response. First, let's look at the normal step choreography of the sexual response.

In order to understand menopausal sex fully, let's review the basics. The fulfilling sexual encounter is preceded by sexual interest. The physiological stages of sexual response were popularized by Virginia Masters and William Johnson. These stages are excitement, plateau, orgasm and resolution (Masters and others, 1970). During the excitement stage of sexual interaction, the vagina is lubricated by secretions that are released from the vaginal walls and there is an increase of muscle tension. During the plateau phase, there is some local constriction in the outer one-third of the vagina and the clitoris becomes elevated somewhat. The orgasm stage is the peak of sexual response, the most enjoyable moment. Physiologically, the outer one-half of the vagina, as well as the uterus, contract in a rhythmic way. During the resolution phase, there is a decrease in vasocongestion and the muscle tension disappears. If orgasm has occurred, then the resolution stage for women is quite quick, but if it has not, then the resolution stage takes a longer amount of time.

It is true that with aging, sexual arousal takes longer for both men and women. One view of this is that women are slower to arouse with age. Another view, however, is that women do not get enough stimulation to become aroused. The net result is that it takes longer for women to become lubricated during foreplay. The explanations for these changes are numerous, including decreased blood flow to the vagina, which makes it less sensitive to stimulation; a change in the neurologic connections, which causes relative numbness; and decreased vaginal lubrication related to estrogen levels.

There is some evidence that there may be a change in the experience of orgasm and a decrease in the frequency of orgasm after menopause. But in fact, the frequency of orgasm has been studied less than the frequency of sexual intercourse. Even Miriam admits to some changes in her orgasms. But as she has said to us, "They may have changed a little, but I'm certainly not going to give them away!"

This change in orgasmic intensity and frequency may be related to the accompanying changes with aging, including the slower ascent to the excitement phase as well as the anatomical changes that are presented in more detail below. Additionally, the uterine contractions which occur with orgasm may be less intense for postmenopausal women. For those women who have experienced hysterectomy, many report a change in the sensation of orgasm related to the complete absence of these uterine contractions.

The anatomical changes that occur with menopause are integrally related to the physiologic changes in sexual response. It is clear that the female sexual organs depend, in part, on estrogen to maintain their anatomy and function. This is not to say that the decrease in estrogen levels at the time of menopause leads to irreparable, inevitable or disastrous changes. Above all, we should take heart in the fact that the only predictable change at menopause is the end of menstrual periods and with it the end of fertility. For many women, this freedom from concerns about pregnancy and female sanitary products is a welcomed change.

The most frequent symptom of sexual changes at menopause is vaginal dryness. Yet, only 25 percent of women actually experience vaginal dryness five years after the last menstrual period. This percentage increases as women get older. But, far fewer women complain of vaginal dryness than hot flashes. Women who become menopausal because of surgery will experience symptoms of vaginal dryness much earlier than women who have natural menopause, whose symptoms may be delayed ten to fifteen years (Nachtigall and Heilman, 1991). Unlike hot flashes, vaginal symptoms may worsen, and not improve with time. Do not despair, however, because there are many good treatments for these symptoms.

The specific changes that occur in the vagina include thinning of the tissue lining called the vaginal epithelium. In premenopausal women, there may be forty to fifty layers of these epithelial cells, but in postmenopausal women, these may be reduced to four or five layers (Sachs, 1991). The end result of this loss of protective coating is that the vagina may become irritated or inflamed more readily. This may be experienced as bleeding or pain at the time of intercourse and burning which can be severe with urination. The medical term used to classify these changes is "atrophic vaginitis." This implies that the vagina is inflamed (itis) and that the lining has thinned (atrophic). The changes that are seen with the lining are attributed to a decrease in estrogen levels. Although estrogen replacement is an effective cure for this condition, it is not the only treatment available. We have also learned from the many women who do not experience these vaginal symptoms that there may be ways to prevent their occurrence.

The vagina also becomes shorter and narrower at the time of menopause. The vagina's elasticity is also reduced as is the fatty tissue in the labia surrounding the vagina. These changes may or may not be bothersome to any individual woman. The specific anatomical changes that occur in the vagina can lead to discomfort with intercourse, known as dyspareunia. This, in particular, is compounded by vaginal dryness. Some women who anticipate painful penetration at the time of intercourse may actually have involuntary spasms at the vaginal opening known as vaginismus.

We often joke among ourselves that the list of gynecological complaints are somewhat "phallocentric." That is to say that many of the anatomical complaints are problematic particularly for male/female intercourse. It is important for a woman to first identify what problems are physically uncomfortable for her alone. After establishing that, she can then understand better what other issues may be particularly difficult with respect to sexual intercourse. Sexual problems among menopausal lesbian women have been detailed less often than those of heterosexual women. However, this may be because lesbian women have been studied even less than heterosexual women at midlife.

❖ URINARY SYMPTOMS

More women than ever before are becoming aware of the possibility of urinary incontinence now that protective shields are routinely advertised on television and radio. The message in these advertisements is that the problem is nearly unique to older women. While it is true that more older women than older men experience incontinence, it is by no means a problem unique to older women. Basically incontinence is the involuntary loss of urine. In general, incontinence is classified into two types. The first is stress incontinence which is the loss of urine, which occurs with anything that can increase abdominal pressure on the bladder including laughing, coughing or bearing down to lift something. This type of incontinence does tend to get worse with age unless preventive measures are taken. The cause of stress incontinence is the weakening and relaxation of the muscles and the ligaments which hold the pelvic organs in place. Like any muscle or ligament, these can weaken with time unless strengthened with exercise. It is also true that estrogen maintains their elasticity and strength. Women who are most prone to this type of incontinence are those who have had multiple pregnancies which can stretch and weaken some of the connecting structures of the pelvic organs.

The second type of incontinence is urge incontinence. This is experienced as an inability to hold the urine when the urge to urinate is felt. Women who have experienced this type of incontinence need to urinate as soon as the urge is felt. Urge incontinence seems to be related to a weakening of the muscle which holds the urine in the bladder or increased tone of the detrusser muscle.

Both the prevention and treatment of incontinence involves specific exercises for the weakened muscles. Like any muscles which may lose strength because of disuse, or in this case because of hormonal changes, this repeated exercise can increase their size and strength. While many of the ligaments and muscles of the urinary tract are not easily exercised, there are specific muscles which can be exercised to control the flow of urine. A simple way to identify the muscles involved in stopping the flow of urine is to voluntarily stop urinating midstream. Once the action that tenses these muscles is identified in this way, the exercise can be repeated at other times. These exercises, called Kegel's, in honor of the surgeon who invented them, are described further in a later section (Kegel, 1951).

The tissue in the bladder and urethra also become thinner during the postmenopausal period. Therefore, they can become irritated more often and open to infections. Symptoms of urinary tract infections (UTIs) are burning with urination, frequent urinating of small amounts and urgency. In the postmenopausal period, it can be difficult to distinguish burning due to infection because of bacteria, from that caused by vaginal atrophy and irritation.

These postmenopausal UTIs can be treated by antibiotics, as we detail in a bit. They can be prevented in a number of ways, including frequent urination to avoid holding urine in the bladder for long periods, drinking plenty of fluids, wiping from front to back, and urinating before and after intercourse.

✦ CHANGES IN THE MALE AT MIDLIFE

We see sexuality as part of the intricate relationships between couples. Janet and Bob's ability to improve their sex life would not have been possible if both of them had not been ready to change. Problems in sexuality at midlife are usually related to both male and female changes. It is important to remember that most menopausal women are married to men who are several years older. One of the changes is that older men take longer to arouse and therefore have erections more slowly. At the same time, their levels of testosterone are lower as well and the daily changes with a peak of testosterone in the morning are less dramatic. This change in testosterone levels may alter the length and desire of a man's sexual experience.

Some authors believe that the changes in sexual experience at midlife have more to do with the fact that men, not women, are less interested in sex. This is based on studies that show that most sexual encounters in male/female couples are determined by male initiation.

Thus if the male loses interest in sex and initiates less often, the couple will have fewer sexual experiences (Blumstein and Schwartz, 1985). So maybe women are reflecting changes in male biology rather than the other way around.

Certain medical conditions in older men also affect sexual behavior. Men who are diabetic often have problems with sexual arousal, as do men who are on medication for hypertension or heart disease. In addition, sexual dysfunction can occur in men who have had prostate surgery. In summary, any assessment of sexual changes in midlife for heterosexual women should look at the male/female biological, as well as psychological and social issues.

✦ How to Deal with All This

Keep at It

In our menopause town meetings, most women want to know, "What can I do about sexual changes?" Our best advice is that practice may not make perfect, but it is important for women who want to maintain their sexuality. Masters and Johnson recommended sex one to two times a week for a continued active sex life. So, if you are in a sexual relationship and it is enjoyable, just keep doing what you have been doing. Use the muscles involved in sexual activity, enjoy intercourse, experience orgasms. All this helps—biologically, psychologically, and interpersonally! If you and your partner have some sexual concerns, try to talk about them, experiment, and share.

Masturbation

Some menopausal women report that partner availability is a major problem. This is often true for women and is a source of sadness for many. But with respect to sexuality, it is important to remember that intercourse is not the only answer. Masturbation can be helpful and can keep you in shape sexually whether or not you have a partner. If you are like our patient Corinne, you might involuntarily flinch or even say "Shh!," upon hearing or reading the word "masturbation." Corinne is a forty-nine-year-old bookkeeper who finds herself in the single world again after twenty-five years of marriage. After working through her feelings about her divorce, she now thinks ahead to the idea of dating. Part of her sexual reawakening was that she wanted to reclaim her sexuality. Given her family history, having been brought up in an Irish, Roman Catholic family, similar to those spoofed in the play *Sister Mary Ignatius Explains It All,* it took us many weeks to even talk to Corinne about masturbation as part of actual conditioning. She had difficulty with the concept because at the age of forty-nine, she had never spoken the word, nor had any of her family members. Corinne is like many women who have been socialized to believe that masturbation is dirty, or even sinful. The truth is that there is nothing wrong with masturbation, and it is helpful in maintaining sexual functioning. Women lubricate during masturbation and use many of the same muscles as they do in other sexual encounters. Masturbation can also reduce tension.

KEGEL EXERCISES

Kegel's exercise can not only improve sexual functioning, but also decrease urinary incontinence. Developed by a surgeon, Dr. Arnold Kegel, in the 1950s, these exercises increase muscle tone in the vaginal area (Kegel, 1951). They involve tensing and relaxing the pubococcygeal muscles around the area of the urethra, vagina and anus. In order to identify these muscles, you can do one of two things. One is to begin to urinate and then stop. The same muscle you use to control urination is the muscle that you will contract then relax during the Kegel exercises. You can also locate and use this muscle by inserting a tampon and squeezing around it. You should hold this muscle for at least five to ten seconds and then release it slowly. After mastering the slow Kegel exercise, you should also do a series of rapid ones. They should be repeated ten to fifteen times, and the whole session should be repeated three to five times per day. Maureen, one of our patients, was delighted to learn these very specific instructions. Previously, she had only heard the part about stopping the flow of urine. She thought that that was the only way to do Kegel's exercise and soon found it to be too difficult and quit. Actually, you can do them anytime you feel like it, anywhere.

There are numerous advantages to the Kegel exercises. First, by developing the muscles around the vaginal area, the woman can have more control and pleasure during the sexual encounter. Second, Kegel exercises can tone up muscles and stop incontinence. Finally, they can build up the muscles in order to counteract any muscle loosening that occurs as a result of menopause. Kegel exercises can be done at any time of the day since they are invisible to the observer. We have read frequently that women can integrate Kegel exercise into any part of their daily routine—like when you are on the elevator, or driving. We have chuckled when we imagine all the women stopped in their cars at various stoplights doing their ten Kegel exercises, and wondered how many minor traffic accidents have resulted! In all seriousness, repetition is important and many women have found that these exercises have had a positive impact on their sex life.

HRT

Many women seriously consider starting HRT because of vaginal dryness. The specifics of HRT are covered in detail in Chapter Six. Estrogen can reverse atrophic vaginitis and this improvement removes a major barrier to satisfying sex. Progesterone, while medically necessary for women with uteri, seems to have no effect on sexual functioning. On the other hand, androgens, the male hormones, seem to affect lipids and sexual responsiveness. There is some evidence that this is particularly true for women who have had surgical menopause (Walling and others, 1990). The use of androgens or testosterone is becoming more common in the U.S. and has been used more extensively in England. Testosterone is sometimes prescribed to treat loss of libido. This positive effect needs to be considered with the potential negative side effects, including facial hair growth, mood changes and acne. Because of this, the dosage needs to be monitored very carefully. Germaine Greer, in her usually provocative fashion, describes feeling overwhelmed by impulses of aggression after taking testosterone, but it is clear that this use of androgens is an area to watch for the future (Greer, 1991).

Because estrogen also reverses the thinning of the area around the bladder, it has been suggested that taking estrogen will reduce the incidence of urinary tract infections. However one recent study suggested that women who take estrogen had a higher rate of urinary tract infections. It is clear that estrogen does reduce painful intercourse, or dyspareunia, because of better lubrication and less irritation.

Many women wish to reverse vaginal dryness but would prefer not to take oral estrogen or use the patch. Vaginal estrogen creams are available and are effective in treating atrophic vaginitis. Even though it is applied locally, the estrogen is still absorbed into the system and carries the same risks as estrogen taken in pill form. The amount absorbed will be relatively low, however, if the cream is used infrequently (two or three times per week) or for short periods of time. There is evidence that at low doses, as little as one-eighth of that usually recommended for vaginal dryness, the estrogen cream can be effective. For women using estrogen cream who have not had a hysterectomy, progesterone may still be necessary to cause menstrual bleeding and prevent uterine cancer.

There are also a number of nonmedicated lubricants including KY jelly, Replense and Astroglide. Some actually work to "plump up" the cells lining the vagina and can work for up to three days, eliminating the need to apply these right before intercourse. Do not use petroleum jelly because it can build up in the vagina and may disguise early symptoms of infection; it has also been reported as a cause of condom breakage. Some women have used vitamin E as a cream or a suppository vaginally.

Many women find the messiness of the cream relatively unacceptable. It is not meant to be used prior to intercourse since it is likely that your partner will absorb the cream as well. The side effects of estrogen are even more unwelcome for men! If added lubricant is needed, then any of the nonmedicated lubricants can be used. For women who cannot use estrogen, there are vaginal creams with 1 to 2 percent testosterone that are also effective in treating atrophic vaginitis (Greenwood, 1984).

Vaginal infections may also develop in the post menopausal period. The symptoms of vaginal infection are easily confused with one of those of atrophic vaginitis, which is characterized by irritation, itching, and discharge. It is important that these symptoms be evaluated so that appropriate treatment can be started. Many vaginal infections yeast infections are the most common type—can be treated topically with antifungal creams. Some require antibiotics taken orally. Infections can be discouraged by altering the vaginal PH with vinegar and water douches, aci-gel or Astroglide. Advice to wear cotton underwear and avoid tight-fitting pants is not a plot to keep you from being sexy but is a way of discouraging yeast overgrowth in the vagina.

CONTRACEPTION

It is true that even in the perimenopausal and early postmenopausal period, the occasional egg can be produced by the ovaries, making birth control a necessary evil for those at potential risk of an unwanted pregnancy. Women should continue to use contraception for a full year after the last menstrual period. The form of contraception really depends on personal preference and medical considerations. Many women and doctors avoid birth control pills in older women (everyone's definition of older is different). It is clearly true that the risks are higher for women who smoke. Barrier methods (diaphragm and condoms) can be very effective when used with spermicidal creams, jellies or foams. IUDs may be more of an option for women who are not worried about future fertility, although they are relatively less favored than other methods. Finally, sterilization is a frequently chosen method for women (tubal ligation) or their partners (vasectomy). For all intents and purposes, these must be considered permanent and irreversible.

SEXUALLY TRANSMITTED DISEASES

We had a lot of fun with our patient Corinne when she went on her first date as a divorced "older" woman. Like many women, when we broached the issue of sexual behavior, her first words were, "I absolutely, positively cannot do this. I was not good at it when I was seventeen and I'm not good at it now!" But after a few sessions of rehearsal, we helped Corinne understand that as a mature woman, she could approach her dating world with much more judgment and maturity and with less to risk. But the world of sexually transmitted diseases and HIV has made the sexual arena a dangerous place. And so we needed to deal with the issues of STDs with Corrine.

The most common diseases of concern include HIV, herpes and genital warts. All of these are caused by viruses and are relatively incurable infections. HIV infection is obviously the worst of the three. A basic rule is that condoms are dress code for all heterosexual encounters. Spermicidal creams, jellies or foams may be partially effective in preventing transmission of HIV and other viruses. Diaphragms may provide yet another barrier to infection. It is here that communication with your partner is critical. Do not allow yourself to be convinced that protection is unnecessary for any reason. Once you have established a long-term monogamous relationship with an individual, this may be an option but not before.

ABSTINENCE

We have met women in our practice who have chosen to give up sexual relationships. This is, of course, a personal choice, and when both parties of a relationship are comfortable with it, it seems to have no ill effects. However, problems can arise for women who have chosen not to engage in sexual activity for many years and who then begin again. The women who have not had hormone replacement therapy or have taken no other preventive actions may meet with some difficulty.

✦ DEALING WITH LOSS OF SEXUAL INTEREST

Sexual interest is a complex topic. Many of the women who complain of this loss also complain of unpleasant symptoms like vaginal dryness and dyspareunia. It seems clear that when sex becomes uncomfortable or even painful, a woman would lose interest. So the first step is often to deal with these anatomic or physiological changes. Some women choose to use hormone replacement therapy, or nonmedicated creams to treat the anatomic changes first. Estrogen does significantly improve these gynecological changes, but as we mentioned earlier, progesterone shows no benefit in this area. The most recent area of development is that of using the male hormones, androgens, to increase sexual interest. But many women find some of the side effects of the androgens to be unpleasant.

A second area of concern is communicating with your partner. Loss of sexual interest may well be interpersonal as well as physiological. So after the anatomic symptoms have been treated, if sexual interest continues to be a problem, you need to discuss this with your partner. Sometimes it is the result of relationship issues that are stressful. Other times a loss of sexual interest can be a result of what some call "habituation," that is, the result of a long-term sexual relationship that can sometimes lead to less variability and ultimately a decrease in sexual interest. Many women and their partners find that when this issue is directly addressed, partners can share their concerns and develop new sexual patterns that are more enjoyable for both of them.

Finally, it is important to note that loss of sexual interest can be a symptom of several psychological problems. Loss of sexual interest is also a symptom of depression. A history of sexual abuse may also be an issue. Other symptoms are detailed in our chapters on stress and depression. If you find that you have some of these symptoms, it is important to get psychological help. Psychological problems can be treated effectively and the sooner you get help the better.

✦ FOCUS ON SENSUALITY

As we discussed earlier, sexual behavior is just part of a sensual relationship. If a relationship has become boring, then of course it is difficult to rekindle sexual interest. Given the fact that many people have more time to share with their partner at menopause, a new sensuality can flourish. Many couples at this point in life take the time to help one another relax by using massage, or taking a bath together. Physical activities like running, golf or playing tennis can bring a couple closer together. Exercise, then, can serve two purposes, keeping a couple physically fit while enhancing their sensuality. Being affectionate, touching, and sharing emotions and experiences are often characteristics which most women associate with a positive sex life.

During the pre-children era, many couples had infinite time to explore their sensuality. When children come along many couples make a point to set aside one night a week to be alone, but even that one night is often sacrificed if another family responsibility arises. All too often this becomes a pattern, where the couple's romance and sensuality is put on hold. If the couple is fortunate enough to reach midlife intact, they can reclaim their romance and sensuality together. Janet and Bob were still watching *Wheel of Fortune,* even though their children were out of the house and they had the opportunity to do just about anything they wanted together.

✦ COMMUNICATION

COMMUNICATING ABOUT SEXUALITY WITH YOUR PARTNER

Many women find this to be extremely difficult. Despite the sexual revolution of the sixties and seventies, sex remains a taboo topic of conversation for many couples, even when they are sexually active. If a couple can be specific and nonjudgmental with one another, they can make sexual changes. For many women the first step is to express their unhappiness to their partner. Many women feel protective of the husband's sexual ego. Janet was afraid of hurting Bob's feelings and making him feel like a bad lover. She actually believed that Bob could become impotent if she were critical of him in any way. Yet this is the very first step in repairing a sexual relationship. Janet and Bob decided to seek sex therapy, but that is often unnecessary if you can learn to communicate as a couple.

Here are some basic communication strategies for approaching this subject with your partner. First, think through what you would like to say. Be specific and practical. Most women do not have difficulty identifying the problem to themselves. You need to directly approach your partner and say that you would like to discuss your sex life. This may not be easy. Other women have had, like Corinne, negative responses to the words penis, vagina, orgasm, masturbation, intercourse, clitoris, and so on. We all need to overcome this early conditioning that makes sex a taboo topic.

Second, identify the problem as a joint venture. This way your partner should not feel criticized and you can create an attitude of sharing and cooperation. For example, Janet could have said, "We enjoyed sex so much in our twenties, I want us to try and make it better now." This would be more effective than by saying "You don't kiss me enough during sex" at the beginning of the conversation. Although your partner may express some initial resistance, you should not give up. You need to ask about your partner's feelings, and most women are experts at doing this.

Third, try to be specific and nonjudgmental. By using sentences that begin "I feel . . ." rather than "You should . . . ," your partner will have the most positive response. For some couples, the husband is less eager and perhaps less able to express his feelings about this subject. For that reason, it is important not to give up easily.

In addition to communication problems, sexual anxiety can make things worse at first. Once you become aware of a sexual problem, anxiety can increase during a sexual encounter. This then leads to a negative experience and therefore the cycle continues. Masters and Johnson refer to this as being a spectator during sex (Masters and others, 1970). A Victoria's Secret negligee may look appealing on the rack but seem ridiculous when you put it on for a sexual encounter. By observing yourself, while at the same time engaging in sex, the pressure to perform is difficult and counterproductive. This is all the more reason to approach your partner and try to deal with sex with a spirit of adventure and a sense of humor.

Some women find romantic and erotic movies to be helpful in getting aroused, or to break out of old routines. Please know that we do not mean common pornography, which is dehumanizing and objectifying to women. If books and videos do not work in helping you to get aroused, you might try inviting Jeff Bridges, Denzel Washington, or k.d. lang over to your house for the afternoon. Seriously, it is important to note whether you cannot get aroused with your partner specifically or by fantasy or if you can feel aroused at all. You also need to be sure that any medical symptoms, like painful intercourse, are being treated properly. If they have been treated successfully and the sexual problems remain, then it is probably time to get help. If the problem is primarily sexual, then sex therapy is in order.

COMMUNICATING WITH YOUR CLINICIAN

Just as sex is a taboo topic in society, and just as sex might be difficult to talk about with your partner, it is often awkward to address with your physician. Yet most clinicians are very comfortable talking about the specific gynecological changes at menopause. After identifying the problem specifically, you can talk it over with your primary care professional. This is one of those times when you will need to talk to your doctor in some depth, rather than asking a few questions after you have had your Pap smear. It is important to set your priorities about what issues you want to discuss, and to do this ahead of time. You might choose to jot them down on a notepad that you can look at before talking to the physician. If your doctor recommends hormone replacement therapy, you should make that decision after reading some of the next few chapters.

Your gynecologist or internist will be able to help you identify the physical problems that are contributing to your problems in sexuality. If your primary problem is lack of sexual interest, or if you feel that it is a relationship problem, then you may also ask your physician for a referral to a psychologist or other mental health professional.

We found that Corinne, who entered the dating world after many years, soon overcame her insecurities. The same woman who had come to our office whispering the word "masturbation," and doubting whether she could go through with a "first date," became a confident, happy, sexually active woman. Corinne developed an openness and willingness to communicate with her doctors and her newfound partner. Corinne had met David, a caring, forty-five-year-old lawyer (and "a younger man!") who interested her in new hobbies like tennis and photography while at the same time accompanying her to her favorite place, the theater. Ultimately, Corinne became more alive sexually at midlife than she would have ever dared to think of before. When Corinne visits us now, she is full of stories about previously uncharted territories and a newfound self-confidence. Descriptions and concerns regarding her sex life are no longer inaudible, we hear her loud and clear.

Talking about sex is often especially difficult for a woman if her clinician is a man. It may make you feel ashamed or vulnerable. This is a natural response to what is a taboo and emotional topic. Try to remember that listening to you talk about sexual issues is a part of your doctor's job and chances are, he has heard it all before. Even if your doctor is a woman, you may be reluctant to discuss sexual problems because you may feel like you are betraying your partner. Your partner will feel better, too, if you both get help. And your clinician is in the best position to get you that help.

Although most clinicians are comfortable in talking about sex, you may be unlucky and have a negative experience. One possibility is that you feel brushed off, that your doctor minimizes your concern. If so, you should restate your concerns clearly. Another possibility is that your doctor strongly recommends HRT, and if you decide against it, he or she may become impatient with your complaints. In that case you should specifically ask, "Are there any other remedies for vaginal dryness?" Or, you may choose to ask about something else that we have recommended in this book.

A less common but more troubling problem is if your doctor seems unusually interested in your sex life. If a doctor, or any other health care professional is making you feel uncomfortable, you should speak up immediately. In some instances, doctors have made sexual advances to patients, or touched their patients inappropriately. If this happens to you, you should terminate your relationship immediately and report the incident to your state Health Department Board of Medical Review. Do not worry about your clinician's feelings and do not blame yourself. It is not your fault, and if the individual acted inappropriately with you, you are probably not the first to experience this clearly unethical behavior.

✦ WHEN TO GET HELP: SEX THERAPY

No matter how many changes you make, it is sometimes necessary to get outside help with a sexual problem. This is as true for menopausal women as it is for women at earlier points and later points in the life cycle.

Sex therapy is a specific and structured approach to treatment and requires specialized education. Most sex therapists are licensed psychologists, social workers or psychiatrists. Beware of self-promoting "sexperts" and be sure the person has the appropriate licensing and credentials.

If the therapist focuses solely on you and the woman's role in appearance and improving her appeal, then you are in the wrong place. Sex therapy, by definition, defines sex as a couple's issue. Sex therapists are usually comfortable working with lesbians as well as heterosexual couples, but you should ask your friends about their reputation in this area. If communication in general is more of a problem, or if you are having too many arguments about other topics, then marital therapy is indicated. Marital therapy is a more general type of therapy that we discuss in our section on depression. Many couples who have sexual problems feel the need to work on the more general marital issues first. So in discussing this resource with your partner, you might try to identify which problem is interfering more in the marriage. Do the sexual problems lead to communication problems, or do they reflect the existing marital problems? If you are unable to make these decisions, you may go see a psychological consultant who can help you sort this out.

We hope you will not do what many couples do; that is, they hope the problems will disappear if they ignore them. Not talking about a problem only makes it worse, it doesn't make it go away. This is particularly true in the area of sexuality, since postmenopausal women who have problems with vaginal dryness and muscle changes tend to get worse over time if they do not get help. Remember, through the eyes of Miriam, "At twenty-five, sex was new and exciting, but let's face it, I didn't have a clue. Now, thirty-three years later, I'm *hot*—pun intended!"

RESOURCES

BOOKS

The field of sex therapy virtually exploded in the late 1960s and 1970s. Consequently, there are many good books that can help you.

For Each Other: Sharing Sexual Intimacy, by Lonnie Barbach, Ph.D. (New York: Signet Penguin Books, 1984), is an excellent and detailed book. Dr. Barbach has also made a videotape titled "Sex After 50: A Guide to Lifelong Sexual Pleasure," available from The Institute for Health and Aging (1-800-866-1000).

Women on Top, by Nancy Friday. This sequel to *My Secret Garden* details women's sexual fantasies (New York: Pocket Books, a Division of Simon & Schuster, 1991).

Intimate Partners: Patterns in Love and Marriage, by Maggie Scarf (New York: Random House, 1987).

The Time of Our Lives: Women Write on Sex After Forty, by Dena Taylor and Amber Coverdale Sumrall. This is an edited book of a variety of women's writings on their sexual experiences after the age of forty (Freedom, CA: Crossing Press, 1993).

ASSOCIATIONS

American Association of Sex Educators, Counselors and Therapists
435 N. Michigan Ave, Suite 1717
Chicago, IL 60611
(312) 644–0828

The American Association of Sex Educators, Counselors and Therapists (AASECT) can help you find a reputable sex therapist: it is a referral service. It also publishes a National Register of Certified Sex Educators and Sex Therapists.

Eve's Garden
119 W. 57th St, #420
NY, NY 10019
(212) 757-8651

A women's erotic mail-order catalog available for $1.

CHAPTER FOUR

Maintaining Our Health: Strong Bones

WE KNOW FROM OUR MENOPAUSE TOWN MEETINGS THAT YOU ARE RE-ally worried about osteoporosis and the possibility of fractures, as well as the dowager's hump. Too many advertisements for estrogen have pictures of that hump! Don't worry, we are not going to include one. You know what it looks like and you don't need more anxiety. High anxiety does not help people change. What you do need is a clear head to process all the new information about preventing osteoporosis. Besides, women entering the menopausal years today have a great opportunity to plan to maintain healthy bones. We can now make changes in our lifestyle that will lead to healthier and happier menopausal years and beyond. Until recently, osteoporosis was another excellent example of a health problem which, having a particular significance for women, had escaped the notice of medical researchers. We now know that this process of bone weakening causes substantial health problems, and can even lead to death for older women. But with appropriate guidance, women now have access to new treatments and preventions that will help avoid many of the heartaches and difficulties suffered by previous generations.

A woman in her menopausal years is likely to carry the responsibility for the care and well-being of elderly members of her family. Quite often, our patients have come to us concerned about the condition of their mothers, having watched them develop back pain or suffer hip fractures. These women begin to see their own future in the suffering of their parents. There can be no greater influence than viewing our parents suffer to make us question our own vulnerabilities. So many of our patients have come to us eager to learn what they can do to prevent it from happening to them. Elaine, a forty-nine-year-old interior decorator is one of those women.

Elaine first came to us because she was experiencing insomnia, headaches and what she thought were hot flashes. After a full evaluation, we learned that she was entering the menopause phase. She was also experiencing tension headaches and was under considerable stress. Elaine is an excellent example of the new generation of women. She came to us not only to address her present problems, but to plan the next phase of her life so that she could maintain her health. Elaine is a competent and self-educated woman in the area of health, the type of woman who listens eagerly to the Thursday morning news on the radio in order to find out what the *New England Journal* had published that week.

As a single parent of two adolescent girls, Elaine was more than busy as she worked full-time in her successful design practice. Elaine's "take charge" attitude had helped her raise her two daughters, since their father had moved to the West Coast and saw them only sporadically. Her divorce had left Elaine somewhat bitter, but over time, those negative feelings had mellowed to a humorous skepticism. Elaine was able to detect phoniness and sentimentality, and able to cut through to the heart of the matter quickly.

Her previously active, seventy-three-year-old mother, Kristina, was always close to Elaine and her family, providing advice and support. She lived nearby in an apartment building and, until recently, had an active and independent life filled with other friends and travel. But recently, Kristina had fallen on the ice and broken her hip. After one complication after another, Kristina had never been able to return to independent living and she had moved into Elaine's house. Although the family was coping, it was not what anyone wanted and was therefore somewhat stressful.

Having witnessed Kristina's condition and inability to care for herself, Elaine was now incredibly motivated. She was particularly dedicated to preventing the development of osteoporosis in herself and had read everything she could find on the subject. We enjoyed meeting with Elaine, but always knew that the sessions with her would be lengthy and detailed. If we had missed anything in the popular press, Elaine could fill us in. She was also worried because she had been told by a previous physician that she had osteoarthritis. She wanted to know if this was related to osteoporosis.

✦ WHAT IS OSTEOPOROSIS?

Osteoporosis is a chronic decrease in bone mass to the point that specific parts of the skeleton are so fragile that they are at great risk of fracturing. Osteoporosis is a significant problem for certain women, primarily white and Asian. For African-American and possibly Hispanic women, the good news is that they develop osteoporosis less frequently. African-American women, in general, attain greater spinal-bone mass than white women and have a lower fracture rate. The major cause of osteoporosis is the decline of estrogen, produced by the ovaries, after menopause. By the time a woman has reached eighty, she may have lost up to 40 percent of her bone substance (Cutler and Garcia, 1992). After menopause, she can lose 1 percent to 3 percent of bone mass per year (Cutler and Garcia, 1992a). The greatest decline in bone mass occurs between the ages of forty-five and seventy (Cutler and Garcia, 1992a). Not surprisingly, as the bone becomes thinner, more and more fractures can occur and many woman are unaware of small fractures that occur in the spine.

Osteoporosis literally means, porous bone. *Osteo-* for bone, and *porosis-* for porous. It is one of the most disabling and common bone disorders. The process of osteoporosis is somewhat complex. The decade of research on osteoporosis shows that osteoporosis is not simply a disease caused by a calcium imbalance. Many other factors are involved, including: genetics, exercise, body frame, and lifestyle, including nutritional issues and other related medical problems. There are two types of bone—cortical and trabecular. Cortical bone is the hard compact *outer* layer of bones (see Figure 4-1). About 80 percent of our skeletal mass is cortical bone. Trabecular bone refers to the spongy, more porous *interior* meshwork of bones that looks a bit like a honeycomb. Trabecular bone accounts for the remaining 20 percent of our bone mass. Each bone has an outer shell of dense cortical bone and a central cavity containing a varying amount of trabecular bone. One study found that if estrogen therapy is begun within the first three years of menopause, an actual modest increase in bone mineral density can be observed within a two-year period (Ettinger and others, 1987).

FIGURE 4-1

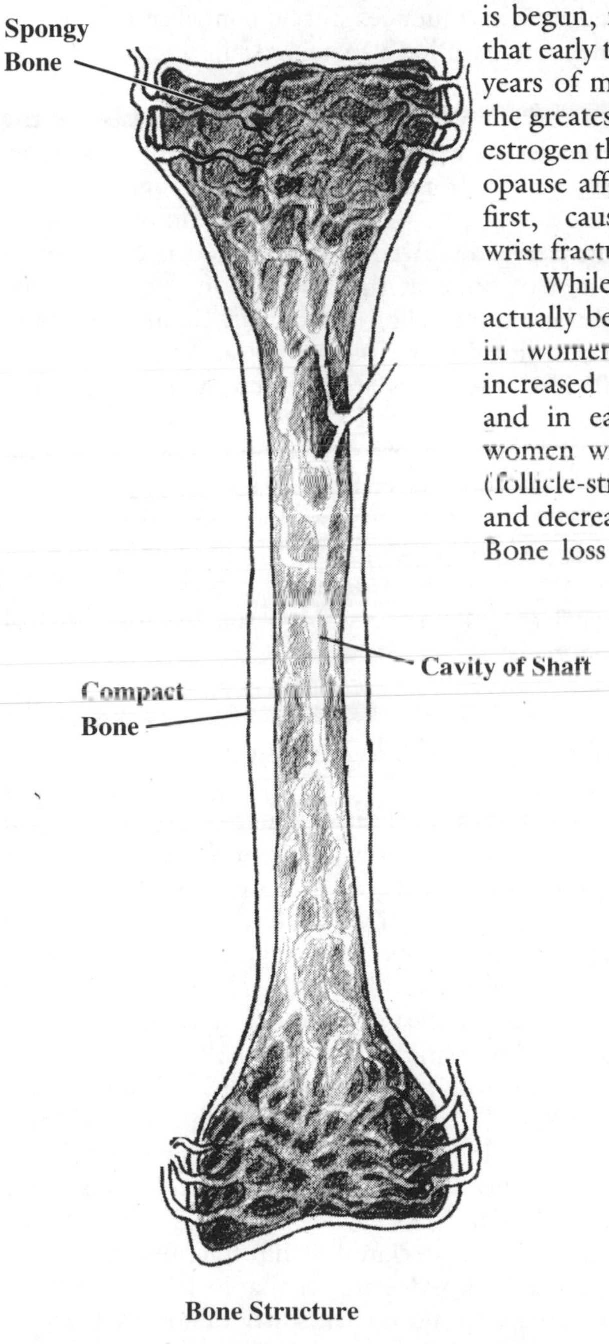

Spongy
Bone

Compact
Bone

Cavity of Shaft

Bone Structure

Although estrogen may protect the skeleton at whatever age it is begun, most experts believe that early therapy (within a few years of menopause) produces the greatest benefit. The loss of estrogen that occurs with menopause affects trabecular bone first, causing vertebral and wrist fractures.

While vertebral bone loss actually begins to occur earlier in women, it is significantly increased in perimenopausal and in early postmenopausal women who have rising FSH (follicle-stimulating hormone) and decreasing estrogen levels. Bone loss from the wrist also increases after menopause. Cortical bone loss occurs at a slower rate throughout postmenopausal life. Cortical bone loss, which occurs later, has even more serious consequences since it contributes to the 40 percent of white women who will have sustained hip fractures by age eighty.

Bone is actually a very active organ system. Osteoclasts are the cells that break down old bones, while osteoblasts build the new bone. Following this process, the new bone is toughened through a process of depositing phosphate and a special calcium. A continuous renovation process with bone being dissolved and reformed is called bone remodeling. The amount of bone in the body at any point in time reflects the balance of these remodeling forces. Dr. Kenneth Cooper refers to these forces as "the demolition squads and the builders." (Cooper, 1989, p. 20) Both processes are affected by many different factors, like a decrease in calcium intake or certain medications.

Osteoarthritis (degenerative arthritis) is another chronic process that wears away the cartilage (protective layer of connecting material) between the bones and leads to joint stiffness and pain. Although osteoporosis and osteoarthritis are both common in women, they are not related. So the presence of one does not mean the existence of the other. Elaine had been alarmed unnecessarily—she had no signs of osteoarthritis or osteoporosis.

✦ THE CONSEQUENCES OF OSTEOPOROSIS

Hip fractures are the most significant consequence of osteoporosis in women. Annually, 250,000 hip fractures occur in the United States (Fleming, 1992). The rate of hip fractures increases dramatically with age in white women, and 80 percent of all hip fractures are associated with osteoporosis. White women have a 15 percent lifetime risk of having a hip fracture (Byyny and Speroff, 1990). These fractures are a particularly significant source of suffering, loss of functioning and even mortality in older women. Surprisingly, between 12 to 20 percent of patients with hip fractures die due to the fracture or its complications within three months (U.S. Congress, 1992). This is because of complications that are life-threatening such as blood clots, pneumonias or heart problems. Of those who survive, many are disabled and may become permanent invalids, like Kristina. According to the National Osteoporosis Foundation, the cost related to hip fractures caused by osteoporosis exceeded seven billion dollars per year in 1990, and these costs are projected to increase to more than thirty billion by the year

2020. All the more reason for all of us to take appropriate precautions and lifestyle changes to promote bone health.

FRACTURES

Fractures of the spine can cause significant back pain. The most common sites for vertebral fractures are in the upper and middle back. The pain with the fracture can be intense but short-lived, decreasing over the following few months. In some cases, it can linger as chronic back pain, due to many factors, including an increasing shift in the spine orientation (thoracic kyphosis). This condition can usually be treated with nonsteroidal anti-inflammatory drugs (NSAIDs) or aspirin and by exercise. On the other hand, many women don't know they have these fractures because they either never experienced symptoms, or did not have symptoms severe enough to cause them to see a physician. They usually find out about their fractures because they are seen on X rays that have been done for other purposes.

Fractures of the forearm bone (the radius) occur earlier in the postmenopausal period than do hip fractures. This risk increases tenfold in white women between the ages of thirty-five and sixty. A white woman has approximately a 15 percent lifetime risk of a wrist fracture, referred to as a Colles' fracture. This is the most common fracture among white women, until age seventy-five, when hip fractures become more common.

Another of Elaine's concerns was her height: her mother had lost several inches and now had the infamous dowager's hump, a permanent curvature of her upper spine. Approximately 50 percent of women over the age of sixty-five will have spinal compression fractures, which cause this shrinking process.

All of us, men and women alike, lose height as we age. This is a result of several factors, including poor posture, some shrinkage of the discs between the bones of our spine and osteoporosis. But remember, most women don't need to worry about actually developing a dowager's hump, but may experience some normal loss of height.

✦ RISK FACTORS FOR OSTEOPOROSIS

Elaine was worried about her personal history as compared to her mother's. There are various factors, including medications and nutritional deficiencies that are risks for osteoporosis. Elaine was right to be concerned about her menopause affecting her risk. By far, the most important risk factor for the development of osteoporosis is loss of estrogen. Seventy-five percent or more of bone loss which occurs in women during the first twenty years after menopause is attributed to estrogen deficiency, rather than to the aging process itself. The risk of having osteoporosis actually depends on two factors—the bone mass that has been achieved prior to menopause (an important point for early prevention) and the subsequent rate of bone loss.

Women who are overweight actually have a decreased risk of developing osteoporosis. This effect is believed to be secondary to the stress that increased weight puts on bones, causing them to remodel rapidly. Maureen, one of our patients who has been struggling with diets all of her life, was delighted to hear this news and said, "Finally, revenge over Nancy Reagan and her size four dresses!"

There are some risk factors that we have no control over such as our sex, family history and ethnic background. That does not mean that we cannot do anything to counterbalance these risks. Elaine was worried because she had a Scandinavian background, as did her mother, Kristina, but, unlike her mother, she was of medium build and slightly overweight. Her mother had also had a hysterectomy at the age of forty, had never been on HRT and had not been a physically active woman. Elaine's lifestyle was far different from her mother's. Her mother had been generally active with her volunteer activities, card games and outings to museums, whereas Elaine's generation had focused a bit more on physical activity. Elaine enjoyed skiing, sailing and jogging, and used physical activity as part of her daily routine throughout the year. In fact, Elaine was sailing so often that we needed to talk to her about over exposure to the sun with respect to skin cancer. On the other hand, her exposure to the sun made it likely that she was getting enough vitamin D, one of the necessary ingredients for bone health. Elaine's physical activity lowered her overall risk a bit. We have more control over some of the risk factors for osteoporosis. And the perimenopausal years are a good time to make some critical changes.

Smoking may be an important risk factor for the development of osteoporosis and it can diminish the effects of any other positive measures that are taken (e.g., hormone replacement therapy or exercise) to prevent osteoporosis. We know that early calcium intake contributes to peak bone mass in young women but for most of us this information comes too late. The good news is that we can still affect our bones with an adequate calcium intake later in life as we will describe in a bit.

Consumption of excessive caffeine and alcohol deplete calcium from our bones and are important risk factors for osteoporosis and fractures. Certain medications can also contribute to osteoporosis, including certain antacids (not calcium carbonate-based), too much thyroid hormone, corticosteroids and antiseizure therapy. But even if you do need to be on these medications, there are ways to minimize these effects.

✦ EVALUATION FOR OSTEOPOROSIS

None of the experts in osteoporosis have suggested that we should screen *all* perimenopausal women in an attempt to select a group of women who are at particularly high risk. This is due to several factors. There is an enormous individual variation in the ability of the body to maintain its bone density. Although measurements of bone mass at different sites of the body may vary, any significant bone loss at any site in the body is important information regarding future risk of fractures. Unfortunately, not all of the equipment at various medical facilities is "state of the art." However, this should not discourage you from getting bone densitometry if your primary care professional suggests it. It is important to check the reputation of the center you are going to.

In the end, about half of menopausal women do not experience any ill effects of menopause on their bones. The ultimate question then becomes: How do we predict the ones that will develop osteoporosis and who should we be testing?

Most experts feel that the additional information that screening will provide is indicated in the following situations. First, it is indicated in any postmenopausal woman whose decision to commit to lifelong HRT will be strongly influenced by the determination of low bone mass. Elaine expressed interest to us regarding HRT therapy because of her risk of developing osteoporosis. Second, testing should be done in any woman with evidence of vertebral compression fractures or thinning of the bones on plain X-ray films. Third, any woman who must receive six months or more of steroid therapy for other medical conditions should have testing.

There are several new procedures that have been developed to measure the density of the bone. The diagnosis of osteoporosis cannot be made by plain X-ray films, unless the osteoporosis is quite advanced. Be wary of any physician who informs you that he or she can tell that you have osteoporosis by looking at a regular chest X ray or hip film. A regular X ray is not an accurate way to assess osteoporosis. At least 30 to 40 percent of bone mineral must be lost before the diagnosis of osteoporosis can be made on X ray. Advances in the assessment of osteoporosis are now happening rapidly. At the present time there are four other methods that are helpful in the diagnosis: Single-photon absorptiometry (SPA), Dual-photon absorptiometry (DPA), Dual-energy X-ray absorptiometry (DEXA) and CT scan. Most centers have been using the DPA and measure the bone mineral density of the lumbar spine, proximal femur and total body to assess the degree of osteoporosis. DEXA is the newest and most common technique. It is faster and has a clearer resolution than the DPA.

Any woman who has apparent osteoporosis should be screened for other conditions that might be causing this process. Some women can develop primary hyperparathyroidism (overactive parathyroid gland), an exaggerated response of one of the glands in the body which produces an elevation in serum parathyroid hormone (PTH). The PTH, in turn, causes release of calcium from the bones. In this case, checking certain blood levels (parathyroid hormone, calcium, phosphorous, and alkaline phosphatase) may be helpful. Thyroid function tests are important as well, since hyperthyroidism is associated with osteoporosis. Assessment of kidney function is important for a so-called secondary hyperparathyroidism that occurs with kidney failure. Blood counts may be ordered, looking for a particular type blood cell malignancy (multiple myeloma) that is associated with some weakness of the bone. Do not be worried about this list of complicated sounding and perhaps frightening diseases. Most women who have osteoporosis are suffering from an unfortunately common disorder that is not caused by any of these conditions, but you should be checked out anyway.

✦ PREVENTING OSTEOPOROSIS

Figure 4-2 is our plan for the prevention of osteoporosis. There is no doubt that exercise and diet have very important effects on bone strength. The earlier in life a woman adopts a nutritional plan to prevent osteoporosis, the greater her chances are of averting the disease. The most essential dietary requirement is adequate daily amounts of calcium. Calcium intake has been shown to be low in both males and females who go on to develop hip fractures. Women with higher calcium diets have lower rates of hip fracture than women with diets that lack adequate calcium.

Individual calcium requirements vary among women due to a variety of factors, including age, dietary habits, drug use, diseases and hormonal status. Rates of calcium absorption can vary as well. Women

FIGURE 4-2

PRESCRIPTION FOR HEALTHY BONES PREVENTION OF OSTEOPOROSIS

MORE	Calcium	Vitamin D	Exercise

and

LESS	Alcohol	Caffeine

and

NO	Smoking or Fasting Diets

Equals

PREVENTING OSTEOPOROSIS

who eat a reasonable diet can expect to absorb approximately 30 to 40 percent of their dietary calcium, but this declines with age. We recommend an intake of 1,000 mg for perimenopausal women, to 1,500 mg per day for postmenopausal women. Unfortunately, this means that a substantial percentage of women in this country are not eating enough calcium. Because of concern about calories and cholesterol, many women have actually conscientiously restricted dairy products from their diet. This may not be a good choice since excessive thinness is associated with an increased risk of osteoporosis. In addition, a woman's risk of osteoporosis may be greater than her risk of developing heart disease from an elevated cholesterol. So a good solution to this dilemma is to eat low-fat dairy products.

There are many foods, including dairy products, sardines, tofu and certain vegetables, like broccoli and collard greens, that are important sources of absorbable dietary calcium. We have found that increasing calcium is one of the easiest and single most important changes that we can make in our lives to prevent osteoporosis. It is shocking that the average amount of calcium taken in by most American women is closer to 450–550 mg a day (Cooper, 1989). By using the list of calcium-rich foods, daily intake can be increased substantially (see Table 4-1). But here is the bind: most women are worried about their calories as well. It seems unlikely to us that women who have avoided dairy products for one reason or another will change their lives by drinking four glasses of skim milk per day. One or two glasses seems possible.

Also, certain women may have lactose (contained in dairy products) intolerance. This occurs because the enzyme that breaks down lactose (lactase) is diminished. They can also eat other foods that are supplemented with calcium. Products like Lactaid may help reduce the gastrointestinal symptoms, or they can eat nondairy foods high in calcium. Calcium supplements are likely to be necessary if this condition is present.

At the same time, calcium supplements can be extremely helpful. In looking at calcium supplements, it is important to consider not only the dosage, but also the amount of calcium that's immediately available to the body. Calcium carbonate appears to deliver the largest percentage of calcium to the body. Over-the-counter antacids are also usually composed of calcium carbonate alone. They contain 250 mg of elemental calcium per tablet. So, two to four tablets a day can increase intake by 500–1000 mg. In general, calcium tablets should be taken with meals and doses above 500 mg should be divided. This process will improve our ability to absorb the calcium. The only contraindication to taking calcium is a personal history of calcium kidney stones. There are, however, some side effects from taking calcium supplements which include bloating and constipation, but these conditions can usually be avoided by increasing fluid intake, dietary fiber, and maintaining regular exercise. The food industry has now made it easier to have a calcium rich diet by supplementing many basic foods such as fruit juices, cereals and breads.

Here is a way to test your calcium supplement. Take a glass and fill it up half with water and half with vinegar. Drop in your supplement and wait a half an hour. At the end of that time, the supplement should be completely dissolved. If it is not, the supplement is not providing your body with the calcium that it needs. This experiment simulates what happens in your stomach. An undissolved tablet will not be absorbed into your bloodstream.

Vitamin D is necessary for us to absorb calcium efficiently. Therefore if we have a deficiency in vitamin D, we will not be able to absorb

Table 4–1

CALCIUM CONTENT IN VARIOUS FOODS

Food Item	Serving Size	Calcium Content (mg)	Calories
Milk			
Whole	8 oz	291	150
Skim	8 oz	302	85
Yogurt (with added milk solids)			
Plain, low-fat	8 oz	415	145
Fruit, low-fat	8 oz	343	230
Frozen, fruit	8 oz	240	223
Frozen, chocolate	8 oz	160	220
Cheese			
Mozzarella, part skim	1 oz	207	80
Muenster	1 oz	203	105
Cheddar	1 oz	204	115
Riccotta, part skim	4 oz	335	190
Cottage, low-fat (2%)	4 oz	78	103
Ice Cream, Vanilla (11% fat)			
Hard	1 cup	176	270
Soft serve	1 cup	236	375
Ice Milk, Vanilla			
Hard (4% fat)	1 cup	176	185
Soft Serve (3% fat)	1 cup	274	223
Fish and Shellfish			
Oysters, raw (13–19 med.)	1 cup	226	160
Sardines, canned in oil drained, including bones	3 oz	372	175
Salmon, pink, canned, including bones	3 oz	167	120
Shrimp, canned, drained	3 oz	98	100
Vegetables			
Bok Choy, raw	1 cup	74	9
Broccoli, cooked, drained, from raw	1 cup	136	40
Soybeans, cooked, drained, from raw	1 cup	131	235
Collards, cooked, drained, from raw	1 cup	357	65
Turnip greens, cooked drained, from raw	1 cup	252	30
Tofu	4 oz	108	85
Almonds	1 oz	75	165

*Adapted from National Osteoporosis Foundation, 1992

calcium well. Vitamin D is generated by exposure of the skin to the sun and a well-balanced diet. We need fifteen minutes per day of sunshine to get enough vitamin D. Therefore, it is possible that some women are not getting enough sunshine on a daily basis. In addition, milk is the only dairy product that is fortified with vitamin D. So you should not believe that you are getting vitamin D by eating cheeses or yogurt that has not been fortified. Finally, there is tremendous variability in the amount of vitamin D fortification in milk. Tests from various dairies found that some milk has too little and other milk has too much vitamin D. Attempts are now being made to standardize this process. If you have health problems that leave you housebound, you may need supplements of between 400 to 800 units of vitamins per day. Anyone with severe liver or kidney impairment may also have a decreased ability to metabolize vitamin D, and may need supplements as well. You should not take vitamin D and calcium supplements without checking with your doctor. This is a situation where the amount of calcium absorbed into your bloodstream could be excessive and dangerous.

If you want to prevent osteoporosis, please try to stop smoking! This is also true if you wish to prevent heart attacks, stroke, lung cancer, wrinkles, early menopause and early aging. We continue this discussion in many of our other chapters.

Moderate alcohol consumption may increase the risk of the development of osteoporosis, and is another compelling reason to restrict alcohol intake. Alcohol works as a diuretic and causes an increase in the loss of calcium from bone. Too much alcohol can also interfere with calcium absorption in the stomach. Women who drink more than one drink per day are at increased risk for the development of osteoporosis. While learning more about Elaine and her daily habits, we discovered that she had one to two glasses of wine at night to relax while she unwound from her busy day. Quite often, she would begin her relaxation with a gin and tonic while fixing dinner, and admitted that her alcohol consumption had risen since her mother moved in. Elaine is not alone. We see many women who use alcohol to cope with stress. We talked with Elaine about her feeling that she deserved some reward at the end of a hard day. Elaine began to understand that alcohol could do more harm than good, especially if her intake increased. We discussed other outlets for relaxation, including a short walk, an herbal bath, or a cup of tea with a good book. In the end, she decided to buy a microwave oven and encouraged her mother to use it to help prepare dinner. This way, Kristina had an activity that made her feel more like a contributing member of the family, and Elaine could pick up that mystery novel that she had been meaning to finish. As Kristina increased her ability to get around, she was able to alternate cooking dinner with Elaine and her two daughters. And, as Elaine cut back on alcohol and the family began to share more of the chores, her headaches began to diminish. This did not surprise us, as headaches are often related to stress and substance abuse. We discuss headaches, as well as stress, in greater detail in Chapter Eight.

Caffeine is also known to act as a diuretic and increases the loss of calcium through the urine so that it is wise to restrict caffeine-containing beverages to one to two per day. There are certain other foods that can affect the absorption of calcium, such as oatmeal and bran. Ironically, high-fiber diets that are seen as healthy to reduce fat and increase bulk can actually interfere with calcium absorption, because they increase the rate at which food is passed through the gastrointestinal tract. Obviously, you don't want to eliminate any of these foods from your diet, as they play an important role in other aspects of prevention. You can maximize your calcium intake by not eating these foods at the same meal as the foods that you take to ensure an adequate supply of calcium.

✦ WHAT ABOUT EXERCISE? IT WORKS!

We need to deal with this exercise issue again. We are surprised that so few women at our town meetings ask about exercise. Then again, why should we be? It turns out that only 22 percent of Americans engage in thirty or more minutes of even light to moderate physical activity five or more times per week. But this is a key issue in maintaining our health, especially our bones.

You have probably noticed that we are referring to "physical activity" and "exercise." Physical activity is any movement resulting in energy expenditure. Exercise, on the other hand, is a leisure-time physical activity that is structured and designed to improve physical fitness. If you are not interested in regular exercise, at least try to be more physically active: It can pay off. Physical inactivity, or a sedentary lifestyle is a health risk for high blood pressure, elevated fats and obesity. In contrast, physical activity is positively related to a longer and healthier life (Blair, 1989).

So, if we know these facts about exercise, why aren't we doing more? There are plenty of reasons. First, it is hard to get going! In addition, most women in the menopausal years grew up with little exposure to enjoyable physical activity or sports. The dreaded gym class in school was the little we got, and it was often combined with "hygiene" (those famous "What every girl should know" pamphlets again). Few of us received any encouragement to explore the role of physical activity, sports or exercise. Many of us felt like klutzes.

Then there is the role of the "cosmetic body." Having little education on the positive aspects of physical activity in our teens, we were then confronted with the demands of "looking right." We spent years feeling inadequate, not thin enough, or buxom enough, or whatever enough. Then came the aerobics movement. We know as many women who were turned off by Jane Fonda's videotape as those who began aerobics. Let's face it: Most of us are not born with a tall and lean body composition like Jane Fonda in the first place.

So what did many of us do? We continued to repress the physical aspects of our lives. We dieted, or did nothing. Why enter a losing battle? Why begin a new activity that will bring back bad memories?

It is time to change all of that. We are women now, not the young girls thrown into gym classes in those awful blue suits. First and foremost, physical activity and exercise is no longer a cosmetic *or* a competitive issue: it is a critical health issue. We do not need to be "good" at it; we do not need to be "attractive"; we just need to do it. This is especially true with respect to bone health.

Weight-bearing exercise, even as little as thirty minutes a day about three times a week, will help. You may well ask: what is a weight-bearing exercise? A weight-bearing activity is one where our bodies must be supported. This would include walking, jogging and many sports activities listed in Table 4-2. Non–weight-bearing activities are those like bike riding, where a bicycle seat supports our body, or swimming, where we are partially supported by the water. As we will describe in our health promotion chapter, an exercise program does not need to be extreme for us to gain health benefits. Table 4-2 also details an exercise program where the target is better bone health. The principle here is to put stress on the bones in a consistent fashion in order to strengthen them. We need to focus exercise on certain areas of the body. Exercises like running or jogging, aerobics, stair climbing and dancing are beneficial for the leg, hip and spine.

Remember that we have arms as well as legs. Since women tend to suffer fractures in the upper arm as well as in the forearm at the wrist, it is important to exercise the upper body as well. These activities would include racket sports, weight training and rowing. (Try some push-ups if you are really tough!) Aerobics classes, of course, can exercise all areas of the body, depending on the specific exercises that are included.

One problem here is that many women enjoy walking and yet

walking apparently does not provide as much stress on the bones and therefore does not harden them as much as jogging. Using the principle of slow but steady change, why not alternate jogging with walking? You are probably walking because you enjoy it and are comfortable, but by increasing the amount of jogging you do, you can also improve your bone health.

The studies that evaluate the effectiveness of exercise on osteoporosis suggest that the exercise needs to be at least *thirty* minutes of duration. Weight training, of course, will vary, depending on the individual's abilities and strengths. With respect to frequency, as little as three days a week can be beneficial.

BEGINNING AN EXERCISE PROGRAM

The first step is to decide that it is important. You and your clinician can work out why you are exercising. Are you exercising primarily to build up your bone strength, or are you interested in maximal cardiovascular fitness? After you have decided your goal, you can choose an exercise plan and setting, as we describe in our chapters on heart health and/or promoting a healthy lifestyle.

The next step is to allot a specific amount of time necessary to accomplish your goals. You might also decide whether you are a solitary exerciser or a social exerciser. The buddy or partner system is often extremely helpful to a woman, as you will learn in a bit. It provides social connection as well as extra motivation. We have also met women who are very active socially and who work long hours who would prefer to use their exercise routine as a private meditation time. So structure your exercise routine according to your individual situation.

There are many barriers to exercise including the weather, being overweight, lack of time, and sometimes the lack of funds to participate in the type of exercise we enjoy most. Time is a difficult issue for menopausal women with multiple roles. That is one of the reasons that we have suggested that exercising with a friend can have multiple benefits. It is also important to know that this might be one of the most important health decisions of your life, for improved bone health, improved cardiovascular fitness and an overall sense of physical well-being.

Women who live in the city face additional problems since they may be worried about safety. Fortunately, many suburban malls now offer mall walking and early-morning exercise programs. Exercise videotapes can also be helpful.

Finances can be a difficult problem. The only real equipment you need for exercise is a good pair of shoes for the appropriate activity or a bicycle if you prefer. Layers of clothing can be developed from your existing wardrobe. Jogging and bike paths are becoming more and more a part of the American landscape and are always available.

Table 4-2 depicts an exercise program for healthy bones. Exercise has to be fun. It has to be a chance to socialize or spend precious time alone, wear comfortable clothes, and do something physical. We can overcome the old ghosts of gym class and the new ghosts of mirrored aerobic classes with youngsters wearing Spandex. The first step is to move exercise to the top of your priority list.

Two other areas related to bone health are often ignored. They

---

Table 4–2

FIT PROGRAM FOR HEALTHY BONES

Purpose: Maintain Bone Health

Frequency:	2–3 times per week
Intensity:	Moderate
Time:	20–30 minutes
Types:	Weight-bearing exercise
	Against gravity
	Increased resistance
	Examples: Weight training
	Rowing
	Stair climbing
	Step machine
	Racquet sports
	Jogging
	Step aerobics

Note: Activities of limited benefit: walking, swimming

are good posture and prevention. It is clear that by straightening our posture, our height can be affected. If we sit up and stand straight (mother was right), we will look taller. In addition, pulling our shoulders back and pulling in our abdominal muscles will improve our posture and bone health and make us feel better overall.

For those of you who have already developed osteoporosis, your first step is to maintain the bone density that you still have. The advantage of early detection, or secondary prevention, is that you can make changes. Your choices here include HRT, calcium-rich diet and some of the medications we have recommended. In addition, if you are beginning to experience pain, it is important to develop a regimen that addresses that pain effectively. Your physician can prescribe nonsteroidal anti-inflammatory drugs like ibuprofen to treat your pain. It is important, also, to maintain your exercise, despite some minimal pain. Try to begin any exercise program with slow stretching in order to warm up and to minimize the actual possibility of injury. If you find an exercise program, whether it be walking, tennis, bicycling or aerobics, it is a good idea to find a partner. It is important to choose someone whose skills and whose health are at about your level. It is unlikely that you will both feel down on the same day and therefore, if one of you has the motivation to keep going, you can help the other. Your partner may also suffer from some of the same problems with osteoporosis, therefore, you can share with her your feelings about this difficult problem. Sharing your feelings with a person who has a similar type of problem is one of the most therapeutic activities. You will feel better, she will feel better and so it goes. Osteoporosis may be a part of aging for many of us, but we can prevent much of it and we can cope with it if we continue an active lifestyle, maintain our bone density, and develop a support system.

Prevention of fractures involves many changes. As we get older, whether we have osteoporosis or not, it is important to reduce our chance of accidents. Here are some suggestions to help prevent injuries and falls: Bend your knees when picking anything up, and avoid lifting heavy objects whenever possible. Women who are beginning to suffer from osteoporosis can organize their household to minimize the possibility of accidents and resulting fractures. Objects that are used frequently should be placed in higher places. Slippery floors and loose floor rugs are also to be avoided, and stairways should include good strong railings. Be especially careful climbing and descending stairs. Stairs and hallways should be properly lit. We should be careful to remove loose wires and cords from the floor. The prevention of falls is yet another good reason to avoid high-heeled shoes.

How Estrogen Can Help

Appropriate estrogen replacement therapy can have a major impact on the risk of osteoporosis with a 50 to 60 percent decrease in fractures in the arm and hip (Lindsay, 1991). Estrogen improves calcium absorption and makes it possible to utilize supplemental calcium in lower doses, reducing the side effects associated with higher doses, such as constipation and flatulence. Estrogen probably has a direct protective mechanism on bone in addition to increasing the absorption of calcium. Estrogen receptors have been isolated in bone cells, suggesting that estrogen directly stimulates bone formation.

This decision about estrogen includes consideration of many risks and benefits for each woman, as we describe in our chapter on hormone replacement therapy. The literature on HRT and osteoporosis is reasonably clear: HRT does reduce the risk of weakening of the bones and subsequent fractures. Elaine was anxious to take HRT because of her experience with her mother. She was also having hot flashes at the time and some sleep disturbances as well, so it was not a difficult decision for her. In contrast, Lauranne, a fifty-one-year-old teacher, whose mother had osteoporosis, also had a sister who was diagnosed with breast cancer at age forty-five. Most experts would agree that the decision to take HRT on a long-term basis should be weighed against the possible increased risk of breast cancer with long-term therapy. We describe this further in the chapter on HRT.

Other Medications

Many women will choose not to take estrogen if they are at risk for breast cancer or for other reasons. Not all these women will, in fact, experience osteoporosis. Good nutrition and weight bearing exercise are the basics here. In addition, there are several other medications that have been investigated. Calcitonin is another substance in the body which stimulates the uptake of calcium by the bone. It has been used either as an injection or as a nasal spray, and both forms can reduce bone loss. Although the nasal spray is not yet approved by the FDA, it may be available in a few years.

We are all familiar with fluoride and its miraculous effect on the decline of dental cavities in this country. There were initial hopes that it would be an effective therapy for osteoporosis. It is a potent stimulator of bone formation, particularly trabecular (spongy) bone, but it appears to decrease cortical (compact) bone and therefore increases fractures. Finally, there is promising data on another medication, etidronate disodium, which has been used, to date, only in clinical studies. It appears to reduce bone weakening and the rate of new vertebral fractures in postmenopausal women, but additional studies are needed.

✦ COMMUNICATION

In choosing a primary care professional, you need to find someone who emphasizes prevention. A primary care physician is, by definition, an internist or a family practitioner who is trained in comprehensive care and prevention. Both fields require board exams. Some gynecologists practice primary care as well. Many primary care offices and group practices have nurse practitioners and physicians assistants who may serve as your primary clinician. These health care professionals are well trained and licensed and some of them may have more interest in and knowledge about preventive care than some physicians. Hospitals can provide you with a list of general internists, family practitioners or general gynecologists who admit to their institution. Such issues as type of insurance accepted, age or gender of the practitioner may be important to you.

Your particular concerns about osteoporosis should be part of any discussion you have with your health care provider about prevention, menopausal symptoms or treatment with HRT. You will want to discuss this subject with the primary care professional who will be following you long-term, making recommendations about diet and exercise, in addition to monitoring any therapy. Many different physicians may have expertise in the area of osteoporosis and can be used as consultants. These include gynecologists, reproductive endocrinologists (a gynecologic subspecialty) and endocrinologists (a subspecialty of internal medicine).

A thorough office visit about prevention of osteoporosis is a good idea. Any discussion with your clinician that is extensive may require extra time. It is a good idea to let the secretary or office manager know that you wish to have a more extensive discussion with your physician at the time of scheduling the appointment. On the day of the appointment, you may choose to call ahead to see if the physician is running on time, so that you can plan your schedule accordingly. By this time you have set up essentially a contract with the office where you know that this will be an extended office visit.

If you are in good health during your menopausal years, then the goal is to maintain your health. If you are concerned about osteoporo--

sis, the first step is obviously to discuss it with your clinician and to work on a prevention plan together. If you find that you are in a very high-risk group, then you might consider the bone densitometry measurements we have suggested. Remember that screening for osteoporosis is not recommended for all menopausal women. Third-party reimbursement may be limited to women who are high-risk when it comes to screening for osteoporosis. This is important because the cost of any bone densitometry can range between $80 and $400, so you should check with your health insurance plan.

If your physician does not take your concerns seriously, your first step is to restate your concerns carefully and clearly and to mention your risk factors. The questionnaire can help you evaluate your risk for osteoporosis. As we mentioned earlier, if your physician recommends a routine X ray, this is not sufficient. You can also ask for a recommendation to an osteoporosis specialist. Most generalists are quite comfortable getting a second opinion. The National Osteoporosis Foundation can also be helpful in providing you with the name of a specialist in your area.

COMMUNICATION WITH YOUR FAMILY

Your prevention program may well require changes in the entire family system. This is true because most women are in charge of the food preparation in families, as unfair as this may be. For example, Barbara, a fifty-three-year-old mother of five, was the energetic hub of her large and active family. Although she had enjoyed sports as a young woman, her family's needs had swallowed up her time and after her hysterectomy, ten years ago, she had gained thirty pounds. She had spent the last twenty years driving her five sons to and from various sporting events and attending as many as she could. This year she created her prevention program and decided to cut down on red meat, increase calcium and ask for a NordicTrack machine for Christmas. Twenty-five years ago, Barbara would serve her family steak and potatoes for dinner. Ten years ago, she focused more on chicken and rice with added vegetables. This year, after meeting with our nutritionist, she carefully prepared a dinner of stir-fried tofu and broccoli in a soy/peanut sauce. She met with mass rebellion. Her five sons, as well as her husband taunted her saying, "Mom's gone veggie!"—as if it were some leftover disease from the sixties—"Tofu, you've got to be kidding!"

Barbara met with our psychologist, as well as our nutritionist, and together they all decided that this was insensitivity and resistance to change, rather than any major family problem. The psychologist sug-

EVALUATING YOUR RISK FOR OSTEOPOROSIS

Do you have these risk factors?

	YES	NO
A. White or Asian		
Family history of osteoporosis		
Slim		
Small-framed		
Early menopause (Before age 40)		
Very fair skin		
B. Smoking		
Alcohol intake of more than five ounces per day		
Low level of exercise		
Diet low in calcium		
C. Medications for		
Thyroid replacement		
Seizures		
Blood clots		
or		
Any steroid		

SCORING: Count each YES answer. A higher score indicates an increased risk for osteoporosis. (Adapted from National Osteoporosis Foundation, 1991.)

gested that Barbara's husband, William, come with her to the next session. There, they could discuss as a family the importance of Barbara changing her habits in order to lose weight and become more physically active. Just this session alone impressed upon William the seriousness of Barbara's commitment. He agreed that if he and the boys did not like her menu planning, they would do their own. At first the family developed a two-tiered system, with Barbara eating more calcium and vegetables in her diet and William and the boys ordering out for pizza. Over time, however, Barbara would sneak in different forms of tofu and the family grew to accept certain of her menus. (Yes, we did suggest that William or the boys do the cooking, but change sometimes takes time!) Most importantly, she uses the NordicTrack machine every evening, and has enjoyed proving them all wrong about her commitment to change. Barbara had not always been comfortable with regular exercise after her hysterectomy, and given the intense demands of her family. When her sons began to see how much happier and alive she seemed, they began to encourage her and of course, ultimately they had to all take turns on the track, with Barbara having first choice.

Barbara's family benefited from her changes in that they began to eat a more healthy diet and began to exercise more too. But Elaine was in the interesting situation of being the mother of teenage daughters and was concerned about their bone health as well as her own. Mia and Karen, age fifteen and seventeen, were typical teenagers. Both were physically active but their diet seemed to fluctuate between fast food, heavy on the grease, to restriction of calories in order to control their weight. Yet we know that peak bone mass is reached between the relatively young ages of twenty-five and thirty-five. So, a teenage girl who has begun to avoid dairy products without replacing them with other sources of calcium is setting up a lifetime habit that can have long-term negative consequences. One study of girls between the ages of fifteen to nineteen found that they only consume about 600 mg of calcium per day (Cooper, 1989). That is considerably less than the 1000–1500 mg that most people recommend. Even the presently recommended daily allowance (RDA) is 800 mg and thus, these teenagers were not even reaching that minimal amount.

The good news is that the younger girls apparently retain more calcium, but still the two girls were setting up bad habits in their teenage years. If you add to that the habits that develop in the late teens and twenties of consuming a lot of caffeine, and drinking perhaps too much alcohol, then the patterns become even worse. Elaine tried to talk to her daughters about these issues and at first, they were reluctant to change. Over time, especially with the example of their grandmother, with whom they were both close, they began to see the necessity to change also. They added some frozen yogurt to their diet and would drink skim milk from time to time. Their mother shared with them the list of calcium-rich foods, including sardines or salmon with the bones left in. They laughed and exclaimed to their mother, "Yeah, right. No way are we gonna munch salmon between meals."

We hope, as time goes on, that Elaine will minimize her risk for osteoporosis and Mia and Karen will build up their bone mass and that her mother, Kristina, will have some alleviation of her suffering.

RESOURCES

National Osteoporosis Foundation
1150 17th Street, NW, Suite 500
Washington, DC 20036
(202) 223-2226

The foundation publishes books and pamphlets on osteoporosis, and puts out a catalog of patient-education materials, including readings and other resources. A $25 membership gets you the quarterly newsletter, "The Osteoporosis Report," with articles on research, medical advances, prevention and treatment. They distribute pamphlets with respect to prevention of osteoporosis and could direct you to your closest treatment center. The National Osteoporosis Foundation publishes one of the best books on osteoporosis called Boning Up on Osteoporosis: A Guide to Prevention and Treatment. *This readable book tells us about risk factors, prevention of osteoporosis and exercise training.*

Ourselves Getting Older *has a chapter on osteoporosis. This book is published by the Boston Women's Health Collective, and it is quite detailed and easy to read. Just as many publications published by the pharmaceutical industry are very pro-hormone replacement therapy, some parts of this book are extremely antihormone replacement therapy. As long as you are aware of this point of view, this chapter can be extremely helpful.*

✦ RESOURCES FOR EXERCISE

With respect to exercise and osteoporosis, we discuss accessing resources in great detail in our final chapter. However, it is important to note that almost any part of the country has either a YWCA or a Jewish Community Center nearby. These types of centers tend to offer low-cost programs in contrast to some of the fancier health clubs and gymnasiums. Many of them also have exercise physiologists who can help you in developing a personalized exercise program. But if all else fails, remember that walking is one of the first steps to maintaining your bones at the menopausal period.

CHAPTER FIVE

Maintaining Our Health: Healthy Hearts

IF YOU ARE LIKE MOST WOMEN, YOU ARE WONDERING, "WHY SHOULD I be concerned about heart disease?" Yet there are several good reasons for you to become knowledgeable about your heart. Cardiovascular disease, which includes heart disease and stroke, is the number one cause of death in all U.S. women over the age of forty. Surprised, are you? It's not cancer, but heart disease that claims more women's lives! African-American women are particularly vulnerable, since their rates of heart disease and stroke are one and a half times greater than those of white women. In all, an estimated 250,000 American women die from heart disease each year (Wenger and others, 1993). Heart disease is an area where health promotion can really pay off. And the menopausal years are ideal for developing a healthier lifestyle.

This chapter will outline for you the most recent information regarding women and the development of cardiovascular disease. Until recently, the risk of cardiovascular disease in women received little attention. A prime example: The Oregon affiliate of the American Heart Association (AHA) organized the first women's health conference on coronary heart disease twenty-five years ago entitled *Hearts and Hus-*

bands. This conference had, as its sole purpose, the education of women concerning the risks of heart disease in their spouses (American Heart Association, 1989). It took that same organization more than twenty years to hold their first conference on women and coronary disease. In contrast to the tremendous amount of attention paid to men and cardiovascular disease, information on the development of coronary disease in women is very limited.

This gender bias in the medical understanding of heart disease has very deep roots. The best known studies of heart disease prevention are the Multiple Risk Factor Intervention Trial (the famous MR FIT study)(Neaton and others, 1984), and the Lipid Research Clinic's Coronary Primary Prevention Trial (LRC-CPPT)(Program, 1984). These two studies are the sources for the belief that if a person lowers his cholesterol by 1 percent, his risk of developing cardiovascular disease is decreased by 2 percent. You can probably guess why we are using the word "his": they only studied men.

While most experts agree that the so-called "traditional risk factors for heart disease" (that is, those identified for men) play a role in the development of heart disease in women, there is still a lot to learn about heart disease in women. Two pioneer studies, The Framingham Heart Study (Eaker and Castelli, 1987) and The Nurses' Health Study (Stampfer and others, 1987) have given us much of the important information available about women and their risk factors for the development of coronary disease. Women lag approximately seven to ten years behind men in the development of coronary artery disease. Some of this discrimination in the research and treatment of women's cardiovascular disease may be due to the way in which our society has valued aging women. Men who have heart attacks are more likely to be perceived as being in their "prime" (midlife), while typically women with heart disease are in their sixties and seventies and, therefore, considered less valuable, economically and otherwise.

We met Ellen in our practice several years ago. She was a respected cardiac care nurse who had quit her job at age fifty-four because of burnout. Ellen had been active in training young nurses for over twenty-five years. Her work on the cardiac unit had always been challenging, but over the previous few years she had found the intense environment less satisfying. She wanted to spend more time pursuing new interests. As a single woman, she also valued her independence. Ellen felt that by taking so much of the job home with her, it was difficult to concentrate on anything else. One day it occurred to her that she could do something else.

She came to us because she discovered that she could not get her own physician to take her newly developed chest pain seriously. She found this particularly infuriating as she had cared for the same physician's patients in the hospital and knew that he had special respect for her clinical judgment. Ellen realized that she needed to take charge of her own health care. She was interested in knowing her own risk of cardiovascular disease and taking steps to maintain her health.

This chapter will help you, like Ellen, assess your own risks for cardiovascular disease. Read the information we have provided and fill out the questionnaire on healthy hearts. This will facilitate conversation between you and your health care provider. The menopausal years are an excellent time to make important changes in lifestyle that can reduce the chance of heart disease later on in life.

✦ WHAT IS ATHEROSCLEROSIS AND CORONARY ARTERY DISEASE?

Coronary heart disease or coronary artery disease (CAD) is defined as the narrowing of one or more of the blood vessels that supply blood flow to the heart. As we age, these arteries accumulate material in a process called atherosclerosis, which decreases the diameter of the vessels supplying blood to the heart. Figure 5-1 depicts a normal and a diseased artery. This narrowing in the diameter of the blood vessels to the heart causes a decrease in the blood flow to the heart muscle. The heart is not able to pump effectively, which causes symptoms such as chest pain or shortness of breath. If a woman develops significant narrowing in the blood vessels that feed her heart, she may experience chest pain from a decreased blood supply of the heart (the technical term is *angina pectoris*). A heart attack occurs when the blood supply to the heart is severely reduced and is called a myocardial infarction. If the heart fails to pump effectively, fluid backs up into the lungs and this is called congestive heart failure. From now on we will refer to coronary heart disease or coronary artery disease as "heart disease," for simplicity.

The obvious question regarding women and heart disease is why are we relatively protected from heart disease before menopause? Why do women, on average, develop significant heart disease a decade later than men do? We know that there are many factors that could account for this sex difference. According to several studies, estrogen has a beneficial effect on serum cholesterol. Estrogen therapy reduces low-density lipoprotein (LDL) cholesterol or the bad cholesterol and increases serum high-density (HDL) cholesterol, or the good

FIGURE 5-1
ATHEROSCLEROSIS —
HARDENING OF THE ARTERIES

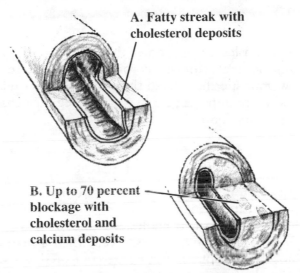

A. Fatty streak with cholesterol deposits

B. Up to 70 percent blockage with cholesterol and calcium deposits

cholesterol (Barrett-Connor and Bush, 1991). There are also theories for why women who take hormones might have less heart disease. There are estrogen receptors in the walls of the arteries, suggesting that estrogen might also have a direct positive effect on the arteries (McGill, 1989). Additionally, estrogen may decrease the formation of harmful clots in the arteries (Ylikorkala and others, 1987).

Another hypothesis for the protective effect of the female gender is that before menopause, women who are premenopausal have lower red blood cell (hematocrit) levels because they are menstruating regularly and, perhaps, lower blood cell count enables better flow through the coronary vessels. Men with high serum iron levels seem to have higher rates of coronary heart disease (Salonen and others, 1992). Maybe the opposite is true, and premenopausal women who are menstruating and have lower serum iron levels than males have decreased rates of coronary heart disease on that basis. Does this mean we should be avoiding vitamins that contain iron? If you are being treated for anemia, it is probably wise to take the iron as prescribed. For women without anemia, whose iron is part of a vitamin supplement, the dose is probably low enough to be harmless. To be on the "safe" side however, ask your health care professional.

One thing is clear: We need much more information about

women and heart disease. We do have enough information now to know that the menopausal years provide us with the ideal time to make changes necessary to prevent heart disease.

✦ RISK FACTORS

Although we know less about women than we do about men, there are many identifiable risk factors for coronary artery disease. It is important to know your specific risks so that you can share them with your physician and more importantly, so you can begin to change the risk factors that you can control.

BIOLOGICAL FACTORS

Biological risk factors for heart disease in women fall into two main groups: The first category is nonhormone related factors, such as diabetes, hypertension, elevated cholesterol and smoking. The second category includes hormonal factors. Even when a man and woman with the same number of risk factors are compared, the man will still have three and a half times the rate of developing heart disease. Clearly, just being male is a risk factor for heart disease. Some biological influence appears to be protecting women as compared to men. Unfortunately, this changes for women as we age.

The presence of *diabetes mellitus* is one of the most significant factors in the development of heart disease in women. Diabetes is a disease that occurs when the body cannot make effective use of insulin, a hormone that processes sugar. This leads to the sugar levels in the blood becoming too high, which has several short- and long-term effects on the body. Diabetes occurs more in women than it does in men, and the presence of diabetes appears to cancel any female advantage in the development of heart disease. Women with even mild diabetes, or what is termed glucose intolerance, have an increased risk of developing heart disease. Diabetes appears to speed up the process of atherosclerosis in the heart. If you have a family history of diabetes or heart disease, a personal history of other cardiac risk factors or symptoms of diabetes (excessive thirst, excessive urination, weight loss or persistent vaginal yeast infections) then you should be screened for diabetes. There are blood and urine tests for diabetes, but the urine tests tend to be much less precise. The diagnosis of diabetes is made in anyone who has one or more fasting blood sugars greater than or equal to 140 mg/dl or anyone who demonstrates sustained blood sugar levels greater than 200 mg/dl during an oral glucose tolerance test.

Hypertension, another risk factor for heart disease, is an elevation of the blood pressure. The development of high blood pressure is a complicated process. Your health care professional measures your blood pressure by two numbers; the higher of which is called the systolic blood pressure and the lower of which is called the diastolic pressure. Normal blood pressure is considered any blood pressure under 140/90 in people under the age of sixty, or 160/90 in people older than sixty. Borderline hypertension is defined as blood pressure 140/90–105, and high blood pressure is when the measure is more than 140/105. Blood pressure should be measured on at least three different office visits to make the diagnosis correctly.

Hypertension is the most common of all cardiac risk factors occurring in up to 20 percent of the entire population. It occurs more in African-Americans and more often in men (both African-American and white) until the age around menopause at which point it starts to be more common in women. Blood pressure can be elevated by even moderate chronic alcohol consumption as well as certain drugs. It frequently occurs with other cardiac risk factors, including obesity and diabetes. In most cases, it can be effectively treated with diet, exercise, and medication.

An elevated *cholesterol* is a common risk factor for the development of coronary heart disease. Cholesterol is divided into two broad classes, high-density lipoprotein (HDL cholesterol) and low-density lipoprotein (LDL cholesterol). HDL, the so called "good cholesterol," removes cholesterol out of the bloodstream, and LDL, the "bad cholesterol," carries cholesterol to the bloodstream.

Younger women have lower total cholesterol levels than men of the same age. This difference is thought to be due to higher estrogen levels. Between the ages of twenty and fifty, a woman's total cholesterol levels and LDL levels are lower than they are in men. But things change after menopause: women develop increasing levels of total serum cholesterol with increases in LDL, the bad cholesterol, and decreases in HDL, the good cholesterol. The higher your HDL cholesterol, the lower your risk of developing heart disease.

Cholesterol values are now frequently obtained as part of routine blood tests. Cholesterol values can vary by as much as 30–50 points for a variety of reasons. Certain factors are known to affect the accuracy of the cholesterol measurement including: recent illness, surgery or heart attack, pregnancy, recent weight gain or loss, new (within four to eight weeks) use of postmenopausal hormones or oral contraceptives and different phases of the menstrual cycle. The quality of the test is important too. Remember that getting tested at your local mall is not as reliable as going to a reputable laboratory.

If your initial cholesterol is found to be elevated, you will probably be asked to give a fasting specimen. This involves fasting for sixteen hours overnight and then having your total cholesterol, HDL-cholesterol, and triglyceride levels measured. Your LDL-cholesterol can be calculated based on these values. Treatment recommendations from your health care professional should always be based on the cholesterol values from this full fasting panel and not on an elevated value for one random (i.e., nonfasting) total cholesterol. This is because it is necessary to know your HDL-cholesterol, LDL-cholesterol and triglycerides before any decisions can be made regarding treatment.

Smoking is probably the most significant risk factor for the development of coronary artery disease in young women (under age forty), and it plays an important role in the development of heart disease in older women as well. It is a disgrace that women were targeted in the 1970s during a period of increased political action for women, in marketing campaigns for cigarettes. Most of you remember "You've come a long way baby," the advertisement that attempted to link political freedom in women with smoking. What they forgot to tell us was that on the way you could get heart disease, lung disease, cancer, earlier menopause and wrinkles! In addition, if you already have a risk of cardiovascular disease due to additional risk factors, smoking will only compound it.

Once you quit smoking, within three to four years, your risk of coronary disease goes back to the same risk as you would have had if you had never smoked. However, if you cut back your smoking to even the lightest amount, one to four cigarettes per day, you would still have a significantly increased of risk of coronary disease. While rates of smoking have dropped in the U.S., this decline has been seen more in males than females. This is most likely because women have different reasons for smoking than men, and therefore varying quit rates. For instance, women are more likely to smoke to relieve stress, to reduce unpleasant feelings and to suppress appetite (Orlandi, 1987). It is only recently that smoking cessation programs have attempted to take these gender differences into account in designing programs for women.

✦ THE GREAT WEIGHT DEBATE

Obesity contributes to the development of coronary disease, but some of its impact may be due to concurrent hypertension, diabetes, or elevated cholesterol (Bush, 1991). (Note: Technically a person can be overweight without being obese. Being overweight is just weighing more than desirable; whereas being obese means an excess of body fat. Some athletes are overweight without being obese. Thus the scale weight does not necessarily reflect being "over-fat." Midlife women who are overweight usually do have an excess of body fat. Nonetheless, we are using the word "overweight" because the word "obese" is almost always used in a pejorative fashion.) Most women who are overweight will develop one or more other factors, including hypertension, diabetes or an elevated cholesterol.

It gets even more difficult to avoid weight gain as we get older because of metabolic changes. Our body metabolism slows down and we need fewer calories to maintain our present weight. Also, as we age, a larger proportion of our weight becomes fat rather than muscle tissue. This is a definite problem, and one that each woman needs to face individually.

The medical attitude toward dieting changes regularly. We know that extra weight is a risk factor for heart disease, but there is little evidence that we can help people lose large amounts of weight. For moderately overweight women, "yo-yo dieting" may be more dangerous than maintaining their present weight. A recent analysis of one study found that people who continue to gain and lose weight more than ten pounds at a time over twenty years (yo-yo dieters), had a higher rate of heart attacks than those whose weight remained constant (Stampfer and others, 1987). So, in addition to our having trouble losing weight, it is clear that the yo-yo dieting problem remains. Psychologist Kelly Brownell of Yale University, a leading obesity researcher, has suggested an approach that we support. He suggests, "I propose that smaller but well-maintained weight losses may well be more beneficial than larger but poorly maintained weight losses" (Keeping Your Weight, 1993). His conclusion is based on decades of research in this area as well as a study of the MR. FIT program, which analyzed over 12,000 men. Many of these men were at risk for heart attacks because they were overweight. Those men whose weight remained constant over time had a lower rate of heart disease than those who lost weight only to regain it. So weight is a complicated health problem.

It is not just what you weigh, but the shape of your body that is important with respect to heart disease. Women who have "pear-shaped," or female-pattern obesity, are less likely to develop high blood pressure, elevated insulin levels and early diabetes than overweight women who are "apple-shaped," or have so-called male-pattern obesity.

Our patient, Ellen, had taught her patients how to follow cardiac diets for twenty years and yet when it came to her own dieting, like many of us, she had really struggled. By the time she had quit her job, she was about twenty to twenty-five pounds overweight. She had been through the hospital-sponsored liquid-diet program twice, regained all of the weight, and became discouraged. She knew that she had a strong family history of diabetes, as well as heart disease, and was determined not to fall into those patterns.

A family history of heart disease predicts heart disease in women as well as men. Having a parent with a history of a heart attack before age sixty increases the risk of heart attack or angina for women. This effect is significant whether the parent is a mother or a father. We do not know if this risk is due to a familial clustering of specific risk factors like hypertension or diabetes, or to some, as yet unidentified, genetic factors. Although we can do nothing about our genetic heritage, we can minimize our other risk factors. For example, Ellen's father died of a heart attack at age forty-six, another reason that her symptoms of chest pain were of such concern to her and why she was so motivated to make changes. We worked with Ellen to cut the fat in her diet, rather than to dramatically cut calories, and this plan of action seemed to work for her.

There has been some research done on the relationship between various *hormonal factors* and the development of heart disease in women. There appears to be no association between age of menstruation, number of pregnancies, age at first pregnancy and the risk of developing heart disease. There is also no evidence that *natural menopause* per se increases a women's risk of heart disease. In other words, in the immediate period after natural menopause there is no abrupt change in the risk of developing heart disease. The risk of heart disease increases gradually with age in the years after menopause.

In contrast, we know there is an association between *early surgical menopause* and risk of heart disease. Early surgical menopause is defined as the removal of the uterus and ovaries prior to the expected age of natural menopause. Because the increased risk of heart disease is well documented in women with early surgical menopause, most physicians agree that they should be on HRT. Most doctors also favor the use of HRT in women who experience early menopause for other reasons like chemotherapy for cancer, or primary ovarian failure.

Should all postmenopausal women be put on *hormone replacement* for this reason? Most of the studies that were done in the 1970s and 1980s placed women on estrogen (ERT) alone, which was the standard of care at that time, not on HRT which combines estrogen with progesterone, so we know little about progesterone's effects. While there have been quite a few studies to date on the subject of ERT, most have been so small and lasted such a short period of time that it has been difficult to draw definite conclusions. *Nonetheless, the majority of studies support the conclusion that there is a reduction in the risk of coronary disease with ERT.*

There has been concern that the addition of progesterone to estrogen therapy would reduce the positive effects of estrogen alone on the heart. This is why most experts advise that the dose of progesterone should be as low as possible to still prevent endometrial cancer while maximizing the positive effects of estrogen on the heart (U.S. Congress, 1992). To the surprise of many, the most recent information suggests that estrogen and progesterone combined may be even more protective than estrogen alone (Nabulsi and others, 1993).

Are you confused? You are not alone. The fact is that this is a key issue in women's health that deserves attention. The good news is that there are several long-term studies underway to further evaluate this. The Women's Health Initiative, a large study of 160,000 women which was started in the fall of 1993, will follow women between the ages of fifty to seventy-nine for twelve years looking for the development of specific types of cancer and cardiovascular disease (Associated Press, 1993). There will also be a smaller group of women within the study who will be treated with different hormone regimens, calcium and vitamin D, as well as a low-fat diet, and followed for changes in their cholesterol, heart disease, cancer rates and osteoporosis.

✦ PSYCHOLOGICAL FACTORS

There has been a great interest in the psychological and social factors that affect the development of coronary heart disease in males. Much has been written about the development of a Type A personality, classically portrayed as the hard-driving individual. First identified in 1959, by Drs. Friedman and Ronsenman, the Type A personality was noted to be frenetic, impatient, high-achieving and competitive. These authors suggested that people with Type A personalities needed to learn to relax and become calmer in order to lower the risks for cardiovascular disease (Friedman and Rosenman, 1974).

Since that time, the relationship between Type A behaviors and risk of heart attacks has been examined. As is frequently the case in behavioral science research, there are problems with the measurements used and the global generalizations that are drawn from the studies. It is the *hostility* of the Type A personality that is most associated with cardiovascular disease. Others hypothesize that it is not Type A behavior, but the personality traits of freneticism and authoritarianism that are the culprits. So, although the Type A question is still somewhat controversial, there is evidence that being hostile is not healthy for our hearts!

Of course, there is another problem with the original research regarding psychological and social factors and coronary heart disease: it was—*surprise!*—limited primarily to white male patients. Now there is a growing body of research on women and minorities with Type A behaviors. Type A behaviors have been associated with stress in African-American men and women. One study of employed white women found that Type A's were less satisfied with their work, worked longer hours, and had been in their current jobs for a shorter time than the Type Bs. In addition, the Type As reported more nervousness in all situations than did the Type Bs. A study of employed African-American women revealed that Type A women were more likely to have higher blood pressure, higher cholesterol and lower coping scores than were Type B.

Some new intriguing studies of sex differences in anger and hostility are now emerging. It seems that men and women experience similar levels of anger, but that men express anger in a more aggressive manner. Women tend to express anger within an interpersonal context, with an emphasis on the specific relationship. Men tend to add the hostility factor. Clearly, this is a new and growing area of research.

✦ SOCIAL FACTORS

Given the acceptance that Type As have more cardiovascular risk, there was concern that as women entered the work force in large numbers there would be increasing numbers of women with heart disease. As women, we were warned against working full-time or pursuing high-powered careers. This fear has been unfounded. In fact, working outside the home *per se* has no effect on the likelihood of developing heart disease, but there are certain characteristics of the work situation which do appear to be important in its development. The clerical, or "pink-collar" workers who have unsupportive bosses, suppressed hostility and decreased job mobility have been shown to have a higher rate of heart disease than other women. It seems that these women are stressed by their lack of control, high level of responsibility and the underutilization of their skills. The group of women at highest risk for heart disease are clerical women who have three or more children and who are married to blue-collar men (Haynes, Feinleib & Kannel, 1980). Their rates of heart disease were as high as those for men in white-collar jobs—the highest-risk occupational group. Perhaps we should worry more about the hostility of some Type A men and how they treat their secretaries than we should about women becoming executives.

Stress itself can cause physiological changes in heart functioning. One study of Swedish women found that women whose jobs were both hectic and monotonous had one and a half times greater risk of developing coronary artery disease over a ten-year period. If you are one of the many women whose jobs are stressful, hectic or monotonous, this is not meant to frighten you. Your feelings should be validated by this knowledge because you already know that stress isn't good for you. Many women feel trapped by their jobs, especially when they're given little credit for their tremendous efforts.

It is not particularly helpful for us to tell you that if you have a difficult job situation, you are more likely to have heart disease, without making some additional suggestions. Once again, we don't want our advice to add stress to your life. So you will see in the following section ways in which you can do the best to change your occupational situation. Many women have found that they have more power than they know, and we want to help you gain access to that power.

✦ Preventing the Development of Heart Disease

Now is the time to make changes in your habits and health care that can decrease your chance of heart disease.

Smoking Cessation

If you smoke, you should now know that stopping is critical to improved heart health. It is absolutely clear that smoking will damage your cardiovascular system; can cause cancers of the head and neck and lungs; and harms those around you who are exposed to your second-hand smoke. We know from our patients who smoke that quitting can be excruciatingly difficult. There is hope, however, as the science of smoking cessation improves. Remember that your risk of heart disease will decline within one to five years of quitting to where it would have been *if you had never smoked*.

There are many programs available. The local chapters of the American Lung Association and the American Heart Association, or your state health department should have listings of these for you. Many hospitals and work sites now run cessation programs. You should try to find out who runs the programs and whether their effectiveness has been evaluated. For example, what are the quit rates of smokers in these programs. Medication, including the nicotine patch or nicotine gum, can be prescribed by your health care professional or as part of the program you join. The best approach is to combine the use of nicotine gum or the transdermal nicotine patch with counseling. Most insurance programs will pay for the gum and at least one trial of the patch. Remember that the goal is to quit. Women are not as successful at quitting as men, but there are several important lessons we can learn from this difference. Because women are more likely to use smoking to control weight or to make them feel better in stressful situations, it is critical to their success that weight control and stress reduction are handled simultaneously. Do not be discouraged if it takes many attempts. As you will see in our chapter on healthy aging, the science of changing behavior is developing rapidly and can help you attack this difficult problem.

COPING WITH JOB STRESS

Problems at work can be a chronic stress on our health. Extremely difficult careers, like Ellen's, can lead to repressed anger or hostility that we know is a risk factor for heart disease. So it's a good idea to develop coping skills for dealing with job stress.

Ellen had left her stressful job behind, but she had a lot of good advice for younger nurses and other women who worked in stressful occupations. One of the best ways Ellen had of coping with her stresses in the cardiac care unit was her involvement with her social network of other nurses and staff members at the hospital.

Ellen and her colleagues at the hospital had developed educational programs for their patients, and eventually for themselves. One of the patient education programs was about the stress of cardiac procedures. In the process of preparing this program, Ellen and her colleagues realized they could also benefit from their own training session in stress management. They asked the hospital's health psychologist to teach them relaxation techniques. They also learned that they could make some small changes to reduce stress and prevent burnout. For example, they helped one another take "time-out" if one of them had a challenging patient or a stressful care situation.

Informal organizations of one or two women can be helpful in providing the social support that we have discussed. By talking about the common problems of the job, women can work together to take control of their own abilities to change. This can be a small step, like better exercise facilities on the job. Women can also organize in order to make more significant changes within their workplace. Ellen helped the younger nurses establish twelve-hour shifts so that they could spend more time with their young families, working fewer days per week. Most women are concerned about greater flexibility and the possibility of family-leave time. Some women employ job sharing for this reason.

Ellen felt "burnt out" by the age of fifty-four, despite all she had been able to accomplish at work. She found it to be extremely helpful to consider her alternatives. She had a partial pension but felt that it was not adequate. She began to think of a way she could work half-time in order to support herself. In addition, this would help her maintain some health insurance benefits, as well as some retirement benefits. For now, she works "per diem," or paid on a daily basis, in a variety of hospital settings. This variety has allowed her to use her substantial skills, meet new people, and view nursing as a profession from a more optimistic and powerful perspective.

PHYSICAL ACTIVITY

For many of us, a lifestyle that included physical activity was not fostered at an early age, but what we may learn is that a daily routine filled with physical activity can be quite pleasurable. You will note that we are not using the word "exercise" at this point. That is because, although exercise, structured and routine physical activity, is important, so is general lifestyle change. Consider this: you can get a lot of benefit for your heart just by beginning to incorporate some modest *physical activity*. Even small amounts of physical activity cannot only be beneficial, but actually fun. Several studies, once again conducted only on men, unfortunately, find that you can reduce the risk of heart attacks by up to 20 percent just by such activities as a fifteen-minute walk each day. There are numerous small changes you can make in your lifestyle as well—taking the stairs instead of the elevator, not looking for the parking place closest to the store, walking rather than driving short distances and so on. For most women we find that this is a basic change in attitude, part of a commitment to become physically active.

In general, women *exercise* much less than men, so it's not surprising that there are fewer studies looking at the role of exercise in the prevention of heart disease in women. At least one study though, suggests that regular exercise may prevent coronary heart disease in women (Douglas and others, 1992). Exercise has a favorable effect on cholesterol, but for women, moderate to intensive efforts may be necessary to produce significant improvements in this area. There also may be some benefit for women who have already had a heart attack.

Maximal cardiovascular fitness requires regular moderate aerobic activity. This can be done, for example, by walking twenty-five to thirty minutes a day or sixty minutes three times a week at 3 to 3.5 miles an hour. Table 5-1 depicts an exercise program for heart health. Other examples of aerobic exercise include low-impact or step aerobics, bicycling, using a stationary bicycle or treadmill. Begin any exercise with a five-minute warm-up time to stretch and limber up to prevent any injuries.

Most importantly, before starting an exercise program, you should consult with your physician. The benefits of exercise for women extend beyond the risk of heart disease. Many women have found that exercise (particularly enjoyable exercise) is also a major stress management tool. Identifying and maintaining an exercise plan is one of the most beneficial decisions that we can make during our menopausal years.

HEART-HEALTHY NUTRITION

When considering a healthy diet to prevent heart disease, as with all diets, we feel that the basic tenets of common sense combined with sensitivity should prevail.

When we talked with Ellen regarding her diet, we concentrated on her concerns to prevent heart disease rather than just focusing on calories alone. We suggested that she try to cut down her total fat intake, specifically saturated fat intake. Saturated fat comes from meat, dairy and certain fish products as well as from vegetable sources including palm oil and coconuts. Saturated fat actually interferes with the body's ability to remove excess cholesterol. Polyunsaturated fats, which include corn, safflower, sunflower and soybean oils, can help the body to remove excess cholesterol.

When Ellen came to see us, she had routine blood work that showed an elevated LDL level. This put her at additional risk for the development of heart disease and really motivated her to develop a diet and exercise program. Specific changes in diet should be considered for any woman with an elevated LDL cholesterol. No restrictions should be recommended without knowledge of the woman's HDL

Table 5–1

FIT PROGRAM FOR
HEALTHY HEARTS

Purpose: Maximum cardiovascular fitness

Frequency: Start: 2–3 times per week
Goal: 3–4 times per week

Intensity: Start: moderate—about 65% maximum
heart rate
Goal: more vigorous 70–80% maximum
heart rate

Time: Start: 2–5 minutes, repeat 2–3 times
Increase about every 2 weeks by 5 minutes
8–10 minutes, repeat 2–3 times
Gradually increase.
Goal: 20–30 minutes continuous activity
per session

Types: Large muscles, continuous repetitive
motion.
Examples: Walking, Biking, Swimming
Low- or high-impact aerobics
Step aerobics
Jogging (after 1–2 months)
Racketball

---

and LDL cholesterol. Many women, even after menopause, will have high HDL (the good) cholesterol levels, which will increase their total cholesterol levels. Your physician's recommendation should be specially tailored to you and your health needs, and not based on some generalizations about ideal body weight or cholesterol values for men.

Ellen was relieved when we did not lecture her about her weight. We shared with her our philosophy that women should not be ashamed of the natural change in their bodies over time. We helped Ellen see that she would do much better at controlling her weight if she focused on physical activity and a low-fat diet, not caloric intake. As women, we have all been conditioned to be preoccupied with our caloric intake while at the same time serving as the main cooks for our families and friends. Men, on the other hand, are less likely to be involved in food preparation and tend to have incorporated exercise into their lifestyle. If, for example, we choose to watch our weight during menopause, we need to focus more on weight-bearing exercises and building muscle mass. These activities may help to get us out of the kitchen, and allow us to worry less about the number of calories consumed. If we continue to exercise and focus on our health, we will not only be in better physical shape, but our psychological attitude toward aging will improve as well.

Ellen was like most people in this country, consuming a diet containing 35 to 42 percent fat. The Surgeon General recommends diets containing less than 30 percent fat with 10 percent from saturated fat and 20 percent from unsaturated fat (Consumer Reports, 1992). However, many experts feel that the percent of fat should be even lower. There are several different nutritional plans to choose from including one from the American Heart Association.

For example, one simple change that Ellen made was to change her snack foods. Ellen tended to munch on potato chips. This is problematic since potato chips have ten times as much fat as pretzels. So, just by switching to pretzels, Ellen reduced her fat intake. Ellen was also surprised to learn that not all pizza is created equal when it comes to fat. For example, one frozen pizza brand contains 50 percent of its calories from fat, and another only 12 percent. All the more reason to read the labels! (Friedman, 1993).

For those of us who are watching our weight, it is important to remember to "let the buyer beware." The diet industry in the United States is a profit-oriented business, and we are likely to be lured by false advertising. A recent study by the New York State Consumer Protection Board found that of five products labeled as "diet" foods, all of them had at least 20 percent more calories than the amount specified. Of twenty products analyzed, sixteen exceeded by anywhere from 2 to 49 percent. This is true despite a federal law prohibiting such deception (Gershoff, 1992). The dramatic "before and after" photos in many television advertisements for diet programs may well be one or two women in a program of one hundred. The diet industry routinely exploits women by making false promises of quick success. A review of all the major diet programs by *Consumer Reports* found very few differences in how much weight people lost, so there's no need to spend a lot of money, in the hopes of a miracle cure (Losing Weight, 1993).

Some notions about nutrition are changing. We now know that sodium restriction is not necessary for everyone. While it is true that women with high blood pressure should restrict salt intake, salt restriction does not maintain heart health for all women. So if you do not have high blood pressure, you do not need to worry that much about restricting your salt intake.

Recent reports from the Nurses' Health Study suggest that adequate vitamin E in your diet may reduce your risk of cardiovascular disease (Stampfer and others, 1993). For this reason, some physicians recommend taking 400 International Units of vitamin E daily.

Moderate alcohol consumption has been found to have a beneficial effect on cholesterol, specifically by raising the HDL cholesterol. There are several reasons for women to be cautious about this information. Most of the earlier data to support this is derived from male populations. So-called "moderate" drinking is also different for males and females. Women cannot drink as much as men; they develop more serious consequences from drinking smaller amounts for shorter periods of time than men do. The evidence that moderate alcohol consumption increases HDL cholesterol in women is actually limited. Beware of advice to drink one to two glasses of wine per day to increase your HDL, because the risks greatly outweigh the potential benefits for women.

◆ WHEN IS MEDICATION INDICATED?

Treating *hypertension* in women has not been evaluated in depth and may involve some racial differences. It is clear that antihypertensive medication benefits black women with high blood pressure, but it is not clear if white women receive the same benefit from treatment of borderline high blood pressure. Clearly, there is a need for new long-term studies of women with hypertension, using some of the newer blood-pressure agents before we can draw meaningful conclusions about medication for hypertension. In the meantime, blood pressure should be treated on an individual basis with diet, exercise and a reduction of alcohol intake. Medication should be discussed with your primary care professional.

Treatment of *diabetes* begins again with diet and exercise. The majority of women who develop diabetes in their forties and fifties have type II diabetes, once called adult onset diabetes, which tends to develop gradually. It is especially responsive to diet and exercise. In some cases, a medication may be added, and less often a woman will need to be treated with insulin.

Most clinicians feel that a total *cholesterol* above 260–300 should be treated. Diet is always the first line of therapy. If diet is not successful in lowering cholesterol in six to nine months, drug therapy should be considered. Further information about the type of medications used is available from the American Heart Association brochures or from your physician.

Studies in men suggest that *aspirin* is an effective medication to prevent heart attacks. It makes sense that aspirin might have this effect since it makes platelets (clotting cells) less likely to form clots. In a Nurses' Health Study report, it was suggested that women who took one to six aspirin per week were less likely to have a fatal heart attack than those who took no aspirin (Manson and others, 1991). However, taking more than seven aspirin per week had no benefit. You should talk this over with your primary care professional to consider your own risks and benefits.

At menopause, *hormone replacement therapy* can be considered to prevent heart disease. The risks and benefits of HRT must be carefully weighed, as we detail in Chapter Six, "Hormone Replacement Therapy." The type of HRT is important when considering heart disease prevention. Much of the information on the beneficial effect of HRT on heart disease is based on studies of estrogen alone. The information on progesterone is conflicting, as we discussed (Grady and others, 1992).

◆ COMMUNICATION

Perhaps Ellen's greatest frustration came when her physician colleague did not take her symptoms seriously. This example is the most ironic, but many women with concerns about cardiovascular disease are faced with the problem of being dismissed when they try to communicate with their health care professional. One way to deal with the situation is to develop a specific and assertive approach.

For their annual visits, many women in their thirties and forties choose to see only an obstetrician/gynecologist who is focused on gynecological problems and prevention of breast and gynecological cancer. As we age, our needs for screening become more complex. If you have not already done so, you should identify a primary care professional who will emphasize prevention, help you to assess your personal risks and determine the lifestyle changes that will be most beneficial to your health.

Most women between the ages of forty-five and fifty-five do not have heart problems, so prevention is the most important aspect of the menopausal years. However, some women do experience chest pain. This symptom may or may not represent serious cardiac disease. For example, palpitations and chest discomfort may occur as part of menopausal symptoms. Your symptoms may be caused by one of the numerous non–heart-related chest-pain syndromes. Whatever the cause, these symptoms can be quite frightening and need to be taken seriously. The first step to getting some answers is to identify an appropriate primary care professional.

Once you have identified a primary care professional whom you trust, you need to consider how to maximize communication. Many features of the current health care system work against this. There is relatively little time scheduled for each patient so you need to come into the office armed with your questions and concerns. You may want to anticipate the answers and be ready with the next level of questions.

In order to prepare yourself for conversation with your clinician, consider the following scenarios:

> Your clinician says something like, "I don't think you are at increased risk for heart disease."
> You may ask, "Why not?"
> He/she says, "Women are less likely to have heart disease."
> You may ask, "What about the role of [any risk factor you have] and my increasing risk of heart disease with age?"

If you need a workup for heart disease, you might consider your needs for medical information. For example, there are two major categories of patients: repressors and sensitizers. Repressors (avoiders) tend to cope with stress by not thinking about it or distracting themselves. These patients do not appear to be anxious. Sensitizers, on the other hand, are anxious and handle the anxiety by gathering information and by paying careful attention to details. You probably already know if you are a sensitizer or a repressor. If you are a repressor, you might want a small amount of general information, and if you are a sensitizer, you'll want more detail. Be sure to let your physician and the rest of the staff know your needs in this area. Medical tests and procedures like cardiac-stress testing can be stressful—psychologically. But the tests are meant to evaluate your cardiovascular system—not stress your psyche! Hospital environments can be intimidating and the high-tech equipment can look and sound frightening. Sometimes health care professionals have grown so accustomed to the environment, that they forget that it is foreign to most other people. We have found that it is important to discuss these tests and procedures in some detail. As a patient, you have a right to know the answers to these questions: What does the test involve? Is it painful? Is it uncomfortable? What will the results mean? What is the cost? Will insurance cover it? When and how will I learn the results? What is the next step if the test is positive? Most studies have found that patients feel less anxious when provided with this information. But others have found that it depends on the needs and personality styles of the individual.

Over time, you will get a sense of whether your physician is taking your symptoms or health concerns seriously. We have found that many of our patients have changed their doctors over the issue of evaluation and treatment of chest pain and even known coronary disease. Ellen had always had a good relationship with her clinician and even worked side by side with him in the coronary care unit, but she came to us thoroughly annoyed when he dismissed her symptoms of chest pain.

COMMUNICATING WITH YOUR FAMILY

Women function as the caretakers of the entire family—the cook, the pill dispenser, the one who finds the health care and the one who remembers the appointments. They often admit to us that they neglect their own health concerns because they feel they already have too much to worry about. Many women in their fifties are experiencing the refilled nest (i.e., their children are moving back in the house again for financial reasons). In some cases, their children are dependent on them for care of the grandchildren. For many reasons family members may not be sensitive to the perimenopausal woman's health and other needs.

Marjorie and her husband sold their profitable gourmet food shop and were fortunate to be able to retire in their early fifties. Marjorie and Jim had been good partners in their business, enjoyed working together and deeply respected one another. When their two children were young, Marjorie had worked in the shop less. Like most women, she took the larger share of family and household responsibilities. Now, she was looking forward to early retirement and the time it would allow her to take off twenty pounds, start exercising regularly and get her blood pressure under control. When Marjorie came back to see us three months after she retired, she was five pounds heavier and her blood pressure was even higher. She told us at that time that she was off to help one of her children paint a new house. When we discussed exercise in order to help her with her weight, as well as her blood pressure, she burst into tears and confessed that she had even less time for herself than she did when she was working! She and her husband had used their savings to help one child start a business and another buy a house, instead of buying the RV they wanted. Although her husband was enjoying golf four times a week, Marjorie found that somehow she had no time to exercise and was eating more. She was frustrated and sad.

When we examined the family dynamics, we all realized that Marjorie and the whole family had raised their expectations of her. Jim was viewed as the "retired exec." who had earned his leisure, whereas Marjorie had become the suddenly available grandmother. She and her children now believed that she should help out with the grandchildren, run errands and be generally available. She felt this way because both her daughter and her daughter-in-law were working full-time in jobs that did not offer as much flexibility as Marjorie had had in the shop. Marjorie, like many women, used food as a quick pick-me-up when she was overcommitted and tired. And we can understand that tendency. Food is tasty, available and a deep part of our female culture. Yet, in this case, it was becoming dangerous to Marjorie's health.

We worked with Marjorie to help her change the family dynamics. We pointed out that her children were now twenty-five and twenty-seven years old and fully able to manage their family lives without so much help from Mom. She could still enjoy being helpful to her two children and their families, without doing quite so much. We then pointed out that the problems needed to be reframed. It was not that her daughter and daughter-in-law worked outside of the home but that *both parents* worked, and therefore both parents needed to look at the responsibilities of the family. We discuss the problems of employed women in our chapter on stress. Besides, Jim was retired now, too, and therefore could be more available. (A little consciousness-raising for two generations at a time!)

We helped Marjorie find a way to explain this to her children. We then encouraged Marjorie to use the same problem-solving skills that she and Jim had used in the business with her weight and exercise concerns. She tried it this way: "Jim, remember how when we expanded the shop, we developed a plan? Well, I need your help now in creating a plan for me to have more time to exercise." This began the conversation. Marjorie was not interested in joining Jim on the golf course. ("Boring!") Marjorie joined the Jewish Community Center where she could swim—an activity she enjoyed as a young adult. (We needed to do a quick session on overcoming exposed-thigh anxiety). Jim cut back his golf to three times a week so he could help more with the house and be available for any grandparenting duties. Marjorie, having met some young mothers at the pool, came home one day and said, "Jim, we didn't co-parent, but we can certainly co-grandparent!"

Now, it wasn't quite that easy all the time. Everyone in the family system, and indeed, all of us expect a lot from mothers and grandmothers. We are particularly busy helping women set limits around the holiday seasons. ("You are the *only one* who can bake the Christmas cookies?" or "You have to do *all* of Passover alone?" You get the picture.) Yet there are many possible ways to change the family dynamics. You need to remember first that you have responded to the needs of your family members and should not feel uncomfortable asking for the same consideration. This is an ideal time in your life to make some changes in your habits and in your family role, but it is not always easy. Family dynamics *can* shift even in the menopausal years. You may well meet some resistance, but push through your initial avoidance of conflict. Changing doesn't mean rejecting your family, it just means changing.

If the direct approach with your family does not work, you can also try asking a family member to come to the physician's office with you. Hearing from your physician or health care provider that changes in the family's schedules, meals or physical activity are *necessary* for your health may make an impact on your spouse or child. If none of these approaches work, you might want to try family counseling, which we describe more in chapters on stress and depression. The menopausal years are a time when it is necessary to make these changes. There is a lot of time left to live, and we need to take some for ourselves in order to maintain and improve our health.

RESOURCES

There are numerous and growing resources for women who have concerns about coronary-artery disease. Additional resources for smoking cessation, nutrition and exercise are listed in the prevention section.

THE FEDERAL GOVERNMENT

National Heart, Lung and Blood Institute (NHLBI)
Information Center
P.O. Box 30105
Bethesda, MD 20824-0105
(301) 951-3260

The NHLBI Information Center provides education materials on high blood pressure, cholesterol, smoking, obesity and heart disease. It publishes an excellent handbook for women on heart disease entitled The Healthy Heart Handbook for Women *as well as many different brochures on risk factors for heart disease. A directory of publications is available.*

Food and Drug Administration (FDA)

Office of Consumer Affairs, HFE-88
5600 Fishers Lane
Rockville, MD 20857
(301) 443-3170

The FDA publishes on diverse topics, including general drug information, medical devices, and food-related subjects, including fiber, fats, sodium, and cholesterol. Their newsletter, FDA Consumer, *has covered such relevant topics as: heart bypass surgery, balloon angioplasty, dieting and nutrition for women. Subscriptions can be ordered through a Consumer Information Center (CIC) catalogue. Educational brochures are also available through the CIC catalog. A free copy of the catalog can be obtained by writing the* **Consumer Information Center, Pueblo, CO 81009.**

Food and Nutrition Information Center (FNIC)

National Agricultural Library
10301 Baltimore Avenue, Room 304
Beltsville, MD 20705-2351
(301) 504-5719

The FNIC answers questions concerning nutrition, foods, and food labeling. They provide bibliographies and resource guides on a wide variety of food and nutrition topics.

Human Nutrition Information Service (HNIS)

Department of Agriculture
6505 Belcrest Road
Room 328A
Hyattsville, MD 20782
(301) 436-8617

HNIS reports results of research on food consumption and dietary guidance in popular publications. A list of DEA publications is available.

Office on Smoking and Health (OSH)
Center for Chronic Disease Prevention and Health Promotion
Mail Stop K-50
Centers for Disease Control
1600 Clifton Road, NE
Atlanta, Georgia 30333
(404) 488-5705

This office provides information and brochures on smoking cessation free of charge to the public.

ASSOCIATIONS

American Heart Association (AHA)
National Center
7320 Greenville Avenue
Dallas, TX 75231
(214) 373-6300

The AHA is probably the most available and well known of all resources. It provides pamphlets and other educational materials not only on heart disease but also on prevention, smoking, nutrition and exercise. In 1989 the AHA held a national meeting in Washington on Women and Coronary Artery Disease which resulted in new educational materials, including a videotape and a brochure entitled Women and Heart Disease: The Silent Epidemic. *Most local offices of the AHA now have a task force on women and heart disease, which, among other activities, will provide speakers on the subject to community groups. Local offices of the AHA offer support groups, classes in CPR, and all of the brochures are free to the individual. This is an important resource for anyone concerned with cardiovascular disease.*

American Lung Association
1740 Broadway
New York, NY 10019-4374
212-315-8700

Local offices of the lung association are an excellent resource for smoking programs that are available in the community as well as for educational materials—videos, manuals and brochures on smoking cessation. You can reach your local office by dialing 1-800-586-4872.

American Diabetes Association
1660 Duke Street
Alexandria, VA 22314
(800) 232-3472; (703)5549-1500

The ADA offers programs and information about diabetes prevention and treatment. Local chapters provide patient and family education activities as well as patient education publications. There is a catalog of publications and products. Membership, which includes a monthly newsletter, "Diabetes Forecast," is $24.

The Women's Health Initiative *is looking for women between the ages of fifty and seventy-nine. This study of 160,00 women is the largest women's health study to date. If you are interested in participating, you can call 301-402-2900 and this office will send you a brief summary of the study and a list of the participating centers. The study, which began in September 1993, will be recruiting patients until late 1995.*

BOOKS

1. *Lowfat Low Cholesterol Cookbook* edited by Scott Grundy, M.D., and Mary Winston, Ed.D. (American Heart Association) (New York: Random House, 1989).
    This book provides creative low-fat recipes, as well as nutritional information.
    2. *Women and Heart Disease:* What You Can Do to Stop the Number One Killer of Women by Edward B. Dietrich and Carol Cohan (New York: Random House, 1992).
    This is a good overview of the subject.
    3. *Our Bodies, Getting Older,* and *Our Bodies, Ourselves,* both published by the Boston Women's Health Book Collective (New York: Simon and Schuster, 1976).
    Both books have chapters on healthy lifestyles. These are two of the best books we know for helping women take charge of their health.

MAGAZINES

Prevention Magazine
Customer Communications
Rodale Press
33 E. Minor St.
Emmaus, PA 18098
(215) 967-5171

PHARMACEUTICAL COMPANY PUBLICATION

CardiSense
P.O. Box 549158
Miami, FL 33054-9875

CardiSense is a free quarterly newsletter published by Marion Merrill Dow, Inc. It includes information about exercise and health promotion.

SELF-HELP GROUPS

Most general medical hospitals with cardiac units provide support groups and educational programs for patients with heart disease and their families. Local chapters of the American Heart Association also sponsor support groups for people who have had heart attacks and their families. We have devoted attention to support groups for exercise and other lifestyle changes in our chapter on promoting a healthy lifestyle (Chapter Ten).

← CHAPTER SIX

Hormone Replacement Therapy

Isn't it ironic that for most of our lives hormones have been blamed for any number of behavioral and mood impairments and are now being touted as the cure-all for what ails us at menopause? It is no wonder that we are a bit leery about estrogen. After all, many of us are the survivors of birth control pills, which initially were promoted as the answer to all of our contraceptive prayers, but later were linked to heart attacks, blood clots and cancer. Nonetheless, for most women who are approaching menopause one of the most significant decisions they will make is whether or not to take estrogen. For some women, the decision is made deliberately after careful consideration of the information available. For others, it is made based on a philosophical stance against tampering with natural events. For still others, it is made by default when the issue is not addressed specifically. Each of these positions has merit, but it is important for everyone to have access to the facts about hormone replacement therapy (HRT). We have found at our menopause town meetings that the question of hormone replacement therapy is at the top of everyone's list. This chapter provides a framework of knowledge for women who are considering HRT.

❧ HORMONAL CHANGES

During the time around menopause, our ovaries' production of the hormone estrogen begins to gradually decline. Estrogen is produced predominantly by the ovaries although it is also produced in smaller amounts by fat tissue and the adrenal glands. When the ovaries are surgically removed, as is often done with hysterectomy, the decline in estrogen is abrupt and complete. The majority of us will experience a gradual decline as we follow the course of natural menopause. As the blood levels of estrogen produced by the ovaries begin to decrease, the brain's pituitary gland senses the lowered levels. In essence, our pituitary gland functions as a thermostat for estrogen, as well as other hormones. When the levels of estrogen fall below the present normal level, the pituitary gland responds by producing stimulating hormones to increase the ovaries' estrogen production.

As the ovaries' ability to produce estrogen continues to diminish, the pituitary gland increases its production of stimulating hormones to stoke the fires of the ovaries. These stimulating hormones are called FSH (follicle-stimulating hormone) and LH (luteinizing hormone). FSH and LH can be measured by a simple blood test. When the level of FSH rises above 40 MIU/ml, this is considered diagnostic of menopause. It may not be entirely obvious to you why FSH and LH are measured to diagnose menopause when the primary problem is decreasing estrogen levels. The reason is that the normal cyclic changes in estrogen levels and the tremendous individual variation make the interpretation of testing estrogen directly difficult. The stimulating hormones give information about the adequacy of estrogen levels for each individual woman as detected by her own pituitary gland. If the estrogen levels are too low, the stimulating hormones will be high, and conversely if estrogen levels are normal, the stimulating hormones will be unusually low.

❧ WHAT IS HORMONE REPLACEMENT THERAPY?

Hormone replacement therapy implies that hormones are being replaced to a level that is considered currently or previously normal. For menopause, the normal levels refer to premenopausal hormone levels. This is extremely important since many of the symptoms of menopause are directly attributable to the lower levels of estrogen produced by the ovaries as compared to the premenopausal levels. Estrogen is the specific hormone which is replaced to a premenopausal level when HRT is used.

Although birth control pills are considered hormone therapy, they do not represent hormone replacement therapy since they are being added to already normal levels of estrogen. Many comparisons have been made between birth control pills and estrogen used for menopausal symptoms, but there is the important distinction between *replacement* in the case of menopause and *addition* in the case of birth control pills. This distinction becomes particularly important when the side effects of estrogen are considered. Menopausal women who are treated with estrogen have blood levels of estrogen at the low-end of normal, in contrast to younger women who are being treated with birth control pills and who have high levels of estrogen. In fact, menopausal women taking the usual dose of estrogen replacement therapy have estrogen levels that would be considered very low for premenopausal women.

The major hormone player in menopause is estrogen. Estrogen has been shown to be highly effective when used for a number of symptoms associated with menopause. This information has led scientists to conclude that conditions such as hot flashes, vaginal dryness and osteoporosis are directly or indirectly related to the extremely low levels of estrogen associated with menopause.

The additional hormone often included in hormone replacement therapy is progesterone. Progesterone is not specifically responsible for the conditions associated with menopause, but is added to estrogen therapy to prevent some of the complications which occur when estrogen is used alone. In the normal premenopausal menstrual cycle, estrogen is the hormone which allows the lining of the uterus to build up in preparation for a potential pregnancy. If the egg does not become fertilized and mature, then progesterone levels increase and cause the shedding of the built-up uterine lining (endometrium), causing menstrual bleeding. In this way, progesterone stops the buildup of the uterine lining, which would otherwise continue if estrogen were the only hormone available.

In the case of hormone replacement with both estrogen and progesterone, it is the estrogen which treats the conditions associated with low estrogen levels, and it is progesterone which prevents the continued buildup of the endometrium. The accumulation of the uterine lining puts women at a greater risk for endometrial cancer. For a woman who has no uterus (i.e., who has had a hysterectomy), the addition of progesterone is unnecessary.

◆ PILLS, POTIONS, PATCHES, PELLETS AND PLANTS

Carolyn is a fifty-year-old waitress who had a hysterectomy at age forty-five for severe bleeding from uterine fibroid tumors. She did not have her ovaries removed at the time of her hysterectomy. Several months before her annual appointment, she had begun to experience hot flashes and was wondering whether she was going through menopause. Carolyn is like almost 30 percent of American women who, because they have no uterus, do not have the usual marker of the absence of their menstrual periods. This makes diagnosing menopause more difficult than it is for a woman who does have her uterus. Carolyn had blood tests drawn, including an FSH and LH. Menopause was diagnosed when Carolyn's FSH returned at 60 MIU/ml. (anything above 40 is consistent with menopause). Carolyn decided that her hot flashes were beginning to interfere with her work and chose to begin therapy with the estrogen patch. She felt that she would probably continue estrogen therapy indefinitely because she was very concerned about osteoporosis, since she had been told on numerous occasions that she was at high risk because she was extremely small, had never consumed adequate amounts of calcium, and did not exercise beyond that which she did at work.

As is often the case, we needed to tinker a bit with her treatment to minimize problems. When Carolyn developed local skin irritation at the site of the patch, we advised her to wave the patch in the air to remove some of the alcohol prior to applying it and to apply it to her buttocks. These simple maneuvers relieved the problem and she continues to use the patch twice weekly.

We can see from Carolyn's example that the manner in which women take the estrogen portion of their hormone replacement therapy can vary. The most well-studied form of estrogen has been estrogen tablets taken by mouth. The estrogen available in these tablets is called conjugated estrogen and the most frequently prescribed form is derived from *pregnant mares' urine* and is called Premarin. The dose of conjugated estrogen necessary to control the symptoms of menopause is usually in the range of 0.625 mg per day to 1.25 mg per day. Some women get relief of hot flashes, specifically, with as little as 0.3 mg per day, but the dose needed to prevent osteoporosis is 0.625 mg per day.

Vaginal estrogen creams have also been used for some time to control vaginal dryness. The creams provide estrogen directly to the area that is symptomatic. We now know that there is also absorption of the estrogen hormone through the vaginal lining into the blood-stream. In this way, women who use vaginal creams absorb estrogen as if they were taking it as a pill. The difference between vaginal creams and pills or patches is that the amounts of estrogen absorbed using the cream are generally lower, but less predictable and more erratic. It is also clear that vaginal estrogen creams have some of the same side effects and complications as oral estrogen taken alone.

The newer form of estrogen is the estrogen transdermal patch which has gained a great deal of popularity. The estrogen patch allows a woman to receive estrogen replacement therapy through the skin. The usual dose of estrogen required by patch is 0.5 mg to 1 mg, re-placed twice a week. Initially, it was feared that some of the cardiovas-cular benefits of estrogen taken orally would be lost if the patch were used instead. This has not been proven in further study. It was, addi-tionally, an early concern that the patch may not have the same benefi-cial effect on osteoporosis since all of the studies of osteoporosis had been done with estrogen taken orally. Not surprisingly, it is now known that estrogen which enters the body through the skin has an equivalent protective effect against osteoporosis.

There are many new forms of estrogen being developed. Estrogen pellets are implanted below the skin and release estrogen continuously, thereby eliminating the need to take a pill every day. However, women who have not had hysterectomies still require progesterone. In very rare circumstances estrogen is injected into the muscle. In Europe, estrogen is now available in a gel which is applied to the abdomen. Soon to be approved is an estrogen tablet which is absorbed through the lining of the cheek into the bloodstream (like smokeless tobacco).

Estrogen also occurs "naturally" in some plants. Ginseng con-tains estrogen and has been promoted as a natural method of treating hot flashes. If this constitutes "natural" or implied "safe" treatment, then estrogen derived from pregnant mare's urine (Premarin) should probably be given the same distinction. Seriously, estrogen from any source carries the same risks and benefits and should be taken as a medication in the proper dose and with appropriate medical evaluation and follow-up.

✦ THE TIMING OF HORMONE REPLACEMENT

Many women begin to think through their own HRT decision well before they are menopausal. Harriet is a forty-six-year-old bookstore salesclerk who was still having regular menstrual periods but wanted to consider the decision about hormone replacement therapy before her periods stopped. She came to us to explore her options. She had a history of debilitating premenstrual symptoms for years, which improved with exercise and diet manipulations. She did not want to experience similarly severe symptoms of menopause if these could be prevented.

Harriet appreciated the opportunity to review in detail her family history and the possible risks and benefits of HRT. A careful review of her history revealed that she was at great risk for having heart disease because she smoked for fifteen years, had a moderately elevated cholesterol, and a mother who had several heart attacks beginning in her fifties. She was also at significant risk for osteoporosis because of her small body frame, her history of smoking, and her mother's history of severe osteoporosis with fractures. There was very little on the downside of taking hormone replacement therapy for Harriet, as she had no family history of cancer and she was not resistant to the idea of continued periods. She decided to begin hormone replacement therapy at menopause.

Menopause typically occurs between the ages of forty-eight and fifty-five, with an average age of approximately fifty-one years. The exact age that any given woman will experience menopause depends on heredity (when her mother and grandmother experienced menopause) and environment (smoking and living at high altitudes lowers the age of menopause). Only 1 percent of women experience premature menopause which is menopause that occurs before the age of forty.

Menopause can occur prematurely if the ovaries are removed (oophorectomy), usually at the time of a hysterectomy (removal of the uterus). In this case, the sudden depletion of estrogen can cause very significant, dramatic symptoms, including severe hot flashes and vaginal dryness. When compared to naturally occurring menopause, surgical menopause produces symptoms that are far more troubling. Many women report similar "estrogen withdrawal" symptoms after childbirth when estrogen levels plummet from the very high levels during pregnancy. Many of our patients can give dramatic descriptions of hot flashes and night sweats, which compounded the sleep deprivation during the early days of motherhood.

The natural history of menopause is that menstrual periods may change in frequency and duration years before the complete cessation of periods. Fertility begins to decline at age thirty but may be present until the last menstrual period when ovarian function has ceased. This is important information for women who would not welcome a "change of life" pregnancy. Indeed, women can experience hot flashes while they are still menstruating, and it is presumed that this represents an early symptom of menopause.

The medical community is divided about the advisability of beginning estrogen therapy while a woman is still having periods but suffering from hot flashes. We tend toward the position of Lila Nachtigall, M.D., as presented in her book *Estrogen: The Facts That Can Change Your Life*. She takes a firm stand against HRT before the very last period. We also know and understand the special circumstances when a woman may be very disabled by menopausal symptoms, and if properly evaluated might be placed on a brief course of therapy (Nachtigall and Heilman, 1991). Others advocate the use of an estrogen-progesterone regimen in women who are still menstruating but who have symptoms of menopause.

✦ The Good News About HRT

Treatment of Symptoms

HOT FLASHES

Let's start with the good news about hormone replacement therapy. First and foremost, estrogen is effective in the treatment of hot flashes. Approximately 98 percent of women experience complete resolution of hot flashes when they take estrogen. For most women, hot flashes are not disabling and may or may not cause enough discomfort to warrant therapy. For those women who do experience severe and unpleasant hot flashes or have significant disruption of their sleep, estrogen therapy represents a welcomed relief.

The dose of estrogen necessary to eliminate hot flashes varies from woman to woman. Some women experience complete resolution of their hot flashes on as little as .3 mg per day of conjugated estrogens, whereas others may need as much as 1.25 mg per day.

As you recall, Carolyn diagnosed her own menopause because she was having severe hot flashes. In fact, her hot flashes had become so disruptive, that her generally sunny disposition had turned to overcast, with threats of storms. In her opinion, her irritability and less-than-pleasant treatment of customers was leading to fewer tips and a major decline in income. Carolyn was inclined to take HRT for the long haul because of her concern about osteoporosis, but many other women choose to replace hormones for a brief time for the treatment of hot flashes only. In this situation, these women can take the lowest possible dose that treats the hot flashes. In general we start Premarin at .3 mg per day in such circumstances. Because hot flashes occur for an indefinite but limited period of time after menopause, the duration of estrogen therapy will also vary from woman to woman. Many physicians attempt to taper the estrogen therapy after six months to a year to determine whether hot flashes will recur. Two things need to be considered in this situation. The first is that once estrogen therapy has been instituted, it is important that it not be stopped suddenly. If this is done, then the symptoms resulting from the sudden drop in blood estrogen levels can be more devastating than the symptoms which prompted the therapy in the first place. More specifically, hot flashes are likely to be much more severe when estrogen is stopped suddenly than when the level of estrogen gradually declines as it does with spontaneous menopause. An analogous situation is the sudden decrease in estrogen levels seen with surgical removal of the ovaries. Some of our patients have unfortunately learned this themselves when they decided to stop their HRT cold turkey.

The second important point is that hormone replacement therapy may be started for one or more reasons. If the sole reason for instituting treatment with estrogen is the relief of hot flashes, then it makes sense to consider stopping the medication once the hot flashes have dissipated and no longer require treatment. On the other hand, as in Carolyn's situation, if therapy was begun for relief of hot flashes as well as the long-term prevention of osteoporosis or heart disease, then treatment—if well tolerated—may be continued indefinitely.

VAGINAL DRYNESS

Another specific symptom which may prompt a woman to consider estrogen replacement therapy is vaginal dryness. This symptom most often becomes noticeable several *years after* the onset of menopause unless, as in the case of surgical menopause, the decrease in estrogen was sudden and complete.

Linda, a bank teller, had a hysterectomy and oophorectomy at age thirty-six because both her mother and grandmother had ovarian cancer and she was estimated to have a fifty-fifty chance of ovarian cancer. After her surgery, she was started on estrogen patches twice weekly. She had no hot flashes but had severe vaginal irritation that did not respond to any of the usual treatments for vaginal inflammation. She was getting discouraged. After some time, we determined that Linda was suffering from estrogen-related vaginal dryness. Her symptoms completely disappeared after a few weeks when her dose of estrogen was doubled.

Linda's case points out the problems of hysterectomy and oophorectomy at a young age. For most women experiencing natural meno-pause, vaginal dryness does not tend to become noticeable until about five years after the last menstrual period. Vaginal dryness may be a problem only during intercourse, in which case lubricants may be used and completely remedy the situation. Many women also suffer from the associated symptoms of vaginal dryness, including irritation of the vaginal lining, which can cause burning and itching. The linings of the urethra (the outlet from the bladder) and bladder can be affected and cause urinary symptoms, including burning, frequent urination, pres-sure to urinate, and ultimately, urinary tract infections. Because these changes are caused by low levels of estrogen, estrogen replacement therapy is highly effective in preventing and reversing them. Estrogen might also be helpful in preventing urinary tract infections, since it restores the bacteria that normally live in the vagina (Byyny and Sper-off, 1990). There is one recent study, however, which contradicts this and suggests that elderly women taking estrogen are actually more prone to urinary tract infections (Orlander and others, 1992). There is, to date, no confirmation of, or explanation for this finding. It could be that women treated with estrogen are more sexually active, and as a result are more susceptible to urinary tract infections.

If estrogen therapy is begun prior to the onset of the symptoms of vaginal dryness and irritation, then it will prevent their occurrence as long as it is continued. If, however, estrogen therapy is begun to treat established symptoms, then it may take months for these to reverse completely. It is important to remember that although symptoms may persist for months after estrogen is begun, in most cases if therapy continues, the symptoms will improve.

Linda chose to take oral estrogen because she was at serious risk of the complications of early surgical menopause and was not solely treat-ing vaginal dryness. Many women opt for vaginal cream to treat the local symptoms of vaginal dryness and irritation. Vaginal estrogen cream constitutes hormone replacement therapy. Even though it is applied locally, it is absorbed into the bloodstream as is the estrogen in tablets or patches. Because of this absorption, vaginal creams carry the same risks as other forms of estrogen therapy and should only be used with a complete understanding of the risks and benefits.

PREVENTION OF THE LONG-TERM COMPLICATIONS OF MENOPAUSE

It is relatively easy for women who are suffering from severe hot flashes or vaginal irritation to see the potential benefit of estrogen therapy. It is much more difficult for women who are having no symptoms related to menopause to see the advantages of beginning therapy. Both osteoporosis and heart disease represent significant health risks for most menopausal women and are not symptomatic until advanced. The greatest benefit to be derived from estrogen therapy, with respect to osteoporosis and heart disease, is when therapy is instituted close to the onset of menopause. This means that women who are feeling well otherwise may want to consider the long-range possibilities of osteoporosis and heart disease and to begin therapy early in order to accrue the greatest benefit. This is not to say that treatment with estrogen therapy years after menopause is without benefit, but rather that the effect is dampened with time. Both osteoporosis and heart disease are described in far more detail in Chapters Four and Five.

Estrogen replacement therapy decreases osteoporotic bone fractures by about 50–60 percent (Lindsay, 1991; U.S. Congress, 1992). Exercise and calcium also have important roles in reducing osteoporosis, but they are less effective than estrogen replacement therapy in improving bone strength.

The more important good news from a public health standpoint is estrogen's protective effect against heart disease. Women who take estrogen have a lower rate of heart disease when compared to those who do not. The combined results of over twenty studies revealed a 44 percent reduction in heart disease with estrogen therapy (U.S. Congress, 1992). These results have been repeatedly challenged by those who claim that the women who are placed on estrogen therapy are most likely to have a lower risk of heart disease, based on the absence of other risk factors. More specifically, it has been claimed that women who smoke and have high blood pressure are less likely to be treated with estrogen than those who do not have these risks.

Perhaps the most compelling data is from the Nurses' Health Study, which has reported a 50 percent reduction in heart disease among the women taking estrogen replacement therapy (Stampfer, 1991). This study is a long-term study which also accounts for all other known risk factors that might influence the development of heart disease.

The way in which estrogen therapy can reduce the occurrence of heart disease is at least partly due to a favorable effect on cholesterol. Estrogen has been consistently shown to increase HDL cholesterol (the good cholesterol) and to lower LDL cholesterol (the bad cholesterol). This change in the ratio of good and bad cholesterol tips the balance to a more favorable ratio which decreases the likelihood that heart disease will develop.

OTHER EFFECTS

Many promoters of estrogen therapy as the miracle cure for aging would have us believe that it will reverse any number of unwanted changes in skin, hair, muscle and energy. The information related to these changes is much scarcer than that related to the clear biological events of heart attacks and osteoporotic fractures and the easily monitored symptoms of hot flashes and vaginal dryness.

There is some evidence that estrogen may improve the ability of the skin to maintain moisture. It is not at all clear that estrogen therapy slows down the skin's natural aging process which results in wrinkles. There are similar claims, which may or may not be true, that estrogen therapy will improve the appearance of the hair.

What we do know is that there is a strong placebo effect of estrogen on some of the symptoms associated with menopause. Any drug, even sugar pills, can reduce a symptom by 10 to 40 percent. It is, therefore, no surprise that estrogen therapy should have a similar beneficial effect on the treatment of menopausal symptoms, particularly since the women who take the therapy have usually been convinced that it will change their lives. This strong placebo effect, however, makes it difficult to assess symptoms such as fatigue, lassitude and irritability, which may be very responsive to the power of suggestion.

To summarize, then, estrogen is extremely effective in treating the most prominent symptoms of menopause, which are hot flashes and vaginal dryness. Estrogen is also highly effective in reducing the risk of osteoporosis, with its associated fractures and complications, as well as reducing the risk of heart disease. There are very few drugs which are as effective as estrogen. Indeed, if there were not side effects or complications of estrogen use, it would be a nearly perfect treatment.

✦ THE BAD NEWS ABOUT HRT

You may ask, Who in their right mind would take a medication which has been clearly associated with cancer to treat a natural physiological event? The answer to this all-important question lies in the real story linking hormone replacement therapy to cancer. During the 1960s and early 1970s, many menopausal women began estrogen treatment for symptoms of menopause. This was coincident with the release of the extremely popular book *Feminine Forever,* by Robert Wilson,

M.D., which extolled the positive effects of HRT. The bubble burst in 1975 when two important studies that linked estrogen therapy with endometrial cancer were reported. In fact, women taking estrogen were four to seven times more likely to develop the cancer than women not taking estrogen therapy (Ernster, 1988). As a result of this information, estrogen use by menopausal women dropped by nearly 30 percent. Much more is now known about the true increased risk of uterine cancer associated with hormone replacement therapy.

It is known definitely that if cancer of the uterus (endometrial cancer) is present at the time estrogen is started, it will respond to the estrogen therapy by enlarging. This reaction to estrogen places endometrial cancer in a category termed "estrogen-responsive tumors." Breast cancer is also considered an estrogen responsive cancer. The symptoms of endometrial cancer include, predominantly, irregularities of menstruation. Irregular periods (usually bleeding between periods) and changes in menstrual blood flow (usually heavier) may be signs of endometrial cancer. At the time of menopause, these changes are very common and can create uncertainty on the part of the physician as to whether the patient is experiencing symptoms of endometrial cancer or normal menopause. When there is sufficient doubt, the physician may recommend an endometrial biopsy. This involves the removal of a small amount of the uterine lining with a small plastic catheter inserted into the cervix. The procedure can be done in the office without general anesthesia. It may be associated with some discomfort when the small plastic catheter is inserted and some crampy abdominal pain thereafter. Many physicians recommend an endometrial biopsy when they initially prescribe estrogen therapy if they have any concern that the patient may have an early endometrial cancer. Endometrial biopsies are not routinely recommended for all women prior to starting hormone replacement therapy. In the circumstance when estrogen alone is used in a menopausal woman who has not had a hysterectomy, then initial and yearly endometrial biopsies are currently recommended.

If hormone replacement therapy is begun and there is preexisting endometrial cancer which has not been detected, there will often be symptoms that should prompt the patient and the physician to consider endometrial biopsy. These include irregular menstrual bleeding at a time not anticipated by the hormone replacement therapy schedule (see Figure 6-1 on p. 159). It is imperative that these abnormalities of menstrual bleeding be reported to the physician so that the appropriate evaluation can be instituted. In fact, many physicians request that patients keep a diary of their hormone replacement therapy schedule with the days of bleeding so that this can be reviewed during office visits.

The only good news about endometrial cancer is that it is a relatively slow-growing cancer which normally causes symptoms before becoming advanced. It is also a relatively rare tumor. Most women who have endometrial cancer can be completely cured with hysterectomy.

Estrogen therapy is also capable of promoting new cases of uterine cancer when none existed before therapy. We now know that estrogen causes a buildup of the lining of the uterus, which in the normal woman would be followed by monthly shedding and menstrual bleeding. When the lining is allowed to continue to build up without being shed, the stage is set for a cancer to develop. The addition of a progestin can completely eliminate the increased risk of uterine cancer associated with estrogen. Progesterone is the hormone that increases in the second half of the menstrual cycle and causes menstrual bleeding. It is also well-known that the addition of progesterone ten days per month will decrease nearly all of the risk of endometrial cancer, and an addition of progesterone for twelve days per month will eliminate all of the additional risk of endometrial cancer that could be conferred by estrogen.

Many women have difficulty getting beyond the word "cancer" in the discussion of potential complications of hormone replacement therapy. Here it is extremely important to recognize that, indeed, estrogen alone has been associated with uterine cancer. It can cause new cancers and increase the growth of preexisting cancers. However, abnormalities of menstrual bleeding will raise suspicion of a preexisting cancer in a woman on hormone replacement therapy, and these cancers can be detected by endometrial biopsy. They are, furthermore, highly treatable tumors which are nearly always curable. Although estrogen can also cause new cancers, this additional risk can be completely eliminated by the use of a progestational agent. So the news is not so bad after all, and needs to be considered carefully by the woman who has concerns about menopausal symptoms or the long-term conditions associated with menopause.

THE BREAST CANCER CONTROVERSY

If the threat of endometrial cancer didn't drive you away from hormone replacement therapy, then brace yourself for the breast cancer story. Breast cancer is now the second-leading cause of death for women with cancer. The lifetime risk of this cancer for United States women is estimated to be one in nine (Henderson and Wender, 1991). It is this alarmingly high rate of breast cancer which has caused such concern over any factor which could raise the risk even slightly. Although this figure has received a lot of attention we must remember that "lifetime" risk refers to a woman's chance of dying at age eighty-five! During the menopausal years, the risk of breast cancer is less. Still, we worry.

Paula's story makes this point particularly well. She was a forty-nine-year-old woman who had breast cancer that was treated with mastectomy and chemotherapy at age forty-eight. Her last menstrual period was shortly after chemotherapy treatment began. Paula married her second husband, Greg, when she was in her early forties. Paula had worked as a volunteer fund-raiser for nonprofit agencies and Greg, who was sixty, was a retired businessman and avid hiker. Both had been unhappily married before, and were cautious about marrying a second time, yet were excited that they each had found someone with whom to share their life. Their relationship became a source of great joy for both of them, and they spent the first seven years of their marriage almost carefree. When Paula discovered that she had cancer, she and Greg were able to work through the issues of her illness and surgery.

If Paula had come to us before her breast cancer, we might have advised against HRT because of her family history of breast cancer. Paula's mother had had breast cancer. This recommendation is somewhat controversial within the medical community, as is the relationship between breast cancer and hormones. Many studies have been done to specifically address the question "Does noncontraceptive estrogen use increase the risk of breast cancer in women?" The results vary widely, from suggesting that estrogen actually reduces the risk of breast cancer to demonstrating that estrogen increases the risk of breast cancer. The study reporting the most dramatic increase in breast cancer risk suggests that women who ever used estrogen are 1.7 times more likely to develop breast cancer than women who have not used estrogen (Mills and others, 1989).

Some studies indicate that there is a trend toward an increased risk of breast cancer with longer duration of estrogen use and with higher doses. Findings have been very inconsistent with regard to the type of estrogen taken (i.e., conjugated versus unconjugated estrogens) and the comparative risk of estrogen used alone versus estrogen used with progestins.

In October 1992, a study was published to help make some sense out of the morass of information currently available. Specifically, the authors combined the results of all of the studies which have been done focusing on postmenopausal estrogen use and breast cancer. The author concludes "there is no compelling evidence that, overall, women who have ever used postmenopausal estrogens are at increased risk of breast cancer" (Henrich, 1992, p. 1902). There were inconsistent and inconclusive findings across the studies, regarding an increased risk of breast cancer in women who had experienced surgical menopause, benign breast disease, family history of breast cancer or had used estrogens for prolonged periods of time. Prior reports had suggested that there was a significant increase in the risk of breast cancer after five years of estrogen use, the highest risk being experienced in women who had used estrogens for at least fifteen years.

For women like Paula, with a family history of breast cancer, the situation is different. It has been demonstrated that there is a significant increase in the risk of breast cancer among women with a family history of breast cancer. Women who have a family history of breast cancer may experience the greatest increase in risk from estrogen use, although this finding has been inconsistent as well. In fact, one review suggests that the risk of breast cancer for women who have taken estrogens and have a family history of breast cancer is three times that of women with a family history of breast cancer who have not taken estrogens. Several studies also suggest that while there may be a slight increase risk of breast cancer among current users of estrogen therapy, that the type of tumors found are less advanced tumors and that, in fact, the women on estrogen replacement therapy experience a lower death rate from breast cancer than those women not on estrogen therapy. It is completely plausible that women who are taking estrogen replacement therapy are more likely to get yearly mammograms and be evaluated for anything suspicious of breast cancer. This increased vigilance in screening for breast cancer could lead to the detection of earlier breast cancers and better outcomes.

So the major problem with estrogen use and breast cancer appears to be if *too much* has been taken for *too long* by someone with a *family history* of breast cancer. Based on what can be gleaned from studies available to us now, we must conclude that there is no clear evidence that postmenopausal estrogen use, in general, increases the risk of breast cancer. There may be a small increased risk of breast cancer for women who have used higher-dosed estrogens (greater than 1.25 mg of conjugated estrogens daily) and for those women who have used estrogens for longer periods of time (greater than fifteen years).

Many breast cancers will grow more rapidly in the presence of estrogen. This is similar to the situation with endometrial cancer and makes it absolutely imperative that all women who are considering beginning estrogen replacement therapy have a breast exam and a mammogram to ensure that no early cancers are present. Thereafter, it is important to continue with yearly mammograms and breast exams in the event that a very early cancer was not detected with mammography. Breast self-examination is recommended monthly and any suspicious changes should be reported immediately to a physician for further evaluation.

Women like Paula, who have had breast cancer prior to menopause, cannot take estrogen replacement therapy. Even if the cancer is completely cured, as we hope it was for Paula, estrogen therapy should not be prescribed. For these women, there continues to be a much greater chance of developing a second breast cancer and any remaining cancer cells could be stimulated to grow with estrogen. Breast cancer is considered an "absolute contraindication" to estrogen replacement therapy. In medicine, however, nothing is really absolute and there are some physicians who feel that for women who have had breast cancer, short-term (one to two years) estrogen therapy is reasonable to treat hot flashes or vaginal dryness. Yearly endometrial biopsies are recommended rather than adding progesterone to the regimen. This is still very controversial, but we tend to take the cautious approach and advise patients with symptoms to try all possible alternative therapies as we will describe later.

As if this were not complicated enough, now we must consider progestin's effect on breast cancer. There is still insufficient evidence to make any conclusions regarding the role of progestins and breast cancer. There has been one study which showed a greatly increased risk of breast cancer in women who use combined estrogen and progestin therapy (Bergkvist and others, 1989). However, there were problems with this study which have made the medical community unwilling to accept these results without confirmation. What is very clear is that we need more information about the use of estrogen and progestin and the occurrence of breast cancer.

If you are concerned about using estrogen replacement therapy, the current information available suggests that:

• if you have had diagnosis of breast cancer, you should not take estrogen (there may be exceptions);
• if you have a family history of breast cancer (in particular in a sister or mother), then you may opt against hormone replacement therapy;
• if you have decided to take hormone replacement therapy, doses of conjugated estrogens in excess of .625 mg per day should be used with caution;

• the potential risk of hormone replacement therapy used for longer than fifteen years needs to be weighed against the potential benefits; and

• if you take hormone replacement therapy, you should be screened for breast cancer on a yearly basis, and any new or suspicious lumps detected from breast self-exams should be reported immediately.

CLOTS

Birth control pills, which have much higher doses of estrogens, have been clearly associated with the development of blood clots. The most frequent site for this type of clotting is in the veins of the leg. These clots in the deep veins of the calf and thigh (deep venous thrombosis) can break off and travel to the lungs (pulmonary embolism). Pulmonary emboli can be fatal and are the basis of the major concern about deep venous thrombosis.

There have been no studies that show that postmenopausal estrogen replacement therapy is associated with an increased risk of this type of clot formation. However, estrogen therapy should be considered potentially risky in women who have had blood clots while on birth control pills or during pregnancy. These women may have underlying conditions which cause them to form clots when estrogen is taken for therapy or when estrogen levels rise during pregnancy. Women who have had deep venous thrombosis with pregnancy or birth control pills in the past are said to have a "relative contraindication" to estrogen replacement therapy. In essence, this suggests that caution must be used in these situations and that potential risk of clot formation needs to be weighed against the potential benefits of treatment.

LIVER AND GALLBLADDER DISEASE

Another potential complication of estrogen therapy relates to the liver and gallbladder. Estrogens which are taken by mouth are absorbed through the intestine and pass into the liver, where they are broken down before entering into the bloodstream. Because of this, estrogen should not be taken by women with active liver disease. This constitutes another "absolute contraindication" to estrogen use.

Women who take estrogen therapy appear to have approximately twice as much gallbladder disease as women who do not (Petitti and others, 1988). It is plausible, but not yet proven, that estrogen therapy which does not require breakdown by the liver (i.e., therapy with patches, pellets or creams) may cause no increase in gallbladder disease. This benefit of alternative forms of estrogen therapy is theoretical and needs to be proven in practice. If women who may be predisposed to gallbladder disease (women who are overweight, have a family history of gallstones, or a prior history of gallstone or gallbladder disease) choose to take estrogen therapy, they may opt for one of the non-oral forms of therapy.

FIBROIDS

Fibroid tumors are benign tumors of the lining of the uterus. They often cause no symptoms whatsoever and may only be detected during an examination of the uterus during an internal or pelvic exam. They may alternatively cause symptoms of lower-abdominal fullness or may cause irregular or heavy menstrual bleeding. Nearly all fibroid tumors can be detected by pelvic ultrasound, but they may need to be distinguished from endometrial cancer, or other causes of bleeding, by an endometrial biopsy. Irregularities of bleeding cannot be assumed to be caused by fibroids until endometrial cancer is excluded as the cause. Estrogen replacement therapy can cause some fibroid tumors to increase in size and cause symptoms where none existed previously.

Women who are known to have fibroid tumors are often cautioned against beginning hormone replacement therapy because the diagnosis of fibroid tumors constitutes a "relative contraindication" to estrogen treatment. As is the case with all relative contraindications, each woman needs to carefully weigh potential benefits of treatment against the possible complications of treatment related to her situation. If fibroids are detected while you are taking hormone replacement therapy and they are causing more symptoms, it may be wise to stop therapy. If the fibroid tumors shrink, it suggests that the estrogen therapy was causing them to increase in size. The plans for continued treatment will need to be carefully considered in light of all of the pros and cons of treatment.

MIGRAINES

Migraine headaches are listed in many references as a relative contraindication to estrogen treatment. Migraine headaches can worsen when women with a history of migraines are started on estrogen replacement therapy. On the other hand, many women's migraine headaches improve at the time of menopause and do not worsen with hormone replacement therapy! As with all of the potential complications of treatment, each individual woman should discuss this with her health care provider and decide for herself.

PERIODS . . .

This may not represent a life-threatening complication of therapy, but it is most certainly an unwanted side effect of cyclic combined therapy with estrogen and progestin. Many women may view this as a cruel plot concocted by male gynecologists or possibly a strategy of the sanitary products companies to improve sales (to the best of our knowledge, neither of these suspicions has foundation). What is clear is that few, if any, women are sad to lose their periods at the time of menopause. The idea of resuming menstruation is particularly unappealing to women who are, frankly, delighted to be freed from monthly menstrual periods. One of our patients summarized her feelings about the options well when she said "I had really been looking forward to menopause and no periods. My daughter even said, 'So menopause means no periods? That sounds great!' So, why on earth would I want to take medication that would guarantee me monthly periods indefinitely. What a stupid idea!" This is, indeed, the sentiment of many women who are faced with the information about hormone replacement therapy. This is not an issue for women who have had their uteri surgically removed.

For those women who do have their uteri, the options are relatively limited. To eliminate the increased risk of uterine cancer, a progestin needs to be added to the estrogen. There is, however, an option to take estrogen alone, but regular endometrial biopsies are essential to find early treatable cancers. In the most traditional method, estrogen and progesterone are cycled to simulate a premenopausal menstrual cycle. This causes shedding of the uterine lining at the end of the twelve day therapy with progestin. This monthly bleeding which, for most women, lasts about four days is usually lighter than premenopausal menstrual periods. The good news is that monthly bleeding will not continue forever with hormone replacement therapy. After some years of therapy, the uterine lining becomes nonfunctioning and thereby fails to build up to a point where it can shed. It can be anticipated that after a few years of therapy, monthly bleeding will stop.

Because so many women opt against hormone replacement therapy based on their unwillingness to continue menstrual periods, alternative methods of combining estrogen and progestins have been introduced. This has the advantage of eliminating the risk of endometrial cancer and yet does not cause monthly menstrual bleeding. Estrogen and progestin are given continuously throughout the month. Progestin is given in much lower doses (e.g., Provera 1–2.5 mg per day) than the dose given for only twelve days out of the month. (e.g.,

Provera 10 mg per day). The daily dose of progestin prevents the uterine lining from building up throughout the month and thereby not only reduces the risk of endometrial cancer but also fails to cause menstrual bleeding. Many women experience irregular spotty bleeding during the first three months of therapy and even thereafter one-third to one-half of women still experience some bleeding. However, the good news is that after one year of therapy, nearly all women are free of any bleeding at all. Still a number of women completely stop treatment prior to this time because of the nuisance of unpredictable spotty bleeding. Because of this unpredictable bleeding, other regimens of HRT are being developed.

So the news is not all bad after all. For women who have had a hysterectomy this is not an issue. For those women who do have uteri, the choices are to grin and bear monthly menstrual bleeding with a combined cyclic therapy for several years, to opt for combined continuous therapy and grin and bear spotty bleeding for three months up to one year, or to take estrogen alone and have yearly endometrial biopsies. The risk of endometrial cancer narrows the choices, but women can still exercise their preferences between bleeding and biopsies.

OTHER SIDE EFFECTS

Women who opt for hormone replacement therapy and fill their prescriptions for estrogen and progestin will certainly take pause when they open the package insert and are faced with the impressive list of complications and side effects of these drugs. Although this is the exact list provided for birth control pills, it is likely that far fewer women who take birth control pills actually read or react to the package insert. It is our suspicion that younger women, feeling far less mortal, adopt a "not me" reaction to this information. As we shall discuss in Chapter Eight, our chapter on midlife and stress, during the menopausal years, we view medical complications and risks in a more serious fashion. What is interesting, of course, is that the warnings are much more pertinent to birth control pills than they are to postmenopausal hormone replacement therapy. This is because the doses of hormones in replacement therapy are far less than those in contraceptive therapy, and they are being given to patients who are hormone-deficient as opposed to premenopausal women who have normal hormone levels. Nonetheless, there are side effects which may be experienced by women taking hormone replacement therapy. Since the occurrence of any side effect associated with estrogen and progestin is very unpredictable, it would be unwise for women who would otherwise take hormone replacement therapy to discount it on the basis of the threat of a particular side effect.

Fluid retention is the most commonly reported side effect of women taking hormone replacement therapy that includes progesterone. In most circumstances, this lasts only a few weeks. If the symptoms of fluid retention continue, a reduction in dietary salt intake may be warranted. Approximately 2 percent of women consider this side effect problematic enough to stop therapy.

Breast tenderness is reported by a number of women, but is nearly always temporary. For those women who continue to be troubled by this, changes in the progestin may help relieve the breast tenderness. The combined continuous form of therapy may be less likely to cause breast tenderness and should be considered as an option for women who find this intolerable.

PMS-like symptoms have been reported in some women during the time that they are taking progesterone in the combined cyclic form of therapy. Women like Harriet who have had severe PMS may be particularly concerned about this possibility. Anxiety, irritability and depressed mood may all be experienced. For many women, these associated symptoms resolve completely after several months of therapy but for some, they may continue to be unbearable. The combined continuous form of therapy may eliminate these symptoms because of the lower dose of progesterone prescribed. Harriet had already decided that at the first sign of problems, she would try the combined continuous schedule.

Some women taking hormone replacement therapy report *weight gain* as an unpleasant side effect. This weight gain may be related to the fluid retention experienced early in the course of hormone replacement therapy. Some of it may be related to the normal decline in metabolism which causes women to gain weight after menopause. Estrogen may also increase the proportion of the body's fat tissue as is does during pregnancy. These effects of estrogen can be reasonably controlled by increasing exercise and decreasing salt in the diet.

A number of *other symptoms* are less frequently reported by women but are, nonetheless, bothersome in any individual woman who experiences them. Nausea, headaches and increased vaginal discharge have all been associated with hormone replacement therapy. Many of these symptoms are fleeting and will disappear completely despite continuation of therapy. Others may need to be controlled in alternative ways or may lead to discontinuation of the treatment if they remain unacceptable.

In all circumstances, it is crucial that a record of symptoms be kept and that these be discussed with the physician prescribing the medications. The list of symptoms associated with hormone replacement therapy presented here is not all inclusive and any symptom which develops in the course of therapy with hormones should be reported. Women who are taking hormone replacement and are experiencing symptoms early in the course of treatment should, in most cases, be encouraged to continue therapy since the odds that the symptom will disappear completely are good.

✦ HORMONE TREATMENT SCHEDULES

Despite the apparent complexity of hormone replacement therapy schedules, there are relatively few methods being used currently. There may be some subtle variations in treatment schedules, but the principles of each method are distinct. Figure 6-1 summarizes the three major hormone replacement schedules.

UNOPPOSED ESTROGEN THERAPY

For women like Carolyn and Linda who have had a hysterectomy, estrogen can be taken alone without the addition of a progestin. Since their uteri have been removed, there is no risk of uterine cancer. This form of therapy is called unopposed estrogen. In the past, it was felt that there may be some rationale to discontinuing estrogen therapy for one week per month. For the most part, this practice has been discontinued since there is no evidence of benefit and many women actually experience hot flashes during the week off estrogen therapy.

For women who still have a uterus, unopposed estrogen therapy without endometrial biopsies is not usually recommended because of the increased risk of endometrial cancer. Some women are so opposed to continued periods and have such potential benefit to be gained by estrogen therapy that they agree to regular endometrial biopsies to detect uterine cancer. All women who have a uterus and are started on unopposed estrogen therapy should have a pretreatment endometrial biopsy and yearly biopsies thereafter while on treatment. There are even some who would advocate biopsies every six months. Any bleeding that is experienced should be reported immediately and should prompt additional endometrial biopsies.

The form of estrogen taken should be based on the patient's

Figure 6–1

Summary of
Hormone Replacement Schedules

Unopposed Estrogen

Day of Months 1 2 3 4 5 6 7 8 9 10 11 12 13 14 15 16 17 18 19 20 21 22 23 24 25 26 27 28 29 30

Estrogen - - - -   ->

Progesterone   none

Bleeding   none

Cyclic Combined

Day of Months 1 2 3 4 5 6 7 8 9 10 11 12 13 14 15 16 17 18 19 20 21 22 23 24 25 26 27 28 29 30

Estrogen ->

Progesterone - - - - - - - - - - - - - - - |

Bleeding |- - - - - - - - - •|

Continuous Combined

Day of Months 1 2 3 4 5 6 7 8 9 10 11 12 13 14 15 16 17 18 19 20 21 22 23 24 25 26 27 28 29 30

Estrogen ->

Progesterone ->

Bleeding   spotting possible for up to one year

preference for route of administration and consideration of the conditions that may favor one form of therapy over another. A woman with a family history of gallbladder disease may opt for estrogen patches as opposed to estrogen pills to decrease the potential of this complication. Many women prefer patches despite the increased cost (as much as ten times the pills) because they can be used twice weekly, rather than pills which need to be taken on a daily basis. As discussed earlier in this chapter, vaginal creams may have somewhat erratic absorption into the bloodstream and may be less desirable because of this.

✦ CYCLIC COMBINATION THERAPY

The method of combining both estrogen and progestin in a cyclic fashion to simulate the premenopausal menstrual cycle is the most frequently used method of hormone replacement. There is absolutely no reason to prescribe hormone replacement in this method to women who have had hysterectomy, because the major reason for using this method is to reduce the risk of endometrial cancer.

Although there are subtle variations in technique, the basic premise in this form of therapy is that estrogen and progestin are combined and the progestin is given for a sufficient number of days during the month to reduce the risk of endometrial cancer. In light of this underlying principle, there are two major ways of dosing the hormone therapy. The first is to prescribe estrogen continuously throughout the month and to add the progestin for the first twelve days of the month. Bleeding which occurs on day twelve of progestin therapy or later is considered normal and requires no further evaluation. If bleeding occurs on day eleven or before, endometrial biopsy is recommended. Likewise, if there is any breakthrough bleeding or heavy withdrawal bleeding, further evaluations should proceed with an endometrial biopsy.

Another method of prescribing cyclic combination therapy is to prescribe the estrogen therapy during days one through twenty-five of the month and the progestin on days fourteen through twenty-five. There is one week per month during which time no hormone replacement therapy is prescribed. With this method, it can be anticipated that menstrual bleeding should begin approximately on day twenty-five and if it begins on day twenty four or before, then endometrial biopsy may be recommended (some physicians biopsy only when bleeding occurs before day twenty-three). Currently, we see no clear reason to discontinue estrogen therapy for one week per month. There is a chance that hot flashes will recur because of the sudden withdrawal of estrogen. Many physicians, however, continue to prescribe hormone replacement therapy in this method based on previous theoretical concerns about continuous estrogen therapy. We did not include this schedule since we do not use it in our practice.

The dose of progesterone prescribed in the cyclic combination therapy method should be high enough to cause menstrual bleeding. In general, medroxyprogesterone is given at a dose of 10 mg per day during the twelve days of treatment. For women who experience unpleasant side effects from progesterone, it may be feasible to decrease the dose to 5 mg per day and continue at that level if monthly menstrual bleeding still occurs. The estrogen portion of hormone replacement therapy can be taken as pills or patches. Pellets have also been used in Europe for this purpose. Vaginal creams are rarely used in combination with progesterone since the absorbed estrogen is unpredictable and would not be consistent enough or sufficient to cause a buildup of the uterine lining.

The cyclic combined form of therapy has been the most widely used and for many women, is very acceptable. It does require that a close record be kept of the timing of menstrual bleeding in order that early bleeding can be investigated further with endometrial biopsy.

✦ CONTINUOUS COMBINED THERAPY

For most of you who abhor the idea of continued menstrual periods, this form of therapy may be appealing. Additionally, women who experience unpleasant side effects from the higher doses of progesterone used with cyclic combined therapy may find this more tolerable. The method of therapy is quite simple and consists of continuous estrogen and progesterone therapy throughout the month. The dose of progesterone is significantly lower than those used in the cyclic combined method: medroxyprogesterone 1 to 2.5 mg per day as opposed to medroxyprogesterone 10 mg per day.

Although the major benefit of this form of therapy is that it does not cause monthly menstrual bleeding, it is frequently associated with irregular bleeding in the first several months. Most women who can continue to take the therapy for one year can expect that all bleeding will stop. Biopsies should be performed for any irregular bleeding during the course of therapy, so most women will get one or more.

As with the other types of treatment, estrogen can be taken in the form of pills, patches or pellets. Careful records should be kept of any bleeding which is experienced during the treatment and reported to the prescribing physician. Some women do experience side effects from the progesterone throughout the month and these symptoms should be reported as well.

✦ ALTERNATIVES TO HORMONE REPLACEMENT THERAPY

There are a number of nonhormonal and nondrug treatments for the symptoms and long-term complications of menopause. Rather than present a shopping list of possible prevention and treatment options here, these alternatives are presented in the individual chapters to which they apply. It is important, however, to recognize that hormone replacement therapy is not the only way to treat and prevent menopausal symptoms and associated conditions.

Paula survived breast cancer and began having hot flashes shortly after her chemotherapy. Because of her breast cancer, she was not a candidate for hormone replacement therapy, but desperately needed relief from her unremitting hot flashes. We met with Paula and worked out a behavioral and non-hormonal plan to deal with her hot flashes. We spoke with her about a comprehensive non-hormonal treatment plan that included self-monitoring triggers, paced respirations, vitamin E and increased physical activity. She did get some relief from our suggestions, and commented on the added benefits she gained with the exercise and physical activity program regarding weight loss and an increase of energy. In fact, Paula told us that she felt that she and Greg had grown even closer since they had worked on the problem together and she expressed an interest in joining him on the hiking trails.

We have been touched by the stories of women who have had the courage to cope with breast cancer, only to face difficult symptoms of menopause. We always wish that we had more to offer, but we are hopeful that new non-hormonal treatment strategies will be developed. Survivors of breast cancer are now taking an active role in making this happen. If you are facing a situation similar to Paula's, you may find helpful *The Menopause Self-Help Book* by Susan M. Lark. This illustrated book focuses on treatments for menopause that are non-hormonal. Dr. Lark is a physician whose book focuses on a healthy diet, vitamins and minerals for menopause, stress reduction, as well as acupuncture and yoga. Although many of the vitamins she recommends have not been tested, most of her advice is practical and sound.

✦ THE BIG PICTURE

There is no "one size fits all" formula to answer the question, "Should I take hormone replacement therapy at menopause?" For any individual woman a particular risk or benefit may take on more importance than all the others. It is well known that each individual places very different values on the consequences of taking or not taking the medication. In the case of hormone replacement therapy, some women have no interest in hearing about the benefit in preventing heart disease once they have heard that they will continue to have menstrual periods. For other women who have experienced the pain and suffering of a relative with osteoporotic bone fractures, the nuisance of menstrual periods may seem very insignificant. As women making this very important decision it is important that we take personal inventory of all of the pros and cons of taking hormone replacement therapy. By necessity, this inventory will need to acknowledge our individual risk for developing the conditions that might be prevented or caused by hormone replacement therapy and set priorities accordingly. Likewise, we will need to specifically assess the consequences of taking or not taking hormone replacement therapy based on our attitudes and past experiences.

It is difficult to determine even the approximate number of women who are currently taking hormone replacement therapy. The Massachusetts Women's Health Study found that 9.2 percent of the women surveyed were being treated with hormone replacement therapy (Avis and McKinlay, 1990). This is in contrast to a survey of women in a California community which demonstrated that 32 percent of the women between ages fifty and sixty-five reported estrogen use with 6 percent reporting progestin use as well (Harris and others, 1990).

Also from the Massachusetts Women's Health Survey, we know that 20–30 percent of women never fill their prescriptions for hormone replacement therapy (Ravnikar, 1987). It is particularly interesting that surveys have shown that nearly all gynecologists would prescribe estrogen therapy for most of their patients (U.S. Congress, 1992). If in fact only between 9 and 30 percent of women actually take hormone replacement therapy, we must assume that the majority of patients for whom hormone replacement therapy is recommended opt against it either before having the prescription written out or filled, or after beginning therapy. Other women may not be able to afford health care or medications. Many women may not be seeking medical attention.

It is also possible that more women are taking hormone replacement therapy, but only for a short time to treat menopausal symptoms. This is supported by a study that looked at women's decision making around the choice of hormone replacement therapy. The authors found that the women studied gave the highest priority to the impact that hormone replacement replacement therapy would have on their lives in the short term as opposed to the impact it would have on their long-term risk of morbidity and mortality. It is particularly disturbing that the women who were surveyed in this study felt that they had inadequate information to make a decision about hormone replacement therapy and that their health care providers did not listen to them (Rothert, 1991).

If you are in the category of women who can consider HRT, you should review your symptoms of hot flashes, vaginal dryness, and your risks of osteoporosis and heart disease. If your symptoms are severe and you are at risk of developing osteoporosis and heart disease, you might seriously consider HRT. This is something to discuss with your health-care professional in depth.

To see how much women can differ, let's take our last look at Pam, a fifty-six-year-old high school guidance counselor who opted against hormone replacement therapy when she suddenly stopped menstruating at age forty-eight. It was Pam's good fortune that she never had a hot flash, nor any vaginal dryness. She had sailed through menopause. When asked to what she attributed her incredibly un-eventful passage through menopause, she said, "I exercise religiously, I eat and sleep well, and I may be a little bizarre, since I never had a single labor pain with either of my two children."

✦ COMMUNICATION

Now that you have reviewed the choices about hormone replacement therapy, you might be feeling overwhelmed. "How in the world am I going to make this decision—one of the most important health care decisions of my life? First of all, don't be intimidated! By now we have explored the various issues with you and we have confidence that you will be able to make this decision. After all, you have probably made numerous other decisions with respect to your own health care, and that of your family members. You have probably, in the past, decided what kind of birth control to use and some of you who are mothers may have made decisions about childbirth and delivery. Any of you who have had surgery for sports injuries know that you had to make that decision and weigh it against other alternative treatment ap-proaches. You will be better able to make this decision by reviewing your risk of heart disease and osteoporosis, and your symptoms like hot flashes and vaginal dryness, and if you follow the strategy that we out-line below. You may notice that we did not include symptoms of stress or depression. This is because hormone replacement therapy is not an appropriate treatment for those problems. We discuss this further in those chapters.

Some of you may be wishing for the good old days, when a benev-olent and paternalistic male physician would take you aside and say, "Dear, just do this." (One of us was actually patted on the head once when she was in her twenties and trying to decide about birth control. Her paternalistic but well-meaning obstetrician/gynecologist told her that she should just get pregnant because he really preferred to deliver babies.) If you have a trusting relationship with your health care professional and feel comfortable with her or his judgment, you may wish to ask what they would do in similar circumstances.

We suggest that you try to take an open-minded approach to this decision. It is important to go into the decision without being encumbered with political or philosophical beliefs. As you know by now, we see estrogen neither as a miracle wonder drug, nor as a dangerous external "chemical" substance. We have tried to present the evidence objectively and we hope that you will be able to utilize it objectively as well.

After reviewing your symptoms and risks, you may want to discuss it with your partner. A person who lives with you can provide a second opinion about the effect of your symptoms on your daily life. Sometimes family members can remember additional details of family history that could be helpful. If your mother, grandmother, or any of your aunts are interested, you might discuss the issue of estrogen with them. Similarly, by talking to sisters and friends, you can get a sense of how estrogen has affected women who have decided to take it. By talking to women who have chosen not to use hormone replacement therapy, you can understand their perspective as well. So by now you should have a sense of your own symptoms and your health needs. In addition, you have gotten some helpful information from women who have made different decisions about estrogen.

It is helpful not to look at this decision as forever. You need not be married to treatment and divorce is always an option. You can make a tentative decision to try hormone replacement therapy and evaluate the consequences. One way to evaluate the effects of hormone replacement therapy is to monitor your symptoms after a trial of several months of hormone replacement therapy. For hot flashes, it may take up to four weeks to assess the effectiveness of treatment and for vaginal dryness it can require months. It is also useful to ask your clinician about the hows and whys of taking hormone replacement therapy, just as you would with any other medication.

Once you start taking HRT, if you have unpleasant side effects, such as bloating or mood changes, you might be inclined to stop hormone replacement therapy. But if you have made the decision to try it in the first place, a better alternative is to discuss the situation with your physician like Carolyn did when she was having difficulties with the patch. Often, she or he can lower the doses of the medication or change the schedule, and the side effects can be managed. It is important to talk it over before making your next decision.

Finally, if your side effects cannot be managed, or if you cannot take hormone replacement therapy because you have a history of breast cancer, or if you choose not to take it in the first place, please remember that you have many alternatives. In every section of this book we have discussed alternative methods that do not involve hormone replacement therapy to cope with symptoms. For example, many women who have hot flashes learn to do paced breathing exercises and relaxation procedures which help them manage. Other women have found that changes in their diet can be helpful. Similarly, topical lubricants can be used to cope with vaginal dryness. It is important for all of us to remember that hormone replacement therapy, albeit an important decision, is not the only choice to improve our health during menopause.

✦ RESOURCES

Communicating with your family members and friends is one way to help you make the hormone replacement therapy decision. A continuing process of communication with your health care provider about hormone replacement therapy is also critical to your health care during the menopausal period. There are numerous other resources that might be useful in this process. First, one of the best uses of our federal tax dollars is *The Menopause: Hormone Therapy Replacement and Women's Health*. This book, although somewhat technically written, is an excellent overview of the pros and cons of hormone replacement therapy. It was written by a consensus panel of leaders in the field and it summarizes what was known in 1992 when it was published. Many of the conclusions are similar to ours. But, you might chose to look at it and to even look at some of the original articles that it references. It is available through the U.S. Bureau of Public Documents.

BOOKS

Many women find the book we discussed earlier helpful—Lila Nachtigall's *Estrogen: The Facts Can Change Your Life*. Another helpful book is Janine O'Leary Cobb's *Understanding Menopause* (New York: A Plume Book, The Penguin Group, 1993).

SELF-HELP

Self-help groups can be extremely beneficial in coping with the decision about hormone replacement therapy. For example, you may not have friends who are struggling with the question to the same extent that you are and by joining a self-help group you can find women with similar concerns. Many of the self-help groups have women who have gone through the menopausal transition and can serve as role models for women who have chosen to take hormone replacement therapy and those who have not. Self-help groups can be extremely powerful because of the intimacy and solidarity that usually develops. If you do not know of a self-help group in your area, you may turn to Chapter Eleven, "Resources," which details your possibilities. Many women's health practices and women's hospitals can be helpful if you call their department of public relations.

PHARMACEUTICAL COMPANIES' PUBLICATIONS

Wyeth-Ayerst Laboratories
P.O. Box 9251
Garden City, NY 11530-9836

Publishes a series of pamphlets called "Life after 45" on menopause, aging, and related issues, with a bias for estrogen therapy. Also Seasons Magazine, *with articles on menopause, health, aging, keeping fit, which is free.*

CIBA Pharmaceutical Company
Division of CIBA-GEIGY Corporation
5566 Morris Avenue
Summit, NJ 07901

Publishes an eight-page booklet on menopause: "Midlife: No Crisis" including definitions, symptoms and treatment, focusing on estrogen therapy.

Mead Johnson Laboratories
Bristol Myers Squibb Company
P.O. Box 4000
Princeton, NJ 08543-4000

Publishes "For the woman approaching menopause," a synopsis of biological and psychological issues.

CHAPTER SEVEN

Myths of Depression

LET'S GET ONE THING STRAIGHT: NATURAL MENOPAUSE IN AND OF IT-self does not cause depression. This may come as a surprise to you because almost everything we read about menopause associates it with depression. As early as 1945, the psychoanalytic view of the menopausal woman was reflected in the work of Helene Deutsch who wrote, "With the cessation of this function, she ends her service to the species, her genital organs become atrophied and the rest of the body gradually shows symptoms of aging" (Deutsch, 1945). This dated theory of the menopausal stage of life has permeated our culture and continues into the 1990s. Articles over the past several years have managed to empha-size this point by consistently describing depression almost exclusively as a problem of midlife women and linking it to a hormonal deficiency.

Certainly when we read these articles we *could become* depressed, but there is one major problem with them. There is no evidence that they are true. Never has a scientific study indicated that menopause alone is a cause of depression. In fact, younger American women tend to have higher rates of depression than older women. Specifically, young women with children under the age of five at home, who are divorced or not getting along with their partner/spouse, are at the greatest risk of depression. Although these factors make a lot of sense, unfortunately we read very little about these women.

The Massachusetts Women's Health Study found that there is no evidence of a menopausal depression when menopause is natural (McKinlay and others, 1987). This study was not limited to women who seek medical attention, but rather included women from the larger community. Menopausal women did not experience depression at the time of menopause any more often than did younger women. The McKinlays found rather consistent rates of depression hovering between 5 and 10 percent for premenopausal, perimenopausal and postmenopausal women, with a slight increase at the perimenopausal period. This group of perimenopausal women may represent women who are experiencing numerous medical symptoms, as we will discuss in a bit.

In this same study, women who had undergone hysterectomies and oophorectomies, on the other hand, had a rate of depression closer to 18 percent. The high rate of depression in this group may have been in response to the *dramatic* drop in hormone production experienced with surgical menopause. In addition, hysterectomy and oophorectomy require major abdominal surgery and a long recovery period. The McKinlays and their associates also suggest that women who are depressed are more likely to suffer from more gynecological symptoms. These women, therefore, might have hysterectomies and oophorectomies more often than nondepressed women (McKinlay and others, 1987). We discuss this in greater detail in Chapter Nine, "Hysterectomy."

Despite these efforts of prominent social scientists to dispel the myth of the menopausal depression, it still flourishes in medical articles and in the popular media. For the most part, the television screen avoids the faces of women in the menopause years. The few women over the age of forty that we see on television on a regular basis are women in their sixties, like Angela Lansbury in *Murder She Wrote*. It was not until recently that we could see Blanche, the youngest member of *The Golden Girls*, and Julia Sugarbaker on *Designing Women* deal with their characters' journey through menopause.

Hollywood, too, has contributed to the myths of menopause that American women absorb. Even the moving film, based on Fannie Flagg's novel *Fried Green Tomatoes at the Whistle Stop Café*, gives an inaccurate message with regard to Evelyn's depression. Evelyn is discouraged and sad, turning only to candy bars and television, when she meets Mrs. Threadgoode. When she describes some of her symptoms,

Mrs. Threadgoode turns to her and says, "Girl, you've got to get yourself some hormones!" The film illustrates that a woman during her menopausal years can develop a more fulfilling and enriching phase of her life. Indeed, the character Evelyn does get those hormones and gets over her "depression." But Evelyn obviously has other stressors in her life that have nothing to do with hormones, including an uninvolved husband, no job or hobbies, a lack of family and social support systems, and practically no physical activity. In fact, she is not only dissatisfied with her situation, but inquisitive and thirsty for a better life. During the film, we watch her break out of old habits and establish a close relationship with a new friend. She begins to exercise regularly, take up new interests and stop asking her husband for permission. It is her exercise regimen, new healthy eating habits and a fulfilling friendship that warrant credit for her escape from "depression," not the hormones alone. One of our favorite and somewhat bizarre examples of television's view of psychological problems during menopause is from the series *Picket Fences,* where they devoted an episode to a woman who became psychotic because of her menopause and ran over her husband with a steamroller! Alas, her insanity defense was not successful. In reality, we haven't come across too many menopausal steamroller operators, and there is no actual increased risk of depression or psychosis at this time of life.

The truth is that even though menopause does not cause depression, depression can still affect many women at menopause. Why? Because depression is the most common mental health problem shared by all American women. It strikes up to one out of ten American women at any point in time. So even though menopause does not cause depression, just this baseline statistic means that many of you are depressed at this moment. Depression is so common in women that it is often called "the common cold" of female psychological problems. The reason that it is so important to make the distinction that some menopausal women are depressed, but that menopause does not cause depression, is that by blaming depression on menopause alone, many women will not get the adequate care they need. The danger here is that serious cases of depression may be dismissed and misdiagnosed as a natural part of menopause. This is particularly troubling since there are now numerous effective treatments for depression.

A tragic result of this misdiagnosis was reported in *New York* magazine in October 1992 (Wolfe, 1992). Theodora Sklover, a former New York City executive, suffered from long-term depression and had experienced many financial reversals. Her friends knew that she was depressed, as she did herself, but ". . . she'd read that menopause could cause depression, and instead of seeking out a psychiatrist for treatment, she went to a physician who gave her estrogen-replacement pills" (Wolfe, 1992, p. 54). The HRT may have helped some of her symptoms of menopause, but it didn't treat her serious case of depression. Theodora Sklover's condition deteriorated, and she eventually jumped to her death from the window of her tenth-story apartment in Manhattan.

Had Sklover had access to more accurate information, she would have known that HRT is not a cure for depression, but that there are many other effective treatments, including antidepressant medication and psychotherapy. It is not hard to understand how women today in Sklover's position may well assume that the symptoms and treatments for depression and menopause are one and the same. HRT for these women is seen as a convenient way to cure depression, more so than beginning psychotherapy. How can we blame menopausal women for this view?

Theodora Sklover's case is just the most dramatic example. The response of Sklover's friends is indicative of the fears that could well continue to fuel the menopause anxiety: "Others panicked. They felt frightened because her death seemed to say something to them about the plight of aging, unattached, professional women in New York" (Wolfe, 1992, p. 47). Sklover's was not a tragedy of aging, menopause or a psychological disease of professional women. Her tragedy was a result of misinformation. Despite the fact that hormones alone do not cause a menopausal depression, millions of women suffering from clinical depression will continue to blame it on this "hormonal imbalance" and not receive the treatment they so desperately need.

A more common case of misinformation regarding the hormone-depression connection is exemplified by Rose, one of our patients. Rose came to see us because of what she described as a "hormonal problem." She was a fifty-two-year-old woman who had worked in a small jewelry factory for the past twenty-five years. Her husband, Ed, was a recovering alcoholic who had been sober for the past ten years. Her three children were grown and lived in nearby communities with their families. Rose was a very funny and insightful woman who was able to cut through to the heart of most matters. She was treasured by her family and at work, for her problem-solving abilities. She also served as a resource in her Baptist church. But something had changed in the way Rose saw the world over the past several years. Ed was a stable and caring man who worked as an accountant and was active in AA. He also tended to spend a lot of time on carpentry, a hobby he loved. Rose's three children relied on her for periodic baby-sitting and were still extremely dependent on her. She was especially close to her thirty-year-old daughter Cathy. Rose had continued to work because she knew the owners well and was able to change her hours to meet her family needs over the years. She was clearly underemployed, even though she recently had been promoted to supervisor.

Rose came to us because her periods were irregular and she had been having severe hot flashes for several years. She was tired, irritable and sad. When we evaluated Rose, we found that she was still perimenopausal since her periods were sporadic and had not stopped completely. Rose represents a category of women who need further attention. Rose, at the age of fifty-two, had experienced a prolonged and difficult perimenopausal period. Although her periods had started to become irregular at the age of forty-eight, they continued. Drs. Peter J. Schmidt and David Rubinow at the National Institute of Mental Health have suggested that this *peri*menopausal period may represent a high-risk time for depression, rather than the *post*menopausal period that has received previous attention (Schmidt and Rubinow, 1991). This would also fit with the Massachusetts Women's Health Study that there was an increase in the rate of depression during the perimenopause (McKinlay and others, 1987). We have found that women whose perimenopausal period is both long and symptomatic may be at risk for depression. This makes perfect sense because difficult symptoms can cause sleep disturbances and a disruption in daily life, which can increase stress. Rose was troubled by her hot flashes, but afraid of HRT because of a family history of cancer.

When we talked with Rose at length, we found that the history of cancer in her family was that of pancreatic cancer. Rose was not aware that the reasons not to take HRT are related to breast or uterine cancer. We discuss this in detail in Chapter Six, "Hormone Replacement Therapy." When Rose started HRT, her hot flashes vanished within weeks and she was greatly relieved.

However, Rose still struggled with her sadness. She had also learned recently that her daughter Cathy was going to be moving out of state. Rose, like many women, remained close to all of her grown children and found that she enjoyed relating to these adults she and Ed had raised. The extended perimenopause was an additional stress, but not the only cause of her symptoms. Since Cathy had been her main support over the past ten years, her moving was potentially a major loss to Rose.

It became apparent to us that Rose had struggled with dysthymia for many years. She was always somewhat pessimistic, expected little from life, and had grown accustomed to the role of being everyone's caretaker. During a course of short-term psychotherapy, we helped

Rose expand her network of friends. We also watched her discover different expectations from her relationship, including more reciprocity. She developed a friendship with a woman at work and initiated more shared activities with Ed.

Rose's story helps us understand that depression during the menopausal years is complicated. Psychological problems, like life, are not that simple. One of the primary reasons we wrote this book was our outrage at the dangerous persistence of both popular and the medical media to portray depression in women as primarily a hormonal problem of midlife women. McKinlay, McKinlay and Brambilla conclude that "menopause as a physiologic process provides a single convenient potentially treatable cause, which is attractive to the busy clinician and avoids the need to consider other, more complex and probably less treatable explanations" (McKinlay and others, 1987, p. 360). It is easier to dismiss menopausal women as suffering from hormonal changes, rather than to examine their complex, social and physical problems.

✦ WHAT IS DEPRESSION?

The epidemiologist Dr. Myrna Weissman suggests that we can view depression as a mood state, a symptom or a syndrome (Weissman, 1980). Depression can also be seen as a continuum of severity, ranging from a "bad day" on the far left of the continuum to a major depressive episode on the far right. Men and women alike have bad days where they feel sad and irritable, and frequently we use the expression "I'm depressed today." But clinical depression is more than fleeting sadness. Depression as a psychological disorder has been studied in great depth. The American Psychiatric Association's *Diagnosis and Statistical Manual, Third Edition Revised,* is a book that describes all major psychiatric problems. There are many different forms of depression. Sometimes a loss, like a divorce, or being fired from a job can precipitate a depressive episode. These reactions to painful or stressful situations are usually called "adjustment reactions." These are usually short-term. To be depressed, of course, is also part of a normal grieving process. One category, "dysthymic disorder," is characterized by at least two years of feelings of low self-esteem, hopelessness, worthlessness, negativism and sadness. This is a long-term problem, and many women may continue to function quite well, despite their personal pain. You can look at Table 7-1 to see whether you might have symptoms of dysthymic disorder (American Psychiatric Association, 1987).

As we move further to the right on the scale, we encounter the

<u>Table 7–1</u>

SYMPTOMS OF
DYSTHYMIC DISORDER

1. Have you had a depressed mood for most of the day, more days than not, for at least two years?

2. Do you have, when you are depressed, at least *two of* the following?
1. poor appetite or overeating
2. insomnia or hypersomnia
3. low energy or fatigue
4. low self-esteem
5. poor concentration or difficulty making decisions
6. feelings of hopelessness

3. Have you ever had a manic episode—overly high amounts of energy, poor judgment. If so, you may have a bipolar disorder.

4. Are you taking medications that can cause depression? If so, check with your primary-care doctor.

•If you have answered YES to questions 1 & 2, and NO to 3 & 4, you may have dysthymia.

Adapted from the *Diagnostic and Statistical Manual of Mental Disorders, Third Edition,* Revised (Washington, DC: American Psychiatric Association, 1987).

more intense and disruptive types of depression. At the far right we find a major depressive episode (as you can see in Table 7-2). A Major Depressive Episode involves frequent and daily symptoms including frequent crying, sadness, loss of interest, inability to concentrate, weight changes, a loss of interest in sex, and may include suicidal plans and suicidal feelings (American Psychiatric Association, 1987). Some women who are already dysthymic may develop more severe symptoms and progress to a Major Depressive Episode also. If suicidal plans become a part of your symptoms, it is crucial to get professional help as soon as possible. Many people have fleeting thoughts of suicide when they are mildly depressed or under severe stress, but when these feelings turn into specific ideas of action or actual impulses toward suicide, it is important to respond immediately. Remember that these feelings can be treated successfully by a mental health professional.

There are several other psychological problems that include depressive symptoms. These include a bipolar disorder or what was once called manic depressive disorder. The essential feature here is that, in addition to episodes of major depression, there are also episodes of manic or extremely active behavior and sometimes euphoric times when the person shows impaired judgment.

✦ WOMEN'S DEPRESSION: THE PSYCHOLOGICAL COMMON COLD

Women are much more likely than men to suffer from depression. Two to three times as many women suffer from depression than do men (Weissman and Klerman, 1985). This stark statistic is almost completely ignored in medical school and psychological training programs and is also overlooked in the ample self-help literature on depression Not surprisingly, formal psychological treatments for depression have often underplayed women's issues as well. It is possible for us as women to get adequate treatment for depression if we approach the situation with care and with the maximum amount of information.

✦ A COMPREHENSIVE APPROACH TO DEPRESSION

BIOLOGICAL CHANGES

The best way to understand depression and why women suffer from it so often is to use a comprehensive approach. Let's look first at the possible biological factors affecting depression. We have just outlined the hormonal change associated with menopause. Another biological factor is heredity. There does seem to be a tendency for major depression to occur in families, generation after generation. If you have a biological relative, such as a mother, father, grandparent, sister or brother, who has been diagnosed as depressed, then you have a greater risk for depression. This does not necessarily mean that you *will* suffer from depression. Yet this is important information for your health care

Table 7-2

THE DEPRESSION CONTINUUM

	"Blues" "Moodiness"	Long-term sadness Negativism Low self-esteem	Sadness Tearfulness Feelings of loss in response to a specific stressor Time limited	Frequent Daily *Symptoms* Tearfulness Loss of interest

Increasing Severity

TRANSIENT FEELINGS	PERSISTENT MOODINESS	DYSTHYMIC DISORDER	ADJUSTMENT OR GRIEF REACTION	MAJOR DEPRESSIVE EPISODE

Table 7-3

SYMPTOMS OF
MAJOR DEPRESSIVE EPISODE

Have you had at least *five* of the following symptoms during the same two-week period, and is this a *change* from your usual functioning?

1. depressed mood most of the day, nearly every day.

-or-

2. markedly diminished interest or pleasure in all, or almost all, activities most of the day, nearly every day.

-and-

3. significant weight loss or weight gain when not dieting (e.g., more than 5 percent of body weight in a month), or decrease or increase in appetite nearly every day.

4. insomnia or hypersomnia nearly every day.

5. psychomotor agitation or retardation nearly every day.

6. fatigue or loss of energy nearly every day.

7. feelings of worthlessness or excessive or inappropriate guilt nearly every day.

8. diminished ability to think or concentrate, or indecisiveness, nearly every day.

9. recurrent thoughts of death (not just fear of dying), recurrent suicidal ideation without a specific plan, or a suicide attempt or a specific plan.

•If you answered YES to 1 or 2 and YES to four items from 3–9, you may be suffering from a major depressive episode.

•Adapted from *The Diagnostic and Statistical Manual of Mental Disorders, Third Edition Rev. 1987.*

provider to have, especially when talking about possible symptoms of mood changes.

A third and important biological change is the experience of hot flashes and other vasomotor symptoms during menopause. When hot flashes or night sweats disrupt a woman's sleep, she can become sleep deprived. This sleep deprivation can lead to a vulnerability to psychological problems like depression. This has been called the "domino effect" of hot flashes (Sherwin, 1993). This domino effect was a problem for Rose and for another of our patients, Joan. Joan was experiencing symptoms of menopause when she came to see us. In addition, she complained of low energy, fatigue and a loss of the ability to concentrate. Because Joan was an accomplished painter and had been very productive, her loss of creative energy was very disturbing to her. At the same time, she informed us that she was experiencing night sweats that would awaken her in the middle of the night. Quite often she found it difficult to return to sleep. The sleep deprivation led to loss of concentration which in turn made Joan feel mildly irritable and frustrated. This indirect result of a biological change associated with menopause is worth exploring further so that it can be clarified.

Joan also felt like she had a "hell of a case of PMS." This is a description that many of our patients use to describe their mood changes during the menopausal years. In fact, if you have suffered from PMS, you may be more likely to have similar symptoms at menopause. What makes Joan's experience and that of other women who feel like they have PMS is that the feelings are usually transient, sometimes cyclical, and more in the category of moodiness or the blues—on the left end of our continuum.

In contrast, women suffering from a major depressive episode like Theodora Sklover tend to feel depressed and sad most of the day, every day for a longer period of time. Depressed women often describe a feeling that they just cannot function anymore. It is important to distinguish the transient PMS-like symptoms from a major depressive episode or dysthymia, because the treatments are quite different.

Joan, for example, decided not to take hormone replacement therapy. She believed that she was at low risk for cardiovascular disease and osteoporosis. Joan benefited from a nonmedical approach to dealing with her hot flashes. She began to wear layers of cotton clothing— and learned paced-breathing exercises. She also reported that taking 400 units of vitamin E was helpful to her. She carried a small fan with her, and soon began to feel better. Joan, a creative woman all the way, decided that she would just get up when she experienced night sweats and do some painting at that time. Joan was fortunate in that she did not have a structured job during the day and could nap when she chose to do so.

Too many other women, like Rose, suffer in silence. They approach their symptoms and sometimes their lives with a quiet sadness. They view menopausal symptoms and even depression as something to live through. We believe that women need to know all their options, from HRT to nonmedical approaches to alleviate hot flashes. They also need to know the different approaches to treating depression. These choices can improve physical and psychological functioning and help women gain control of their lives.

PSYCHOLOGICAL CHANGES

We have seen that many of the psychological changes are positive. Women who tend toward depression, however, often have problems with self-esteem. Self-esteem is defined as the general feeling of worth and importance, separate from the present situation. Thus self-esteem is something we each carry within us as individuals. Although much has been written about self-esteem and depression in general, less attention has been paid to how women specifically define our self-esteem. We still psychologically *organize* our lives around family and relationship issues. Alexandra Kaplan and others at the Stone Center at Wellesley College have developed new literature looking at women's psychological development. These scholars suggest that the best way to understand women's adult development is through a *self-in-relationship model*. Unlike models of male development, a female model of development postulates that women define themselves *primarily* through relationships with others—family members, friends, lovers, children. Thus, any attempt to understand women's development, and especially depression, must place relationship issues at the *center* (Kaplan, 1986).

One of our patients, Rebecca, was a fifty-year-old woman who came to see us because of a difficult divorce. Rebecca's divorce had been traumatic; she discovered that her husband had been in an extramarital affair for many years. She had raised her fifteen-year-old daughter essentially alone because her husband had always traveled extensively on business. However, during the divorce, her husband suddenly filed for sole custody, and therefore suggested that he should keep the family home. When this strategy failed, he filed for bankruptcy during the divorce itself, only to reemerge two years later doing quite well. Rebecca, however, took on private tutoring in addition to her teaching, and managed to provide well for herself and her daughter, although they had a modest lifestyle.

Rebecca had always worked as a reading specialist in a school and was very invested in her career. Nevertheless, she always felt that it was not very worthwhile, because she made so much less money than did her financially successful husband. Rebecca's family history only bolstered her view that a woman's importance was related to her marriage alone. Her father was also a successful businessman and was devoted to her mother. Her mother, however, was very protective of her father and insisted that Rebecca and her younger sister be extremely quiet when their father was around so they wouldn't bother him. She painted an image of two little girls playing in their room with dolls while the mother and father talked quietly over cocktails in the living room. Thus, "being quiet and dutiful" was an important part of Rebecca's self-esteem. We also discovered through our work together that Rebecca's mother had abused alcohol for many years and essentially had anesthetized herself into a quiet and subservient position. After a course of psychotherapy, it became clear to Rebecca that she would live through her traumatic divorce.

SOCIAL CHANGES

In the past, most of the writing about menopause emphasized one sociological factor labeled, "the empty-nest syndrome." The empty-nest syndrome was defined as women feeling sad and a sense of loss when their children moved out of the home. Although the empty nest has received a tremendous amount of attention, it may or may not affect menopausal women. This becomes clear when we trace the history of the use of the term "empty-nest syndrome."

The "empty-nest syndrome" was first used in a study in 1966 in the *American Journal of Psychiatry* (Deykin, 1966). The study, rather than examining large numbers of women in American society, looked at eleven women in a psychiatric hospital in Boston, who were suffering from major depressive episodes. Among these eleven women, nine were found to have had conflicted relationships with their adult children (Deykin, 1966, p. 1422). Hence the empty-nest syndrome was hatched! There are several problems with this simplistic analysis. One of the most destructive effects of the popularization of psychology is that frequently people generalize from a very small group to a large group. The very fact that these women were hospitalized sets them apart from the majority of women at midlife, and yet the empty nest has been generalized as a syndrome for most midlife women. If they had examined a more representative group of women in midlife who had children, they would have found that these women may or may not have had primarily sad feelings about their children moving out. We discuss this more in Chapter Eight, "Realities of Stress." Whether or not the empty-nest syndrome exists, it certainly would not affect all women at menopause. Some women bear children in their early twenties, and their children have been out of the home for ten years before they reach menopause. Other women have teenagers still at home. The empty-nest syndrome serves as an example of how all midlife women have been lumped together in one handy waste-basket category.

Another problem with emphasis on the empty-nest syndrome is that women now work outside of the home in record numbers. Our sources of satisfaction are not as restricted as they once were. One study found, not surprisingly, that the lowest rates of depression occurred in women who were both employed and had low employment strain as well as low strain in their marriage. Conversely, the highest level of depression occurred in women who had only one source of gratification, that is women who were not employed outside of the home and who were also experiencing a high level of stress in their marriage (Aneshensel, 1986).

RACIAL ISSUES

Minority women have higher rates of depression too, with one study finding that African-American women had 42 percent higher rates of depression than white women (Russo and Olmedo, 1983). Latin women and Asian-American women also suffer from depression more than men (Loo, 1988). Native American women have rates of suicide twice as high as other American women, and their rate of death from alcoholism is six times as high. Most importantly, their rate of treatment for these problems is lower than that of other groups (U.S. Department, 1988). This is undoubtedly a result of less access to mental health services. These increased rates do not surprise us because depression in menopausal women has been linked to multiple sources of worry, and being a member of a minority group can add another level of concerns, from discrimination to harassment.

A related sociological issue for depression is that of poverty. The economic struggles for women in the 1980s worsened the situation dramatically. Most people on welfare in the United States are mothers and their children. Many of them receive virtually no financial support for these children from the fathers. The skyrocketing divorce rate has also left additional women in a state of poverty, creating a new term, "the feminization of poverty." Others have pointed out that many women are just "one divorce away from poverty." In addition, many married women have husbands who have been either laid off from their jobs, or whose financial situation did not develop as the family had hoped. These economic losses become an additional reason for some women to work outside of the home. And remember, women still suffer from unequal pay for equal work. It is clear that poverty and its associated stress is a risk factor for depression as well as numerous other mental health problems. For any woman, menopausal or not, these economic stresses can precipitate depressions.

The severity of pain from relationships can also be seen in the divorce rate of 40 to 50 percent of all American marriages; and divorce during midlife can be a powerful trigger for depression. Pressures relating to extramarital affairs, as in the case of Rebecca, are common when divorce occurs during the menopausal years. The breakup of a long-term relationship may be particularly threatening to a woman struggling with issues of aging and a heightened awareness of potential loss. For many midlife women like Rebecca, betrayal comes as a sudden and traumatic shock, profoundly threatening self-esteem.

The Massachusetts Women's Health Study documents that these social changes at midlife are powerful among women who do become depressed. There was an association between depression and *multiple sources of worry*. Another important factor was the actual number of people who were worrying the depressed woman. Women who were worried about someone, usually a member of their family, were *three times* more likely to be depressed than other women. They were usually concerned about issues involving their husband, partner or children (McKinlay and others, 1987b).

The authors also revealed that women who had less than a high school education and who were widowed, separated or divorced had a rate of depression approaching 23 percent, more than twice the rate of depression in all other categories (McKinlay and others, 1987). This finding underscores two important issues. First, women need strong relationships in their lives. Women who are widowed, separated or divorced may be lacking that relationship, as are women like Rebecca who are struggling in a difficult marriage. Education is also an important factor in women's well-being. Women with less than a high school education are most likely to suffer from the effects of poverty and job discrimination. The low rate of depression among women who had never been married has been consistently reported in literature on depression in women (so much for the old-maid myth).

In summary, there are multiple biological, psychological and sociological changes that affect women during the menopausal years. Much evidence suggests that effects of the psychological and sociological changes at midlife are in fact stronger than the biological changes alone that are associated with menopause. That still leaves us with menopausal women suffering from a depression rate of between 5 and 10 percent. We need to concern ourselves with the complicated assessment and treatment issues.

❦ TREATMENT FOR DEPRESSION

The most important thing to remember about the treatment of depression is that there is a variety of effective treatments available to you. First, if you look at the tables on depression, and find that you are suffering from dysthymia or a major depressive episode, you should seek psychological treatment. There are many types of qualified mental health professionals. The most important issue is that the person be experienced in treating depressed women. Depression is usually depression, and responds to specific types of psychotherapy, as we will describe shortly. Many other women choose to go to their primary care clinicians, who may be a family practitioner, general internist, gynecologist, or nurse practitioner to be diagnosed. Any woman seeking medical advice regarding depression needs to be as explicit as possible. For example, if there is a family member who has been depressed, your primary care clinician should know about it. Also, if there are problems in your marriage or relationship, that is significant information, not a cause for shame. Alcohol consumption, prescription and over-the-counter medications that you might be taking also need to be discussed.

Many drugs are commonly associated with depressive symptoms. The most common culprits are alcohol, benzodiazepines like Valium and Xanax, drugs used to treat hypertension and oral contraceptives. So, if you take any of these medications and you are depressed, you should discuss the situation with your physician.

Some women become depressed after starting HRT. It is the progesterone, not estrogen, that is the problem. If you have had previous problems with depression in response to oral contraceptives, you should inform your physician when trying to make a decision about hormone replacement therapy. The hormones used in earlier forms of birth control pills were at significantly higher doses than those used today in hormone replacement therapy. In addition, our situation at menopause leaves us in a state of estrogen deficiency. In other words, before menopause we were adding hormones to hormones when using birth control pills. During menopause, we are lacking in estrogen, so the body's response is different. Nonetheless, a previous depressive episode in association with oral contraceptive use should be discussed with a physician in order to provide the best care.

At Women's Health Associates, we work as a team in order to provide a comprehensive assessment of a patient's problem. Many women can clearly identify their depression and can pinpoint a psychosocial factor that is responsible for the depression. It is always important to be as thorough in diagnosis as possible. We have found, from time to time, that a woman who presents with depression actually has hypothyroidism (an underactive thyroid gland) or another medical problem. Similarly, some women go to their physicians for problems such as chronic back pain or headaches, and turn out to have depression associated with marital or other family or relationship problems. The overlap and interaction between medical and psychological problems is complicated. Research indicates that somewhere between 30 to 50 percent of depressions are misdiagnosed (Goldberg, 1988). At the same time, as we have reviewed, sometimes depression may be a part of a medical condition. We find that we present the biopsychosocial model to a woman and she can understand that there are numerous approaches to her depression, just as their are numerous factors causing the depression.

DEPRESSION VERSUS EXHAUSTION?

Many of our patients are working outside of the home, as well as bearing the largest share of the burden of household duties and remaining responsibilities for teens or adult children. It is for these women that we evaluate the difference between exhaustion and clinical depression. A recent national panel on sleep disorder reiterated that most Americans require seven to eight hours of sleep per night. However, most Americans do not get this much sleep. We have found that for many of our patients, giving up sleep is one of their first strategies for coping with an inordinately stressful and busy schedule. We have our patients fill out diaries tracking the amount of sleep they get, the intake of caffeine and sugar, and the amount of individual exercise. Here is Rebecca's schedule, before her divorce.

6:00 a.m.	Wake up, shower and get dressed
6:45 a.m.	Tidy up the house

7:15 a.m.	See that daughter is awake
7:30 a.m.	Prepare breakfast for family
8:00 a.m.	Phone call to mother
8:30 to 5:00 p.m.	Work
5:30 to 6:00 p.m.	Pick up daughter from sports, pick up groceries, return home
6:00 to 6:30 p.m.	Make dinner
6:30 to 6:45 p.m.	Eat dinner
6:45 to 7:30 p.m.	Clean up dishes, kitchen
7:30 to 8:30 p.m.	Call family members, regarding mother
8:30 to 9:30 p.m.	Tidy up the house
9:30 to 10:00 p.m.	Try to talk to daughter
10:00 to 10:05 p.m.	Talk to husband when he comes home
10:30 to 11:00 p.m.	Exhausted, both physically and mentally, attempt to read or engage in some form of personal relaxation
11:00 p.m.	Go to bed

If this hectic schedule looks familiar to you, you may be living the *Second Shift*, a term created by author Arlie Hochschild (Hochschild, 1989) for women who are employed and work one shift at work and another at home. We are never surprised that a woman with such a schedule might consume large amounts of caffeine and sugar to keep going during the day, or consume alcohol or be tempted by Valium or other drugs to relax at night. You might try filling out a daily diary to see how your own schedule measures up. Given these stresses, food and alcohol are two substances that women often use to help them get by.

THE DIETING DEPRESSION

With so many women dieting, the associated depression is understandable. It is clear that women's reactions to dieting are significant and may include irritability, anxiety and depression (Stunkard and Rush, 1974). Since women have been socialized from an early age to see food as nurturing and as something for which we are responsible, food has a primary role in women's lives. In addition, many women we see who are under severe stress use food, particularly simple sugars and carbohydrates, to feel better quickly. Indeed, the ingestion of sugar and carbohydrates can lead to a dramatic increase in blood sugar, which can make a woman feel much better. This is only temporary, because just as the blood sugar rises quickly, it drops quickly, precipitating symptoms of shakiness, fatigue, hunger and creating a vicious cycle. In this situation, dieting can be associated with feelings of deprivation and loss, which can in turn lead to sadness and chronic irritability. Chronic dieters are hyper-responsive to anxiety and other emotions (Polivy and Herman, 1985). Although a full-blown clinical depression, or major depressive episode, is not a typical response to dieting, such feelings of chronic sadness and irritability are quite common in women who are dieting. In this situation, we often find it helpful to adjust a woman's nutritional regimen by working with a nutritionist to move away from dieting as a lifestyle. We emphasize the positive role of exercise and a low-fat, not necessarily low-calorie diet.

ALCOHOL AND DEPRESSION

Many women turn to alcohol to reduce stress. In our practice, we've seen many women who use alcohol to treat their own sleep disturbances—one of the classic signs of anxiety or depression. This provides only short-term relief. In small amounts, alcohol does work as a sedative, but over time, consistent and heavy use can cause or worsen sleep problems. Alcohol and depression in women need to be evaluated. Dr. Barbara McCrady, Professor of Psychology and Clinical Director of the Center of Alcohol Studies at Rutgers University, suggests that 25 percent of alcoholic women have suffered from depression. A woman who abuses alcohol may find her depressive moods are worsened by the guilt and shame she feels about drinking (Tamerin and others, 1976). Dr. McCrady adds that after a month period of abstinence, if a woman is still depressed, or if it is clear that depression preceded alcohol abuse, then the depression should be treated (McCrady, 1988).

We work with women who have numerous responsibilities and stressors to try to help identify a part of their day during which they can reserve quality time for themselves. Even a half hour of quiet isolation, reading a book or taking a walk with a friend, can make all the difference. It is clear that women continue to provide the bulk of household work, as well as family obligations. This is true for most societies, despite the fact that women have continued to enter and stay in the workforce in record numbers.

✦ PSYCHOTHERAPY

Whether a woman is experiencing an adjustment problem, dysthymia or a major depression, as we discussed earlier, the most important thing to remember is that psychotherapy can usually provide effective and rapid treatment.

Psychotherapy is a structured process that is aimed at alleviating psychological pain. Most psychotherapy involves individual weekly sessions that are approximately forty-five to fifty minutes long. Psychotherapy is extremely effective in treating depression and is usually covered to some extent by health insurance.

There are many ways to find a good psychotherapist: The first step is to collect some names of qualified mental health professionals. A psychotherapist who specializes in treating depression is preferable. You will be surprised how many people have had contact with mental health professionals. Friends and relatives and members of the clergy can often give you referrals and may even be able to share with you a personal experience of psychotherapy. Usually, psychotherapists do not see *best* friends or close relatives of their present patients, but in that case, your friend's psychotherapist can recommend someone else.

Your family physician or health care provider may be another good resource and usually is familiar with qualified mental health professionals in your area. Remember to be clear if you ask them for a referral, and specify that you are interested in "psychotherapy." Some physicians hear a request for relief as a request for medication. Medication may not be necessary, and in fact could be counterproductive for some.

After getting names of good psychotherapists, you should make sure that person is a licensed health care professional. This is important in providing you with well-trained professionals, but also is often used by insurance companies in deciding whether your psychotherapy will be reimbursed. In addition, each state has a Board of Health that licenses health care providers, including psychiatrists, psychologists, social workers and psychiatric nurses. If there have been documented ethical complaints about a provider, the Board of Health often has that information. There is a pamphlet available, "Choosing a Psychotherapist," from the American Psychological Association, listed in the resource section of our book.

If you are seeking psychotherapy and you are a member of a minority group, it is often helpful to find a therapist from a similar background. Many women prefer to see a female psychotherapist. If that is not possible, however, it is often possible that a sensitive therapist of any background or gender can be helpful. Some of the best therapists we know take an approach that they will learn about the cultural differences from their patients, while being able to provide their own knowledge about treatment of depression.

Once you have found a psychotherapist, the next step is the initial consultation. During the first consultation it is very common to spend most of the time talking about symptoms and life issues. These life issues may involve your partner, parents and children, as well as recent life experiences. You should try to reveal any history of sexual abuse, physical abuse or neglect, and alcohol and drug abuse so that your therapist can be helpful to you. It is essential to discuss any suicidal thoughts or feelings that you may be having. Toward the end of the session, it is quite appropriate for you to ask the psychotherapist what they think will be helpful to you. If you are not comfortable with either the psychotherapist or the treatment plan, there is no reason to schedule a second session without at least getting a consultation from another psychotherapist. It is very common in psychotherapy for people to schedule first appointments, but to later decide that they would work better with another mental health professional. You should not feel nervous about changing if you find another psychotherapist with whom you feel more comfortable.

You will probably be apprehensive about your first consultation and that is okay. Once, years ago, Dr. Landau had an office in a building that housed several other psychotherapists as well. She was scheduled to see a new client. At the appointed hour, she went out to the waiting room and said, "Ms. Joanne Jones?" A woman in the waiting area answered, and Dr. Landau then introduced herself. The interview proceeded, but after several minutes, the woman's story did not sound like the one Dr. Landau remembered from their earlier phone conversation: Ever the astute clinician, Dr. Landau interrupted, "Excuse me, are you Joanne Jones?"

The anxious client responded, "No, but I'm so nervous I would have said 'yes' to anything!"

After showing her upstairs to another psychologist's office, Dr. Landau went back out into the waiting room—then fifteen minutes late—to find a mildly irritated but equally anxious Joanne Jones!

Whatever form of health insurance you may have, it usually includes some psychotherapy as part of the benefit package. We hope that ample mental health services with freedom of choice will be provided in any new health care reforms and that all Americans will have health insurance. If you have no health insurance, psychotherapy can be expensive, with hourly fees anywhere from $50 to over $100 per session. However, everyone can go to a local community mental health center. You may not be seen weekly on a long-term basis, but crisis intervention is usually available. In addition, there are agencies funded by religious groups and by the United Way, like Family Service Agencies, that also provide counseling and psychotherapy at an affordable cost. If you are not familiar with your local community mental health center, you can also contact the local branch of your National Association for Mental Health.

The types of psychotherapy that are most effective for depression have several factors in common. They focus on providing a depressed woman with alternatives to her feelings of hopelessness. In addition, most of these programs involve an active psychotherapist and are quite structured. Some psychotherapists tend to listen and reflect back to the client as the major treatment technique. This technique alone is not usually helpful when dealing with depression. After one or two sessions of gathering information, you should expect the psychotherapist to be interactive and focus on change. One of the best guides to one form of psychotherapy is Dr. David Burns' *Feeling Good, The New Mood Therapy.* This book, described in resources, details cognitive behavior therapy, which focuses on specific short-term goals and negative-thinking patterns that can both lead to depression and keep a woman depressed (Burns, 1980).

Other forms of individual psychotherapy that have proven to be effective with depressed woman are interpersonal psychotherapy, behavior therapy and feminist psychotherapy. If you want more detail about these forms of psychotherapy, the American Psychological Association publishes *Women and Depression: Risk Factors and Treatment Issues.* This book, edited by a group of eminent women psychologists, is the most up to date review of treatments for depression as they apply to women (McGrath and others, 1990).

If your problem is primarily marital (and most women know when this is the case), then you can consider marital therapy. An unhappy marriage can certainly either precipitate or worsen a depression. As women, we all too often accept most of the responsibility for a problematic relationship. By participating in long-term individual psychotherapy without addressing the problems of the marriage, it is clear that a woman will suffer unnecessarily. At times, women are so depressed and unable to function, that they are not able to address the marital problems right away. In that case, a course of individual psychotherapy, followed by marital psychotherapy, may well be beneficial.

✦ ANTIDEPRESSANT MEDICATION

Antidepressant medication can often be used to treat depression. Medication is best used in combination with psychotherapy. This has been supported by the work of many researchers. You are most likely to respond well to a medication when you have the symptoms of a major depression that we outlined earlier—if your depression is severe, if you have a family history of depression, or if you have responded well to medication in the past (Burns, 1980).

It is important not to see treatment for depression as either/or. Some people are unable to engage in psychotherapy without some medication to treat the biological symptoms such as sleep disturbance or weight loss. Many psychotherapists will see a woman individually for eight weeks before recommending medication. If you see a psychiatrist, she or he can prescribe antidepressant medication. Otherwise, your psychotherapist often works with a consulting psychiatrist. In some situations, your primary care physician may be comfortable prescribing an antidepressant medication. In both cases, it is important for your physician to remain in contact with your psychotherapist to provide the best coordinated health care.

There are dozens of different medications for depression. The first generation of antidepressants was the group of tricyclic antidepressants, so named because of their chemical structure. They had the advantage of being able to treat depression effectively and they are not expensive. The best way to take a tricyclic medication is to start with a small dose and work up to a larger dose as necessary. Many women report that they have taken tricyclics such as amitriptyline (Elavil) in the past, but that they had no positive response. In that case it is helpful for you to remember the highest dosage ever taken and the duration it was taken, because many women have been prescribed an inadequate amount for an inadequate time.

The medication receiving the most recent attention is fluoxetine, or Prozac. In a matter of two years, Prozac went from being newly introduced to the market to being the most frequently prescribed antidepressant medication in the country. One of the reasons that Prozac is so popular is that it is quite effective. In addition, it does not have some of the common side effects of the tricyclic antidepressants, including dry mouth, constipation, bladder problems and dizziness. In some cases, women feel agitated on Prozac. Prozac does occasionally have a side effect of making a person feel somewhat anxious or "hyper." Some of our patients who have had a negative reaction to Prozac describe feeling as if they have been consuming too much caffeine. If this feeling does not disappear over a matter of days, it should be discussed with your physician. Prozac has been seen as a wonder drug that not only treats women for depression but also helps them lose weight. An informal poll of the health providers at Women's Health Associates revealed that no one knew a woman who had actually lost weight on Prozac. On the other hand, none of the women treated with Prozac had gained weight, a common reaction to the tricyclic antidepressants!

There are many other types of antidepressant medications. One of the most important things to remember is that with modern medicine, if you are suffering from a severe depression, the combination of psychotherapy and medication can be extremely effective. It is important not to quit if either one or both of these attempts should fail the first time. You must not give up hope. With the wide range of psychotherapies and psychotherapists available, you should be able to get relief from depression. Other long-term problems may well take longer to change, but you can get relatively quick relief from your serious symptoms of depression within a matter of ten to twelve weeks.

✦ WHAT NOT TO DO WHEN YOU ARE DEPRESSED

The tragedy is that many women do nothing when they are suffering from depression. Most psychological problems are treated by primary care physicians, not mental health professionals, if they are treated at all. We as women are often more comfortable getting help for others than for ourselves. Reaching out for support from other women and from a mental health professional are the most effective steps you can take.

Just as there are social factors that might cause depression, so can social factors alleviate depression. One of the most important things to fight, especially at the beginning of the depressive episode, is a tendency toward isolation. If you feel depressed, *do not remain isolated and brood*. Depression can make you feel so bad that you don't feel you are even worthy of other people's time. Do not cut yourself off from friends and family. Doing so will not help you "sort things out," it will make you feel worse. Many women are particularly reticent about revealing their problems, because the problem often involves their husbands. They worry about betrayal, or their husbands have told them explicitly not to confide in anyone. This is not acceptable. You can find a trustworthy friend, family member, member of the clergy or doctor who may be helpful. Also, these resources can recommend a psychotherapist, if you decide to see one. On the other hand, if you can get over your initial lethargy and tendency toward being alone, talking with a close friend can be one of the most important outlets for depression. A study by Drs. Brown and Harris in Great Britain found that the presence of a close and confiding intimate person in a woman's life could protect her from depression when she would otherwise be likely to succumb (Brown and others, 1986).

Do not self-medicate with alcohol and other drugs. As we discussed before, many women try to treat themselves for fatigue by using large quantities of sugar and caffeine during the day. At night they may relax with a glass or two of wine, or perhaps a prescribed tranquilizer. These are dangerous habits and once started are very difficult to terminate. The studies on alcohol we discuss further in Chapter Eight reveal that even two drinks of alcohol per day can lead to medical problems in women (Tuyns and Pequinot, 1984). Alcohol may relax you and help you sleep—at first. However, after four hours or so, you will awaken because alcohol causes a sleep disturbance. Alcohol worsens depression, and you will be gaining another problem.

Xanax, a benzodiazepine, was first introduced as a wonder drug, able to treat both anxiety and depression. Over the long run, it has proven to be addictive. We have seen many women suffer tremendously from Xanax withdrawal. Valium, Librium and Ativan are also tranquilizers that should be used cautiously to treat anxiety, not depression.

An intriguing review article by Susan Nolen-Hoeksema of Stanford University helps us understand the isolation of depression when she links social and psychological factors. She suggests that when women begin to feel depressed, we turn inward, and by taking responsibility for relationships, often blame ourselves. Men, on the other hand, may tend to turn outward more, that is become involved with sports and other hobbies and distract themselves. Thus, they may have better ways of coping with depression than do women (Nolen-Hoeksema, 1987). Our work suggests that the female tendency toward analyzing relationships, combined with little power to create change in those relationships, can lead to feelings of helplessness and depression. These two separate styles of possible coping mechanisms for depression put women and men at cross purposes and relationship stress can follow.

Susan Nolen-Hoeksema's work suggests that men, who distract themselves by exercising or playing sports, may have a good idea here (Nolen-Hoeksema, 1987). *Do not remain sedentary if you are depressed.* Of course, if your sleep pattern has been disruptive, it is hard to maintain even your normal activities, and indeed this is one of the signs of depression. Some studies on running found that the release of endorphins was helpful in coping with depression. However, to the extent that you can control your behavior, the possibility of increased activity can be extremely successful. If you are like some of us and have never managed to experience this "runner's high," don't worry, try something else like walking, a dance class, basketball, or rollerblading. We discuss exercise in our chapter on health promotion, Chapter Ten.

We will leave you with one thought about treatment for depression—if you are feeling depressed, get some help and fight against the tendency to remain alone! Don't become one of all too many women who fail to receive help even though it is there.

✦ COMMUNICATION WITH YOUR HEALTH PROFESSIONAL

It is important to be as detailed as possible in talking with your physician. Your symptoms of depression may be elicited by your health professional. It is important to be as direct as possible about other issues. Some of the issues patients often have difficulty talking about include: sexual abuse, eating disorders, early childhood neglect and abuse, drug or alcohol abuse, sexual problems in a relationship, homosexuality and domestic violence. This information can provoke shame, and many people are reluctant to disclose it. The physician or other health care professional who is trying to assess your situation and make appropriate recommendations needs to know any permanent history.

You are most likely to get the best treatment if you are direct and open with your physician or health care provider. However, physicians are human, often make mistakes and may not be as sensitive as we would like them to be. For example, suppose you have been waiting for your physician for over a half hour. He or she comes into the examining room and in a hurried fashion, apologizes, and looks preoccupied. You try to bring up your issue of depression but you feel "brushed off" or minimized. It is important for you to be as direct as possible and to state, "I'm concerned that I've been depressed." Sometimes physicians in their attempt to be supportive, minimize problems. If this is the case, it is important to state again, ". . . but I know I'm having a problem here, and I think I could use a referral to a psychotherapist."

If after one or two attempts you feel that you are not being heard, you have several choices. First, you can try to make an appointment for another day, assuming that your physician may have had a couple of unusually busy days. Or, you could try to talk to your physician on the phone. If these approaches do not work, you could consider changing physicians. Some physicians are only comfortable in the biological sphere and are less comfortable in the psychosocial sphere. In that case, you might want to continue to work with your provider, but use other resources for obtaining psychological care.

✦ COMMUNICATION WITH YOUR FAMILY

We define family as people who are committed to one another, who love one another and who may or may not live together. A depressed member of a family can have a powerful negative effect on the family system. At the same time, an unresponsive family can increase a person's feeling of isolation, worthlessness, hopelessness and ultimately increase depression. One of the tragedies of depression is that a person feels completely isolated and this can become a self-fulfilling problem. This isolation leads to brooding, the brooding leads to further isolation, family members often become alienated from one another and the situation deteriorates. When we see a depressed person, we often have her family member join us for at least one visit. This helps us assess the situation and often helps to attempt to make changes in the family patterns.

Some of the simple strategies we use involve creating a situation where each member of the family can try to state clearly how they feel in the other's presence. In many marriages, or relationships of a long duration, the partners have stopped listening to one another or stopped talking. One of the most important and basic parts of communication is that of empathy, that is, not just stating you are sorry, but trying to actually understand how the other person feels, "putting yourself in their shoes." We recommend that a person try to respond with their feelings and not with judgments. Similarly, we encourage direct rather than indirect statements.

Using strategies based on the work of Deborah Tannen and others, we find that it is important for one spouse to be able to tell the other *exactly* what she needs. For example, many women want to have that empathic connection just to be heard and for their husband to understand them, rather than a quick solution. Many men, on the other hand, who are used to "report talk" as opposed to "rapport talk," try to solve the problem, by giving their wife a suggestion rather than an empathic connection (Tannen, 1990).

It is important to remember the children in a family suffering from depression. If a woman is feeling sad and hopeless, and continues to have the major amount of responsibility for her family—her work and the welfare of her children, as well as the care of the house—it is clear that something has to give. Children, even teenagers (especially teen-agers!), are often particularly sensitive to the moods of their mother and will pick up feelings of depression. Similarly, marital problems, that are often associated with depression, will affect children very directly. If you are concerned about your children, it is important to mention your worries to your psychotherapist or health care provider in order to discuss the situation more fully.

Lesbian women have a specific set of needs with respect to depression. One of the most important problems for lesbian women is that of social isolation. When heterosexual women have problems, they may have an extended network to rely on, but some lesbian women who are closeted have fewer connections with which to explore their relationship issues. It is also clear that lesbians suffer from discrimination and prejudice. These additional factors can undoubtedly lead to increased stress. One of the few studies of lesbians, the National Lesbian Health Care Survey, found that half of the women seeking therapy saw depression as their major problem (National Institute of Mental Health, 1987). Just as with heterosexual women, involvement in a positive relationship with a partner has been related to low levels of depression in lesbian women. Similarly, the loss of a relationship is a risk factor for depression. This could be especially true for lesbians who may not be able to grieve openly and who have less social support. Communication problems are not absent from the lesbian community and in situations where the depressed person feels criticized by her partner, the patterns of isolation and hopelessness can be similarly devastating.

It is also important to explain depression to members of your family and close friends, and to remember that family members may have misinformation about depression as well. They might give you well-intentioned, but ineffective advice like "just pull yourself together and cope." Just pulling yourself together, still burdened with the same sociological, relationship and biological stressors, will only intensify your depression and make coping impossible. Communication, then, can be the first step toward obtaining support and breaking the cycle of depression.

✦ COMMUNICATING WITH FRIENDS

Studies of marriage reveal a paradox. In many marriages, a husband will be asked who his best friend is, only to reply that it is his wife. His wife, when asked the same question, will come back with the name of a woman friend. This is a generalization, but it is true for many women. In times of stress, they need to turn to someone who can share their feelings, who can help them solve problems and to whom they can feel connected. Unfortunately, in some marriages, the husband is not able, or willing, to participate in an intimate relationship to the same extent as his wife. Thus, women often turn to other women for emotional support. In other situations, a woman feels very well connected with her husband, but is in need of additional support also. It is this feeling of connectedness, as well as reciprocal problem solving, that can be a lifeline for many women. Many other mental health professionals have found that just helping a depressed woman reach out and develop new friendships is a powerful tool. Not only does it allow feelings of social support, but a woman may gain independence from her family and begin to feel more competent and effective outside of the home. In addition, she may get another perspective from someone who sees things in a slightly different fashion. Finally, this feeling of connectedness has the added benefit of increased social activity, as usually the women will begin to do things together—from walking to going to concerts, dropping by just to say hello and so on. Generations of women at home have found this connection through the coffee-klatsch of the 1950s, to the support groups or "networking" of the 1990s.

For many women suffering from poverty and discrimination, it is their connection with friends, usually other women and family members, that has gotten them through difficult times. Many single mothers develop cooperative relationships with other mothers in order to help provide emotionally for their children and for themselves. Women working outside of the home often find that if they have just one female colleague in their department or office, they can accomplish a lot of problem solving and benefit from mutual moral support. On numerous occasions, one of our colleagues has come into the conference room and closed the door quietly only to throw up her hands and say, "You won't believe what just happened!" This sharing of problems is not "male bashing," but a more general sharing of feelings and the difficulties in any particular job situation. This is particularly important in male-dominated settings, like medicine or architecture, or in settings where there are many women, such as libraries or schools that are populated by women but usually controlled by men.

We know that sharing your feelings of depression can often be difficult. Similarly, the process of psychotherapy is frightening to some. But if you break the cycle of secrecy and isolation, you can connect with friends and family or a psychotherapist, and you can recover from depression.

Psychotherapy can be difficult, but it can also change your life.

Rebecca's psychotherapy continued for several years. After some individual work, we referred her to a women's group and she came to see us less often. We have watched as she no longer defines herself as a failure and has grown more assertive, self-confident and comfortable with many newly discovered aspects of her personality. Just recently, during an individual session, she shared her feelings about her mother's recent death. Rebecca had cleaned out the family home, sorting through furniture, clothing and boxes. During this session, Rebecca brought out two photographs of her mother that she had found while cleaning. One was of her mother stepping out of a car on her wedding day. In this image, her mother appeared elegant, surrounded by onlookers, as she approached the church where the ceremony would take place. On her face, though, was an expression of profound sadness and fear. "But look at this," Rebecca added, and handed us the second picture.

The second photograph was of her mother during her high school years, participating in the long-jump during a track meet. Rebecca handled this snapshot very carefully, as if she were holding on to something precious. Even in the slightly faded black-and-white image, her mother's strong arms and legs, stretching out as she soared, offered the viewer a clear picture of her energetic joy. Rebecca, now at the age of fifty-five, is reclaiming her mother's spirit.

RESOURCES

In addition to communicating with your health care professional, family and friends about depression, there are numerous pamphlets available from a variety of mental health associations. For example, "Choosing a Therapist Who Is Right for You" is available from the American Psychological Association. The APA also publishes an excellent short book, *Women and Depression: Risk Factors and Treatment Issues*. The National Institute of Mental Health publishes a pamphlet on depression as does the National Association for Mental Health.

Reading many of these brochures can help you understand in greater depth both the nature of your depression and the resources available to you.

BOOKS

When Feeling Bad Is Good by Ellen McGrath, Ph.D. (New York: Henry Holt & Company, 1992). Dr. McGrath's *When Feeling Bad Is Good* is a great contribution to the field of self-help for depression. She is one of the psychologists who edited the American Psychological Association's Task Force on Depression. Her book is thorough and inclusive and deals with many women's issues directly.

Harriet Lerner's *The Dance of Anger, The Dance of Intimacy* and *The Dance of Deception* are transforming books. Many psychoanalytic, or psychodynamic, theorists believe that depression is anger turned inward. Although that is a somewhat simplistic assessment, it is clear that for women in particular, expressing feelings of anger directly is often not possible. Thus, sometimes we can become overwhelmed with feelings of hopelessness and inability to be effective. At other times we might be indirect in our anger. Dr. Lerner's books not only analyze these patterns but provide hopeful strategies for changing these behaviors.

ASSOCIATIONS

American Psychological Association
750 1st Street, NE
Washington, DC 20002-4242
(202) 336-5500

The APA publishes a short book, Women and Depression: Risk Factors and Treatment Issues, *which is available through their order department, as is a listing of their other publications, including pamphlets, books and journals. They also publish a pamphlet "Choosing a Psychotherapist." For referrals to psychologists, call your state psychological association.*

American Association for Marital and Family Therapists (AAMFT)
1100 17th St., NW, 10th Floor
Washington, DC 20036
(800) 374-2638

The AAMFT can provide you with a list of certified marital or family therapists in your area.

FEDERAL GOVERNMENT

National Institute of Mental Health
5600 Fishers Lane
Rockville, MD 20857
(301) 443-4513

NIMH publishes a number of free brochures on various mental health issues, including many on depression, in English and Spanish, as well as a listing of available books and pamphlets. They sponsor The Depression Awareness, Recognition, and Treatment (D/ART) Program, educating physicians and the public about depressive illness through educational materials and community outreach.

National Mental Health Association
Information Center
1021 Prince St.
Alexandria, VA 22314-2971
(703) 684-7722 or (800) 969-6642

Association with national affiliates that give information, referrals, and support concerning mental health issues. They have more than forty educational publications and a newsletter.

CHAPTER EIGHT

The Realities of Stress

LET'S FACE IT: YOU DON'T HAVE TO BE MENOPAUSAL TO KNOW STRESS. Much of the fuss about the stress during menopausal years has been exaggerated. Our approach is different. We know that there are some major transitions that occur during the menopausal years. But these transitions and changes are not crises. Moreover, solutions to stress can be quite pleasurable. For many women, midlife can be a time of self-discovery and fulfillment, a time to enjoy our past successes, make new plans and take more time for relaxing activities. In this chapter we will explore first the realities of the unique stresses today of menopausal women. We will outline the important connections between health and stress. By understanding the relationship between your health and personal stress, you will be better able to *enjoy* the middle years.

Each woman has a unique life plan. Some of us may be grand-mothers at menopause, others may still have children in grammar school. Some of us will be advanced in a career, others may just be starting to work outside the home. Still others may continue or resume their education. If we are not what American society has dictated as the norm—that is, white, married women and mothers—we may meet with additional pressures from society. Some of us are women of color.

Some of us are lesbian women. Some of us are single parents or widows. All of us face adjustments and changes in midlife and can face stress. But none of this suggests that the transition of menopause has to be a crisis.

Our work with menopausal women has taught us about the positive force that women can mobilize at midlife. Stress can be an opportunity for change and growth. By the time we reach the menopausal years, our experiences, such as intimate relationships, childbirth, child-rearing, work issues, as well as sexual harassment and discrimination (just to name a few), have given us the coping skills to tackle almost any challenge. Many women are unaware of the depth of their strengths and abilities. For these women, the menopausal years can serve to activate their true powers.

The next time you are feeling stressed, you might remember the experience of Lorraine Lengkeek and how she rose to the occasion. Lorraine was hiking with her husband down a trail in Glacier National Park, singing "How Great Thou Art," when her husband was attacked by a grizzly bear. Lorraine, a woman in her fifties, might well have felt stressed at this point; but Lorraine, a new menopausal heroine, fought off the bear by whacking it on the nose with her binoculars and then used her bra as a tourniquet to stop her husband's bleeding! We found this example in one of the Timex magazine advertisements, most of which we don't like because they involve stories of people being stuck on carnival rides and being inverted for a half hour at a time. But this one strikes us as a great example of a woman rising to deal with true adversity.

For most of us though, the psychological issues of midlife are certainly less dramatic than Lorraine's. Robin's story is more typical. Robin was a fifty-six-year-old woman who originally came to see us for her high blood pressure. She worked in her husband's construction business. With the declining economy of the late 1980s, she and her husband, James, were forced to sell the business. She went to work in another office but James could not find work. On January 1, 1990, when the governor of Rhode Island closed all the state savings and loans and froze all the accounts, Robin and James were left without access to their life savings. Her daughter divorced her husband and moved back home with two small children. James, still out of work, started to build a small addition to the house for the extra family but suffered a heart attack. Robin was left as the sole breadwinner of her family and spent her time worrying about finances, James, his health, her daughter, her grandchildren and the unfinished addition. We'll tell you more about Robin later.

Robin's situation of economic hardship and family worries is just one of the many possible problems of the menopausal years. The fact is that there is no one predictable pattern for women in the menopausal years. We have learned this by listening to the many different experiences of our patients. There is one thing we can expect during the menopausal years and that is change! Depending on your life plan, during this decade you may well: change jobs; see your children get married; become a grandparent; tend to the needs of elderly relatives; get a promotion. By understanding that these changes are part of the natural life process, you can use your internal and external resources to help you cope.

One study of midlife issues found that women's lives are more affected by the original choices they made with respect to their families. Women who had children when they were younger experienced a lessening of family burdens and some shifts in their outlook at midlife. On the other hand, if women had delayed childbearing, they might be grappling with some of the issues of childrearing and family concerns in their early and middle forties and might be dealing with their children's adolescence in their fifties. So these days the nest is not necessarily empty at menopause.

Many of our patients, heterosexual and lesbian, have no children and are in long-term relationships, growing old together as equal partners in life. "Reproductive versus nonreproductive life" has no meaning for them. More important dichotomies for most menopausal women include underpaid versus fairly paid, powerless versus powerful, employed versus unemployed or in a happy relationship versus in an abusive relationship.

Even the term "midlife crisis" has always been a controversial term, based more on theory rather than reality. Another problematic issue is the definition of midlife. While one writer, Elliot Jaques, suggested that age thirty-five is the beginning of the midlife crisis, others have written about people in their forties and early fifties (Jaques, 1965). Another way to look at midlife is not to use age as a marker, but rather a shift in outlook. This shift is moving away from viewing life as infinite to a focus on the time we have left.

For women, with an average life span being approximately eighty-two years, a chronological midpoint would be approximately in the early forties. If many women begin to struggle with midlife issues in their forties, by age fifty they have already made adjustments in their lives! Lynn, one of our patients, told us that at age fifty-three, "The forties were a hassle for me. My two children were coming and going, my husband was bored at work and I wanted time for *me*—to be myself, to get back to work. Now that I'm in my fifties, things have settled down. The kids moved away, my husband decided to work less and is volunteering at a vocational school and I'm teaching part-time. *Much* better!" A recent study of menopausal women reveals that women in their fifties feel better than they did in their forties. The women experienced a decrease in dependence and self-criticism, while simultaneously experiencing an increase in their self-confidence and ability to make decisions (Helson and Wink, 1992). So by the time of menopause, many women have experienced positive rather than negative changes.

✦ SYMPTOMS AS STRESSES

There are numerous biological changes that are common during midlife. The biological changes at midlife can trigger psychological issues. We have detailed the real changes that are a result of hormone changes during menopause. As we have discussed earlier, many of the biological changes are actually associated with aging and have little to do with estrogen deficiency and menopause. For example, over time our eyesight changes so that most of us need reading glasses by the time we are in our forties. Similarly, our hair begins to turn gray and we begin to develop wrinkles. All of this is true for men also. For some midlife women, the aging process is unacceptable.

Erik Erikson described the primary conflict around the biological issues as generativity versus self-absorption. Generativity is the process of transmitting values to the next generation. Erikson did not limit this to parenting or grandparenting exclusively, but included the activities of teaching and contributing to the younger generation through mentoring or other work. Erikson believed that at midlife we can lapse into self-absorption if this task of generativity is not mastered (Erikson, 1970). Preoccupation with too much attention to personal needs and possible changes in physical health can lead to brooding and turning inward. Then the biological changes can precipitate sadness and fear. On the other hand, if a midlife woman or man shifts toward generativity, an increased sense of command and contribution to society will follow. We have found that the more committed a woman is to her life, whether it's career, relationship or a political issue, the less she worries about the aging process.

Women's ability to focus on others allows us to have deeper, more intimate relationships and may lead us to be more naturally inclined toward generativity. The connectedness with family members allows our transitions at midlife to be more positive. These close relationships can serve as a counterpoint to the self-absorption that can take place at midlife. After all, the moments of closeness and intimacy, whether they come from parents, children, friends or lovers, are some of life's most meaningful. By the time we reach our menopausal years, we have become experts in relationships, and we can continue to benefit from them. Many modern psychologists place this ability to connect to others at the core of our development as women.

Self-absorption, on the other hand, begins when we try to fight the aging process. Jung noted that paying more attention to the inner world is a natural tendency during midlife. By this he meant the world of ideas and feelings, not the external physical and individual changes. Of course, a preoccupation with physical appearance is a natural tendency for women due to the intense media attention and socialization toward youthful sexuality. Although we completely understand when our patients come to us wanting a referral for cosmetic surgery, we have our doubts. Some magazine articles recommend that cosmetic eye surgery needs to begin in the early thirties. We have also seen young women who have had breast implants more than once by the time they are twenty. These women, at menopause, may be on their second, if not third generation of cosmetic surgery. All of us know the struggles we have with appearance, and few women are exempt from this worry. We also know that experimenting with appearance and makeup can be a creative activity for many women or an experience of "female bonding." Cosmetic surgery is quite different because it usually involves general anesthesia, with all of the risks of a major surgery, for the sake of delayed wrinkles. It seems that women are being exploited to see cosmetic surgery as a vehicle to permanent youthfulness.

The onset of symptoms of medical problems can also lead to anxiety. Here again, we have found that flexibility can be a woman's greatest coping strategy.

Samantha, one of our forty-five-year-old patients, had been diagnosed with multiple sclerosis ten years earlier. When the disease worsened, she did not panic. A single parent, she had raised her son alone despite tremendous financial turmoil and little support from the boy's father. Carl, her son, was off to college when Samantha was faced with her plans for her future. She quietly sold her home that had beautiful curving—but challenging—Victorian staircases. Even though she loved the aesthetics of her house, Samantha bought a new house with two apartments, had the first floor rebuilt to accommodate any possible change in her motor skills and used the second floor as an income property. She refers proudly to her recent project as, "my retirement plan." Samantha's flexibility and ability to face what her future may bring is just one dramatic example of the strengths of midlife women. Her ability to think about retirement in the face of severe illness reflected the coping skills she had developed all those years as a single parent. Certainly, Samantha faced a potential midlife crisis, but she is using her problem-solving skills and her psychological resources to face each new challenge.

Certainly coping with multiple sclerosis is a particularly difficult situation. The more common biological stressors of midlife tend to be minor, yet troubling nonetheless. These may include changes in vision, early osteoarthritis, higher blood pressure, decreased caloric needs and reduced stamina. Most women adjust to these changes well. It is important to realize that social pressures that fight against graceful aging only add stress to the menopausal woman's life. We hope that as women continue to gain positions of power in the media, in government and in health care, that the social pressures will change. There are also a number of other social and sociological issues that can create stress during this developmental phase.

Some of the symptoms of menopause, usually hot flashes, can provide additional stress to a woman who is just barely able to manage the multiple roles she must juggle. Gloria came to see us because her twenty-three-year-old son was still demanding money from his parents and was unable to make a career choice. At the same time, her elderly mother needed to enter a nursing home, and Gloria was having difficulty arranging for the appropriate level of care. When she began to have unpredictable night sweats, she couldn't sleep and she felt completely "burnt out." Gloria had always been the family's "helper," but she began to suffer from role overload, as a wife, a parent and a daughter with tremendous demands. She found the hot flashes associated with menopause to be a terrible burden. Through our team approach, we helped her find appropriate resources for her mother and short term psychotherapy in order to help her set more limits with her son. She also decided to take a short term course of hormonal replacement therapy to manage her hot flashes.

◆ SOCIAL ISSUES

THE JUGGLING ACT

Most menopausal women juggle work, family, friendship and leisure roles. At menopause, many women reevaluate the importance of these roles in their lives. Women who have functioned within a specific role for many years may decide to make changes at midlife. Juggling the different tasks within one job or role can be difficult enough and this is called "intra-role conflict." Not all changes within jobs lead to intrarole conflict, though. Some of the most pleasurable jobs allow different types of work. This protects an individual from boredom and allows for flexibility, creativity and a variety of interests. For example, Gail was a university professor who came to see us complaining of "post-tenure letdown." A quiet and diligent scholar, she had worked productively for over fifteen years, publishing a great deal of research. She had finally been promoted to full professor and had received tenure at a major university. She was now finding it difficult to concentrate and was beginning to question the validity of her previous choices that centered on research rather than on teaching. Fortunately her job was quite flexible and she was able to shift gears and devote more attention to her graduate students and undergraduates. By working with graduate students to develop their own research strategies, she became a major mentor and role model. This made her feel that she was making a contribution, within her larger career choice, but in a slightly different way.

A more common role conflict involves "inter-role conflict," that is when tensions occur between our *different* functions. Many women are so emotionally debilitated by family problems that it interferes with their work functioning. In other situations, the demands of a high-stress job leave a woman emotionally depleted and fatigued at the end of a long work day. This is particularly true for women who have careers that require tremendous amounts of responsibility without much financial reward. They are filling the "pink-collar" positions that make up the majority of the female workforce in this country. The women who hold these positions find their situation difficult to change and have an increased risk of heart disease that we discuss in Chapter Five, "Maintaining Our Health."

The plight of these stressed "pink-collar" workers is illustrated by one of our local manufacturers. This manufacturer had a large number of employees on strike, picketing daily outside the factory. Those with the signs, catchy phrases and bullhorns were not the female "pink collars" fed up with unfair treatment, but the male forklift workers who were determined to receive higher wages and an expanded benefits package. The others who deserved a pay increase and expanded benefits package remained inside the building, overworked, typing, answering the phone, correcting their boss's letters, making coffee, often doing their boss's personal chores and sundry other related tasks. These secretaries were being paid significantly less than the forklift workers. When a local resident near the factory was questioned as to why he thought the forklift workers, often with less education, were paid so much more, he responded, "They make the money for the company. Every time they lift a box to ship to a customer the company is making money." The company makes a lot of money from the secretary who processed the order, fixed the Xerox machine and produced the annual report.

The truth of the matter is that secretaries often have the very same financial responsibilities as forklift operators. Many of them are single, divorced or have husbands who are out of work, and most are struggling to make ends meet. The heavy workload these women handle on the job, combined with their barely livable salaries and numerous family responsibilities, leave them exhausted and stressed.

The multiple stresses experienced by clerical workers became clear to us recently when we met Claudette. Claudette was a fifty-five-year-old postmenopausal woman who came to us in a panic. She was referred by the Employee Assistance Program at a medical-secretarial agency, where she worked as a transcriptionist. The local business had recently merged with a larger company, and Claudette's job now required her to produce a certain number of typed lines per day. She had always been an extremely accurate typist, but was a bit slower than her colleagues. She made up for this shortcoming by helping others proofread and by working longer hours from time to time. Her new boss found this unacceptable and was quite critical of Claudette. Claudette was usually an accepting and cheerful woman who was a devout Roman Catholic; she was suffering from moderate hot flashes at night but had coped well, until recently when she felt increasingly anxious. When we first met her, her thinking was hard to follow and she was extremely tense and worried. Her blood pressure, usually a bit low, was now high, 140/102.

As a team we saw Claudette and learned the following: Claudette had untreated hyperthyroidism, which significantly increased her feelings of anxiety. In addition, she was separated from her husband, Louis, who had been laid off as a laborer in a warehouse, because of back problems. She had finally left him after thirty-three years because she "just couldn't take it anymore." They had experienced marital problems for many years, after they lost a three-year-old daughter to leukemia. Both she and her husband had been devastated by this tragedy, but Louis, always a quiet man, withdrew further and refused to get help. When she went to a pastoral counselor, Claudette became increasingly aware of her own neglected needs. This counseling relationship had restored her faith. Years earlier, when she went to her parish priest for help, he had only instructed her to pray and she became disillusioned. Over time, Louis began to drink too much, and became increasingly critical and possessive of Claudette. He questioned her every move and tried to prevent her from talking with her friends on the phone—her lifeline to support. She did not believe in divorce and she was terrified for both of them, because if she lost her job, neither of them would have health insurance.

Claudette's three children were struggling with their own families, and her youngest daughter had recently been traumatized when her husband beat her. The crisis at work had just "put [Claudette] over the edge." We helped Claudette take a short leave of absence, treated her thyroid condition, and saw her for a few sessions of psychotherapy. Claudette surprised us at how quickly she developed a more assertive manner. When we told her that we were so pleased with her quick change, Claudette reminded us that change often comes after extensive deliberation. "Getting something more for myself has been on my mind for years. You're just helping me act on these hopes. About five years ago, I realized that I don't have to be this way. I don't have to be the one to always take the overcooked part of the meat!" We met with her husband, and Claudette negotiated the conditions under which she would return home. He would have to agree to joint counseling, and she could use the telephone without his criticism. We referred Claudette and Louis to a family service agency.

We also referred Claudette's daughter to a domestic violence hotline. It would be easy to see Claudette's daughter as an unusual story, but unfortunately it is not. Many women have been battered, with an estimated 16 percent of women experiencing violence at home (Foley and Nechas, 1993). Most communities now have women's shelters and domestic-violence hotlines, so no longer do women need to suffer alone.

We also helped Claudette negotiate with her new boss, but the efforts were unsuccessful. She ultimately managed to find another job in a smaller company, where she could work at her own pace. Claudette's case is just one from our busy practice, and we know many other women who are trying to deal with inflexible jobs, problematic marriages and needy families.

THE SUPPORT GAP AND THE SANDWICH

Women are the emotional glue for most families. We serve as the support and confidantes for our friends and family members alike. Unfortunately, in some male-female relationships, this is a one-sided interaction, with women providing most of the emotional support but receiving much less. Women in relationships with men and sometimes even in relationships with other women, often suffer from a support gap, that is, they provide more support than they receive. Although many women feel connected to the men in their lives because the men confide in them, all too often there is little reciprocity. We have seen many women who go home after a long day's work to inquire about their husband's day, when the same question is never asked of them. The research on social support suggests that social support can be a major buffer to stress and can protect women from such stressful psychological conditions as depression (Brown and others, 1986). The cornerstone of social support is mutuality and expressiveness, where both partners have a meaningful relationship and commitment to one another. This is unfortunately not true for some women in their relationships with men. But, things are looking up as many men and women begin to change.

The issue of social support is also important for lesbian women. We have found that many lesbian women have strong social support networks within their relationships and within the lesbian community. However, being in a minority, they suffer additional social pressures, as well as discrimination and harassment. Women who have not "come out" often live in a certain amount of fear because of the possibility of exposure and resulting discrimination, and even losing their jobs.

The support gap often strikes women more intensely at the time of menopause, culminating in the problems of the "sandwich generation." Often, menopausal women have children who still need encouragement and support, and most women are happy to provide that support (especially if the child is now living outside the home). At the same time, women may be struggling to take care of elderly parents and in-laws. A woman in such a situation becomes "sandwiched" between the needs of the parents and children.

Gina, a recent patient of ours, is typical of the sandwich generation. Gina is a fifty-five-year-old courageous postmenopausal woman who was trying to keep her ninety-year-old mother out of a nursing home. Gina and Richard are a hardworking couple who are devoted to one another. Gina showed us many of her creative solutions to caring for her mother, who was suffering from Alzheimer's disease. She did orientation exercises with her mother, created skirts with rubber linings out of concern for her mother's incontinence, and coordinated a tremendous amount of social support for her mother. Gina was having additional difficulty comforting her newly divorced daughter, who was trying to support two children on a salary from Burger King. Like all too many women, her daughter was only receiving sporadic child-support payments of $50 a week. Gina was so sandwiched between the needs of her mother and her daughter that the main purpose of one of her office visits was to help gain access to social services from the Visiting Nurses Association for her mother and a community mental health center for her daughter.

Our staff meetings are full of descriptions of women, like Gina, who struggle to take care of their families and friends. Before the national family-leave policy, many women were forced to take time off from work to help find nursing homes for their parents or to take care of family members themselves. Although most women want to be helpful to their family, their goals are often unsupported by employment policies and by other family members. We know many women, forced to take time off from work, who find themselves punished. When they return, their responsibilities are often downgraded. Fortunately, the new federal legislation is beginning to change this situation, but many women are still perceived as not "committed to their careers" if they care for their families. Women provide the vast majority of care for the elderly. It is quite common for one sibling in a family, usually a daughter, to take on a larger proportion of the care for elderly parents, while others do very little.

THE POSITIVE SIDE OF JUGGLING

The work-home conflict, then, is a real one for many menopausal women. We should remember though, that we can all enjoy having multiple roles. Although a tremendous amount of attention has been given to the stress of work for women, there are many positive qualities of work. The majority of studies of women find that women enjoy work and enjoy the flexibility, autonomy and the independence that it offers them (Barnett and others, 1987).

Similarly, most women enjoy their children. Adjustment to midlife and the issue of adult children is often quite variable. Women have different feelings about their grown children based on many factors—how they feel as mothers, the nature of their relationships with their adult children and finally, the way the children leave home. Indeed, women have mixed feelings about the "empty nest." For many women, their children have filled the intimacy gap in their marriages. Other women raise their children alone. Still others have a solid relationship with their spouse or partner, but also have been very child-centered. The close connection with young children is emotionally exhausting but also intense and loving. Sue Miller, in her insightful novel, *For Love,* describes the change for one woman, a single mother watching her son become a man:

> "What she'd felt in recent years, though, particularly since Ryan had gone off to college, was how absolute the ending to that mother-child romance was. It astonished her, given how central it had been in her life, given how much of her emotion had been taken up by Ryan—by love for him and anger at him and sadness with him and pride in him—how suddenly gone he was. All of that world was. She'd had a sense, the last few times he'd been home for a stretch, that there was some new relationship unfolding, something that, with luck, might look finally like a friendship. But mostly what she felt was the absence in herself of the old mothering emotions. Not that she loved him less. Not that at all. But that the kind of love was different. Less consuming . . . She was, on the whole, glad for this" (Miller, 1993 p. 80).

As we have discussed in the previous chapter, this does not mean that women become clinically depressed when their children leave home. Just that life changes. Some children leave home to go to college at age eighteen and then work for a few years and either establish a career track or return to graduate school. The entire family may see this as a positive change and an accomplishment. On the other hand, children who are not college-bound must struggle with the issues of careers at an early age and their separation may be less predictable. Sometimes they can find secure and well-paid jobs, but sometimes they can't. Given the recent crises in economics in America, it can be difficult for these children to find work and the stress on the entire family multiplies; and it is often the mother who bears the major responsibility for supporting the family through these changes.

In fact, the returns to the nest or "boomerangers" account for some eleven million young men and women in their twenties who try to leave home and then decide to come back. Although 34 percent of them are students, others are single people with full- or part-time jobs or are unemployed. One of the issues here is delayed marriage. The median age of marriage is at present twenty-six years for men and twenty-four years for women, a full four years later than the same statistics of the 1960s (Quinn, 1993). So, actually, many menopausal women are still helping their boomerang children.

❧ CRISES OF MIDLIFE

DEATH OF A SPOUSE

Conflicts at work and home can usually be managed. Most women overcome their anxieties about midlife and enjoy aging. The normal psychology and stresses of midlife are usually a series of small changes and most women do not find them to be particularly traumatic. Yet, there are some crises at midlife that can be traumatic and difficult. One such crisis is the death of a spouse or partner. Since women tend to marry older men, widowhood is something that many women begin to confront during the menopausal years. For women who become widowed, they often lose instrumental support, that is help with their pragmatic details of life, as well as emotional support. For many women, they also lose the social structure of couples that have held their social life together. The phases of grief and loss include numbness, yearning, protest, despair and recovery (Kübler-Ross, 1982). Although all women do not experience the stages in that order, they do tend to be common in the grieving process. Pathological grief that does not resolve after a couple of years can often turn into a midlife depression, and depression can be successfully treated with the proper combination of assessment and psychotherapy. We describe this in detail in Chapter Seven.

Gladys, the women you met in our first chapter, lost her husband to a heart attack three years after we first met. Even though Gladys had a good job and a supportive extended family, she went through a difficult time, financially and psychologically. About eighteen months after her husband died, she told us, "I guess I know I can get by now, but it's still hard, every single day."

There are now numerous support groups for widows that we have detailed in our section on resources. The social support provided by other women can help in coping with the feelings of loss and detachment. Support groups can be very beneficial in providing practical issues also. Women tend to share resources and problem-solving strategies and can be very creative in their work together.

Lesbian women who lose their partners often find that society at large does not allow them to experience the same grieving process. This was dramatic in a case where one woman who was suffering from a serious stroke was not allowed access to her lover when her family discovered their relationship. It took a protracted legal battle for these women to be able to live out the rest of their days together. Disruption of this grieving process can also make the loss more difficult for women recovering from the death of their partner. Most recently, some religious institutions have reached out to gay people to allow these rituals and social transitions to be truly inclusive.

Most menopausal women, however, do not experience widowhood but begin to worry about the health problems of their husband. The thought of widowhood becomes a reality for the first time. This was true in the case of Robin who needed to nurse her husband after his heart attack and had to confront her fears of possible loss.

DIVORCE/MARITAL ALIENATION

A more common problem during midlife is marital alienation and divorce. Longitudinal studies of marriages find that the highest peak time for divorce is seven years into a marriage. This usually occurs in the thirties, since most Americans still marry in their mid-twenties. There is, however, a second peak time for divorce, and that is around midlife. While good marriages tend to get better over time, problematic marriages often cannot tolerate the stresses associated with developmental life changes. One study of divorce found that the most frequent reason for divorce during midlife is extramarital affairs, either long-term or more recent in nature. Seventy-five percent of the people in the same study reported long term difficulties but waited for either the children to leave or for other social changes to occur before the divorce took place (Kaslow, 1981).

A less dramatic but more common change is marital alienation. This alienation may involve a woman whose identity has been centered on raising the children, and who may not have received enough credit for it, from her husband or from the larger society. The lack of validation, combined with the loss of emotional connection to children, may make the adjustment to the menopausal transition more difficult. This situation can lead to sadness about the "empty nest" unless the couple make some adjustments.

Another similar pattern involves the changing needs of the midlife husband. Having accomplished his career goals, he may look to his wife for more shared leisure time. The wife may be freed from the burden of the children (sometimes), and want to go off to college, or open a business, or continue her career path. If a couple cannot negotiate these different expectations, marital stress can be debilitating. As people grow and face the changes of midlife, there are often changes in the original marital contract. The most common change is that when the couple married, the woman agreed to stay home and take care of the children. As the children grew older, however, the woman wanted more contact outside the home and had career goals. Often these changes necessitate changes in the marital contract—who does the housework, who does the grocery shopping and so on. Couples who are flexible take a logical approach to this and problem-solve together. Gina and Richard have used this problem-solving approach to their family life over the years.

Other couples, who have never been able to negotiate problems, find such changes too difficult and the marriage deteriorates. This is extremely problematic since so many people reevaluate their lives at midlife, and this naturally leads to changes in the marital contract. Too many of our midlife depressed women have husbands who are extremely rigid and unyielding, resistant to such changes. In other couples, the partners drift apart quietly and without conflict, each of them aware of their alienation, but not knowing what to do about it. Sophia and Preston, a midlife couple, are trapped in a rigid marriage in Whitney Otto's book *How to Make an American Quilt*. Sophia can't seem to escape from her inflexibility with her family and turns to other women, quietly:

> "Sophia wants to tell Preston that she loves him, wants to be less rule-bound with her children, but instead she spends one night a week piecing together bits of fabric with a group of women. As if she could piece together all the things she feels inside, stitch them together and make everything seem whole and right" (Otto, 1991, p. 76).

FINANCIAL DIFFICULTIES

Financial difficulties have become an increasingly prevalent problem in American society. This has been true for single women, single mothers and for the legions of women who have jobs where they are subject to sexual discrimination and harassment. Many of the women who are "pink-collar" workers are married to men who are "blue-collar" workers. We have found that many women in this situation have come to us, experiencing extreme stress related to their husband's work problems or unemployment.

Many of their husbands have been let go from their jobs unexpectedly. This can be particularly difficult for a single-career family where the men are employed and the women work at home. Gina's husband, Richard, has been a foreman in a rug-weaving plant for twenty-five years, and was looking forward to five more years before his retirement. Richard and Gina both believed that the company would take care of them, as it had their parents before them, but it was sold to a larger company and moved to Georgia. Richard and Gina could not leave their multiple responsibilities, and they were left without his full retirement pay. We find that many men and women like Gina and Richard face a new world of mergers and escalating health care costs. Many of the men are unemployed with few new job skills and with tremendous burdens for the financial security of their family.

Unemployment has a negative effect not only on the man who may be the single wage earner, but on the family as well. In many families, women are willing to go back to work and do so. This often has a beneficial effect on the family system. The husband feels relieved and both partners feel that they can share in the responsibilities for family finances. Yet in others, it is difficult for the man to accept his wife's work. Some men see this as a threat to their masculinity, or they begrudgingly *allow* their wives to "work outside the home," but do nothing to participate in the maintenance of family responsibilities, such as household chores, shopping and so on. Claudette's husband, Louis, became more controlling and jealous with her after he lost his job. Open communication and the ability to problem-solve play the key factors here in helping families contend with the changes of financial and employment difficulties.

Retirement and unemployment are not just men's issues. Married women, as well as single women, need the money they earn. Since many women have taken time off from work over the years because of their families, they have less Social Security and less income to save for retirement. According to *The Women's Encyclopedia of Health and Emotional Healing*, the average age that an American woman is widowed is fifty-six but does not become eligible for Social Security's widow's benefits until age sixty (Foley and Nechas, 1993). Even though many of us are intimidated by financial planning, the time to plan for retirement is now.

HISTORY OF PREVIOUS TRAUMA

As we spent more time with Claudette, she revealed to us something she had never told anyone in all of her fifty-five years—that she was sexually molested by a neighbor when she was eleven. This trauma had affected almost every aspect of her life, from her sexuality to her raising her children to dealing with authority. New research has found histories of sexual and physical trauma in women who come for treatment of substance abuse, chronic pain, sexual problems and a number of psychological disorders. Since most women never get psychotherapy and since these experiences are associated with guilt and shame, many women cannot reveal their pain at all, or wait until their middle years to do so. This may be especially true for women in their forties or fifties today with early experiences of abuse, when they had essentially no formal resources for help during childhood.

Judith Lewis Herman, a psychiatrist at Harvard Medical School, has written an eloquent, moving and informative book, *Trauma and Recovery*. It was our patient Claudette who first brought in Dr. Herman's book. This was a welcomed reference, since we were already familiar with Dr. Herman's work in the area of sexual abuse (Herman, 1992). Bringing us the book also made it easier for Claudette to tell us about her own story.

✦ STRESS MANAGEMENT

Any of you who have read women's magazines or health magazines in the past ten years can now be called stress experts. Stress management ranks up there with topics like "ten new luscious chocolate desserts" and "trim five inches from your thighs" as popular cover stories. The double bind created by placing these two stories on the same magazine cover is bound to increase stress in all of us, but that is another story (see our discussion of weight problems). Articles about women who have totally managed their stress down to the smallest detail have become burdensome in themselves. Even Candice Bergen in a televised interview in 1991 revealed that she had felt better immediately once she had stopped reading articles about how well Jane Pauley manages her life!

The first step in coping with stress is to identify it. We help our patients by providing them with assessments, using several questionnaires and strategies. These self-analysis tools provide new knowledge, and as you know by now, one of our strongest beliefs is that knowledge is power. So many women come to us with vague feelings of uneasiness or physical complaints. They know something is wrong, but they don't know what. One of our first steps in working together is to find out what specific stresses affect them. One helpful exercise is the pie chart. First, a woman lists the ways she may spend her time—work, spending time with family members, household chores, friends, leisure activities, self-improvement. The next step is to create a pie chart with sections devoted to how much time is spent per week on each activity. After that, the woman rank orders these behaviors as to their importance in her life. A second pie chart represents the way she would like to spend her time based on her values.

You might try this exercise yourself after referring to Molly's pie chart in Table 8-1. Molly was a forty-eight-year-old woman who was beginning to have hot flashes and entered psychotherapy because she felt "spacey and disconnected." Molly indeed was entering the menopausal phase but was not interested in hormone replacement therapy at the time. After she was evaluated medically, she began to see one of our psychologists. We found that although Molly was the mother of four teenage children, she also worked twenty hours a week. In addition, her husband, who was a highly paid, alcoholic executive, firmly believed that work was fine as long as "Molly did what she was supposed to do first." When we looked at Molly's pie chart we found that she was spending long hours outside her paid job, tidying up the house, preparing dinner, and waiting for her husband to come home. He often was late, without calling to let her know when he would be home.

Molly found that a full 75 percent of her time was devoted to working, taking care of the house, doing chores, preparing meals and waiting for her husband. Only 25 percent of her time remained for her other roles as colleague, friend, family member and person interested in maintaining her health. By actually looking at how she now spent her time, Molly realized the discrepancies between it and what she really wanted to do. Her priorities were to pull away from the lives of her children and husband. Her children had moved on to late adolescence and were beginning college. Her husband, despite her numerous attempts to involve him in therapy, continued to live an isolated and alcoholic existence. These discrepancies helped Molly examine the choices she needed to make to enter the next phase of her life.

It was a long process for Molly to come to the shocking realization that she had spent so much of her time on other people's needs without receiving much in return. Not that she didn't value taking care of her husband and children, but the extent to which she neglected her own needs had never been so apparent. She had been suffering from dysthymia, a chronic type of depression, for many years but merely added that to the list of negative feelings about herself, rather than being able to take charge of her life and make some significant changes. However, with continued psychotherapy, she was able to join an Al-Anon group, spend more time with her women friends and examine her dependence—financial and emotional—on her husband.

TABLE 8-1
MOLLY'S PIE CHARTS

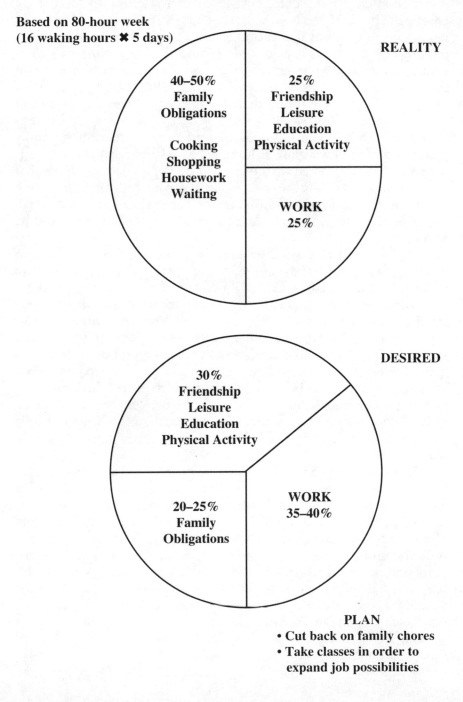

Based on 80-hour week
(16 waking hours ✖ 5 days)

REALITY

40–50%
Family
Obligations

Cooking
Shopping
Housework
Waiting

25%
Friendship
Leisure
Education
Physical Activity

WORK
25%

DESIRED

30%
Friendship
Leisure
Education
Physical Activity

20–25%
Family
Obligations

WORK
35–40%

PLAN
• Cut back on family chores
• Take classes in order to
  expand job possibilities

✦ THE MIND/BODY CONNECTION

We see stress management as an integral part of our practice. This is because we do not engage in the typical mind verses body dichotomy, but see the mind/body connection every day in our practice. It is now very clear that stress can affect health negatively. This is not just some fuzzy philosophical belief but a growing area of medical science. People who have been widowed or suffered the death of their partner have a higher likelihood of dying during the six months after that loss. Six months after a divorce or marital separation is a time of more frequent visits to physicians and to emergency rooms. The link between the mind and the body may well be our immune system that controls the body and protects us against the possibility of infection or viruses. The relatively new field of psychoneuroimmunology (longest word in the book) has lead to medical breakthroughs in understanding this connection. In *Healing and the Mind,* Bill Moyers interviews numerous researchers who have shown the connection between stress and the immune system, where increased stress can interfere with the immune system's ability to work (Moyers, 1993). Similarly, decreasing stress can improve health. There are numerous stress management strategies. Here are but a few:

Deep muscle relaxation involves at least two components. First, it involves taking slow, deep breaths in order to control the rhythm of your breathing. You will be surprised at how relaxing it can be to take a few minutes for yourself and just think "Breathe in—pause—breathe out." You then consecutively and systematically tense and relax the various muscle groups throughout your body. Meditation often leads to relaxation. Meditation is a sense of complete concentration. It usually involves deep relaxation first and then includes trying to close your eyes and focus completely on a single word that you repeat over and over.

We are fond of using imagery as a technique. It, too, involves deep breathing exercises but adds a visual image that you can conjure up by concentrating. This is essentially a form of creative memory. You try to remember a time when you experienced either complete relaxation or joy. By conjuring up the physical details of that memory and even perhaps the smells and feelings that go along with it, you can create a state of intense relaxation.

Biofeedback is a way of measuring relaxation. The biofeedback machine involves measuring your heart, blood pressure and skin response. Bill Moyers describes his experience of being hooked up to a biofeedback machine. In working with Doctor Karen Olness, professor of pediatrics at Case Western Reserve University, she asks him to recite the Gettysburg address and when he stumbles after several sentences, he sees the line measuring his heart rate bouncing. She then asks him to imagine a comfortable scene and he does so: "I close my eyes again, in my mind I am standing on a peak near the Western slope of the Rockies. I have been to this spot only once a dozen years ago but the experience is as immediate and exhilarating in my mind's eye as it was that day when my friend and I paused to catch our breath and found ourselves silently, slowly, turning in a circle, complete circle—black elk's great hoop—and seeing as far as one could see nothing but sky and clouds and mountains, a 360-degree prospect as pure as Eden, as peaceful as a baby's breath . . . I look, the little white line moves serenely across the screen like a sailboat on the waveless horizon" (Moyers, 1993, p. 173). The biofeedback machine then was able to let him know how he had reached a state of relaxation. Now, few of us have such a rich and evocative way to recall experiences, but relaxation techniques like biofeedback can be helpful to everyone.

Any number of these techniques can improve your ability to cope with stress and you need to find the one that works best for you. Many women prefer the less structured and more interpersonal approach available in psychotherapy. Psychotherapy can often provide tremendous relief from stress and is discussed in great detail in our chapter on depression. Short term psychotherapy can help a woman identify her stressors and take a direct and problem-solving approach. Many women accomplish this in ten sessions or less.

In addition to the specific techniques of coping, there are many *attitudes* and psychological attributes that we need to add to our lifestyle to cope with stress. We have suggested several possible books and tapes in our resource section. Here are some of the attitudes and techniques then that we use with women in our practice. A few of them are very common; others are contrary to what you might expect.

ATTITUDE

Stress management should not be stressful. Review what you have learned about yourself in the pie chart or in discussions with a friend or psychotherapist and make some small adjustments first. In fact, an overly detailed and *heroic* approach to stress is counterproductive. Flexibility is the key. When we try to do too much of the "right thing," whether it is lowering cholesterol or reducing stress, we can become too rigid, preoccupied and more stressed.

Although stress can be difficult during menopause, women who directly confront their particular stresses feel more in control and more powerful. An attitude of taking control and making small changes can be most beneficial. You can be creative and imaginative in changing your life. The last thing we want to do is to increase your stress with our stress management advice. So think about our suggestions, but use them in combination with your own good common sense.

FLEXIBILITY

Our belief in flexibility dictates that we need to avoid an "either/or" approach. This "either/or" thinking is associated with stress in a number of ways. One of the most common areas is women and their weight. Judith Rodin, a psychologist and president of the University of Pennsylvania, has described women's weight issues as a "chronic stressor" in women's lives (Rodin and others, 1985, p. 267). Our preoccupation with what we eat, our weight, and how we look, can lead to a vicious cycle of dieting and bingeing or alternating between dieting and thinking of normal eating as "breaking a diet." Thus, many of us are either "on a diet" or "off a diet." It is this type of either/or thinking that is sure to destroy any hope for normal eating behavior.

An inflexible either/or approach can make your life worse! This is related to the superwoman role. Let's face it, most of us are not superwoman. There are many successful women who are hard driving, organized and who pay great attention to detail. This drive is related to the Type A personality that we discussed in the healthy hearts chapter. But other times this behavior is a woman's best attempt at coping with the many different jobs in her life. It is not helpful for us to tell you to stop if this lifestyle is working for you. On the other hand, many women who are superorganized suffer from being perfectionists and too self-critical. Their either/or system leads them to feel that they are either on top of things or failing.

DECREASING PERFECTIONISM

Many of us suffer from perfectionism. This can be a particular challenge to menopausal women. How can we manage our household responsibilities, deal with elderly family members, work and relate to our own friends and family? There is no way we can all be perfect at all these roles. There is no reason we have to have a perfectly clean house or apartment. Nor can we be perfectly available to our children and friends, particularly if needs are competing. One of the ways to correct this thinking is to ask ourselves, "What is the worst thing that could happen if I don't do this perfectly?" By applying this test, very few tasks will be as important as we think. The worst thing that can happen if we don't have a clean house is that there will be some extra dust. The worst thing that can happen if we don't complete a report in a day is that it will be a day late.

It is more difficult to change our thinking about relationships. Being perfectionistic about our relationships can be extremely damaging. Among other things, we do not have total control over our relationships. As women we somehow take the rap for the behavior of our grown children, as if we had total control of their environment as they were growing up. Children in their late teens and twenties are now individuals who have their own behaviors and these behaviors lead to many consequences, most of which we cannot control. When we combine our perfectionism with our feeling of total responsibility for the family's welfare we can easily become overwhelmed. We must divest ourselves of it.

We mentioned Gloria, earlier, who felt sandwiched between her son and her mother. Gloria is an example of a woman who was preoccupied with her grown children's lives. We understand her worries because that's what good mothers are supposed to do, of course! And it's hard to turn off these concerns when a child reaches some arbitrary age. But Gloria was still worrying about her thirty-year-old daughter, who was overweight and not married. After discussing the family situation with her, it became clear that her daughter Janet was probably the happiest of the three siblings. She had a well-paid, highly innovative job that allowed her to travel. She had many friends and was quite active in community theater. Yet, Gloria was struggling with the belief that not only should all her children be married, but that she had the responsibility for making this happen.

We need to work together as women to get rid of our perfectionism and need to be superwomen. These are difficult times and most women are just trying to get by. Let's move beyond "having it all." Nobody "has it all." The myriad of articles in magazines that promise the ability to have a high-paying job with an easy family life and few stresses promise more than society has been able to deliver. The implication here is that if we don't have it all, it may be our fault. Susan Faludi in her groundbreaking book *Backlash* has documented that for many of us liberation has not arrived and yet is being blamed for a tremendous amount of social ills (Faludi, 1991). This focus on women who "have it all" only fosters competition among women. We need to stop competing with one another and continue to cooperatively solve problems.

SENSE OF HUMOR

Numerous writers from Norman Cousins to Joan Borysenko (as well as Joan Rivers) have suggested that laughter is often our best medicine. Laughter reduces stress both psychologically and physiologically. There is probably nothing better in alleviating stress than a good dose of laughter. It can help us cope from everyday life to serious illness. In *On Women Turning Fifty,* Cathleen Rountree talks with Ruth Zaporah, a teacher and dancer. Zaporah has had previous struggles with migraine headaches, depression and divorce. Here's what she says about her fifties: "In my fifties I feel ripely quiet. Life seems much simpler: I am more appreciative. More of life seems funny to me, humorous and light. I consistently have a good time. It hasn't always been like that" (Rountree, 1993, p. 59).

So, why not rent the videotape or read the screenplay of Jane Wagner and Lily Tomlin's *The Search for Intelligent Life in the Universe?* Or, watch "The Mary Tyler Moore Show." Or, if you're a more scholarly type, read one of Shakespeare's comedies. Or, go see a performance artist, like Julie Goell in *Women in a Suitcase.* Read social and political essays, like Barbara Ehrenreich's hilarious *The Worst Years of Our Lives.* We hope you're beginning to add to the list.

One night, after giving a seminar on menopause, the three of us were completely exhausted, having gone through a long day of numerous family, teaching, and clinical responsibilities. At the end of the session, just when all of the women from the audience had left, one of us literally collapsed to the floor in order to demonstrate her fatigue, sending the other two into peals of laughter. This released all of our stress from the evening and prompted us to spend another half hour together talking, laughing and sharing the day's news.

WORK CAN BE FUN

Enjoy work. Here is a surprise. Most of what we read about women's work stress suggests that work is an "add on" that women do only after meeting all other family responsibilities. All too often that is the case. Work is also usually described as something that is inherently stressful and inherently in conflict with our roles as mothers. Yet sociologists Roselyn C. Barnett and Grace Baruch describe how multiple roles can actually be helpful to women. This supposedly negative role of women as workers is in contrast to the real data. Being a paid employee is associated with positive mental health and general health benefits for women (Barnett and others, 1987).

Women who are employed usually enjoy the challenges of their careers. All too often, women have more control over their work life than they do over their home life. Although we love our families, it is very common for women to comment that going to work is a vacation compared to family responsibilities! Remember Robin, the woman whose husband lost the construction business? Over time, she obtained a bookkeeping job in a small firm. She came to love the new work and social contacts she made and as she grew more independent, helped her family deal with their financial crises. She and her family are still struggling financially, but psychologically, they are coping well.

EDUCATION

Many women do not choose to work outside the home after their children are grown. They continue their involvement in educational activities and social-service or volunteer organizations and are happy doing so. Others feel a sense of malaise or emptiness during the menopausal period. For many women, the menopausal years are a time for a renewed interest in education. After Gloria began to give up her worries about her children, she looked to do more with her spare time. After so many years out of paid employment, however, Gloria felt particularly inferior compared to other women in the adult education programs she would attend. She finally found a book club that was small and included many women whom she knew. After several months, she gained self-confidence and re-enrolled in an undergraduate program in liberal arts. Many universities now have special programs for women who are returning to school, like Brown University's Resumed Undergraduate Education program. Education of any type can be helpful to many women at menopause and provides roles and benefits similar to those of paid employment.

EXPAND YOUR LEISURE AND CREATIVE ACTIVITIES

Reading alone can be a pleasant distraction from the stresses of everyday life. We've mentioned many books already. Many of our patients have also enjoyed Amy Tan's *The Kitchen God's Wife*, classics like *Tar Baby* or anything written by Toni Morrison, mysteries by Sue Grafton and Amanda Cross and nonfiction, like Gloria Steinem's *Revolution from Within*. Joining a book club is also a way to combine meeting new people with expanding your reading list.

Music is one of life's most powerful stress relievers. Writing this book has, of course, been stressful at times. We discovered a new coffee house where the sound of jazz fills the room. Often we meet there to discuss the book, and at other times one of us may go there alone and jot down some notes while sipping coffee and listening to Ella Fitzgerald. You might prefer classical, folk or rock. Whatever you do, if you find that the music has the calm and relaxing, or passionate and exciting feeling that we can all identify with, then you are not stressed at that time.

Writing can be a soothing and creative pastime. It can be yours alone or you might want to share it. Keep a journal, write down a story, even a play or a poem. Don't worry about whether it's "good" or not; it's yours.

Other creative arts can serve as a relief and an alternative force to stress. Explore painting, sketching, sculpture; put some rhinestones on an old T-shirt! One of our patients discovered pottery at menopause. She described the incredible relaxing quality of the hum of the potter's wheel and the feel of the clay.

We discuss physical activity in our chapter on healthy aging, and remember that any physical activity is beneficial and can be pleasurable. The artist Coeleen Kiebert started bodysurfing in her fifties (Rountree, 1993). You do not need to bodysurf or even jog three miles, you can walk. None of these activities work of course, unless you give yourself the time. Enjoying leisure activities, on a regular basis, can be as effective at managing stress as a formal program.

THE IMPORTANCE OF RELIGIOUS BELIEFS AND COMMITMENT

Many women in midlife are searching for depth and meaning, as well as for intimacy. Many reevaluate the role of formal religion at midlife. This seems to come with wisdom and with the inevitable confrontation with the reality of the limits of human life. Some spiritual life helps us with the confrontation with death and suffering that we experience more as we get older. With the generation of our parents now dying or near the end of the natural life span, we are now becoming the senior and responsible generation.

Herbert Benson, after writing *The Relaxation Response,* published *Beyond the Relaxation Response,* because the previous book neglected the issue of commitment. Stress management can be very effective, but most people at midlife also benefit from a deeply felt set of values and beliefs. These commitments can be formal religion, a sense of spirituality, a devotion to a humanitarian cause or to the larger community. Many women return to their religious traditions or find new types of commitments when confronted by illness and mortality. Gloria became more active in her synagogue, especially the Social Action Committee. As she worked, she began to feel her considerable energies in a new, deeper way. She also enjoyed the time spent with other clergy and lay members of the synagogue.

Healing and the Mind pays a great deal of attention to eastern religions only, but the fact is that prayer and meditation are major components of most religions. From the prayers of Christianity and Judaism to those of Islam, Buddhism and other eastern religions, contemplation and peaceful meditation are seen as important (Moyers, 1993). Having or developing an awareness of a larger reality is one way of understanding that the individual life has meaning and significance beyond the actual years of active living. Such a sense of meaning and or the spiritual dimension of life is valuable and helpful for many people.

Much of the writing about midlife has a religious and existential focus. Erik Erikson, for example, wrote that healthy children will not fear life if their elders have enough integrity not to fear death (Erikson, 1950). The poet Audre Lorde fought a fourteen-year struggle with cancer and died while we were writing this book. Throughout her ordeal, Audre Lorde continued to write poetry. She described herself as ''a Black, Lesbian, Feminist, Warrior Poet, fighting the good fight in spite of all'' (Morgan, 1993, p. 58).

KNOWING WHEN TO GET ADDITIONAL HELP

Despite all of our efforts, stress can become too much. Although most of us suffer from a certain amount of normal stress, at some point stress can become severe. Many women experience severe physical tension. Quite a few women come to see us, suffering from tension headaches, gastrointestinal problems and backaches. Many medical conditions like asthma, headaches and irritable bowel syndrome are exacerbated by stress. Since part of our evaluation has always been to combine the medical with the psychological, here are some of the symptoms that may suggest your stress level is too high.

HEADACHES

By far, the most common stress-related problem we see is the headache. In fact, Gloria originally came to us because of her headaches. Headaches are a problem for many menopausal women. Although the hormonal changes may be a factor for some women, stress also plays a role. Headaches are common in men, too. There are several categories of headaches. *Tension* headaches are the most common type of headache and are a result of the contraction of neck, scalp and facial muscles. Most people describe the pain as feeling like pressure is being applied to their head or sometimes their neck. These headaches also tend to coincide with periods of stress. If tension headaches become routine, they can then become *chronic*. These muscle-contraction headaches can also be caused by depression, anxiety, or other emotional factors.

A full 60 to 75 percent of people suffering from headaches are women (Andrasik and Kabela, 1988). Women suffer more often from *migraine* headaches than do men. A *classic migraine* headache is preceded by an "aura," or a warning that may be in the form of flashing lights or a temporary loss of vision which occurs between ten and thirty minutes before the headache begins. A *common migraine,* named so because it is much more common than classic migraines, is not preceded by an aura. The migraine process is not completely understood. It is believed that people who get migraine headaches have blood vessels that overreact or overdilate to certain triggers. These triggers can include stress as well as eating certain foods like chocolate, or the additive monosodium glutamate (MSG). It is the dilation that causes the throbbing pain of migraines. During the headache, many women will try to find a quiet, dark place to sleep. Both light and loud noise typically worsen the pain and sleeping seems to help. For some women, nausea and vomiting may also accompany the headache.

Gloria suffered from common migraine headaches. Some migraines reoccur around the time of menstrual periods and increase in frequency around the menopausal period. But the precise relationship between hormones and migraines is unclear. In some situations, the hormone progesterone can cause headaches. So, if your headaches began after you started a course of HRT, you should discuss them with your physician.

Migraine headaches may tend to occur in the pre- or perimenopausal periods rather than the postmenopausal period. Women who are between the ages of thirty and forty-nine and from lower-income households are at the highest risk for experiencing migraine headaches. The stress factor plays an important role once again.

Gloria got some relief of her migraine headaches by taking a medication that counteracts the vasodilation that occurs during the painful stage of the headache. These medications, the most common of which is ergotamine, should be taken during the early stages of a migraine headache. Ergotamine will not be effective if the migraine has been in progress for some time and it is contraindicated in certain medical conditions. For women who are troubled by severe and frequent migraines, preventive medications can be used, including propranolol and other Beta-blockers, medications that are also used to treat high blood pressure. One study at a headache clinic found that the most useful combination treatment for migraine headaches was propranolol and biofeedback (Margolis and Moses, 1992).

An international symposium of the World Health Organization and the World Psychiatric Association found that many people who had headaches also experienced a depression at the same time. It is not clear whether the depression caused the headache or whether the headache caused the depression, but it is clear that severe headaches tend to be associated with depression. Tricyclic antidepressant medication can be useful for some people with frequent headaches. Psychological consultation could be helpful to women either in sorting out the depression or in developing pain management strategies.

The treatment of tension or muscle-contraction headaches includes muscle relaxation, and many of the stress management procedures we outline in a bit. Nonsteroidal anti-inflammatory drugs (NSAIDs) like ibuprofen can be effective also. If you suffer from chronic headaches, try to become involved in a comprehensive program that will evaluate medical, nutritional and psychological factors. Be sure to avoid addictive painkillers like codeine and Percodan. They may work in the short run, but over time you will have a second problem—that of prescription drug abuse. A study of substance abusers found that almost 90 percent of them experience some type of headache. Of these substance abusers, women who had migraine headaches tended to develop their headaches first and then begin to crave pain medication. Others, who experienced tension headaches, tended to develop these headaches after using substances. Thus it is possible that substance abuse may cause tension headaches and that some of these headaches are caused by hangovers or withdrawal from prescription drugs (Andrasik and Kabela, 1988; El-Mallakh and Rif, 1987).

AVOID SELF-MEDICATION

In addition to prescription medication, sometimes women turn to alcohol to relieve headaches, stress, or anxiety. This is particularly problematic for women, who experience the adverse affects of alcohol more readily than men. Women have higher blood alcohol levels than men after drinking the same amount of alcohol even when weight differences are considered (Jones and Jones, 1976). Partially as a consequence of this, women develop such alcohol-related diseases as liver disease and hypertension earlier than men (Tuyns and Pequinot, 1984). Most women find it shocking to discover that as little as two alcoholic drinks per day can be dangerous. The real danger in using alcohol for stress is that it works, at least in the short run. It is, after all, a depressant, not unlike Valium. The use of alcohol to reduce stress or to get to sleep is risky not only because of the biological consequences, but also because of psychological dependence. Many women start drinking at particularly stressful times, for example during a divorce. The pattern of drinking continues well after the stressful period has passed. We often ask our patients if they use alcohol to alleviate stress. If they do, this is a real warning of a possible problem, and we suggest other stress-management strategies.

✦ UNPRODUCTIVE WORRYING

Stress also affects the cognitive realm—the way we think. We have discussed some of the thinking problems above, such as the either/or problem or the problem of perfectionism. Psychologist Albert Ellis suggests that it is not the events that happen to us that cause stress, but our *thinking* about the event. Albert Ellis calls this the ABC model, where A is an activating event, B is our thinking about the event and C are the feelings and behaviors that result (Ellis and Harper, 1975). We see many women who are suffering from their thoughts about an event. For example, a secretary in one of the hospitals was severely chastised by one of her bosses on a regular basis. Lucy was in the category of pink-collar worker who was at greater risk of cardiovascular disease because her job required lots of responsibility but gave her little power. She came to us with severe feelings of worthlessness and stress. She felt anxiety before going to work and was finding herself drinking two daily gin and tonics to unwind after work. When we talked to her at length, we found that her intervening thinking, the B of the ABC model, was that surely if she were a better secretary, her boss would not reprimand her (see Figure 8-1). Surely if she were more organized this wouldn't happen. Lucy began to learn that when she talked more and more about her boss's behavior, the behavior had less to do with her than it did with her boss. We helped her change her thinking pattern to, "I've done a decent job, this is an unacceptable reprimand." Over time, Lucy began to talk to other people and understand the unrealistic demands of her job. She was transferred to another department with a more collaborative management, continues to work effectively, and no longer needs alcohol to relax after work.

Many women with cognitive stress become burdened with preoccupation that can become obsessive and brooding. This occurs when

FIGURE 8-1

LUCY'S FAULTY THINKING

A ⟶ **B** ⟶ **C**

Activating Event	Belief System	Emotional Consequences
Boss harshly reprimands Lucy ⟶	Lucy thinks: "If I were a better secretary he wouldn't do this" ⟶	Stress Anxiety Worthlessness

Lucy begins to drink to reduce stress

CORRECTION TO FAULTY THINKING

Boss harshly reprimands Lucy ⟶ "This is unacceptable. I have done nothing wrong." ⟶ No anxiety

Lucy looks for support

you continue to think about a problem over and over without making any headway. For some women with these cognitive problems, their mind is actually too active and too busy for them to relax enough to engage in muscle-relaxation procedures. They find it difficult to concentrate on the tapes. In this situation, there are other possibilities. Alternative activities like exercise, music or dance can engage the mind and distract a woman from her worries.

Closely related to unproductive worrying is one of the most common psychological problems for women, *anxiety*. Anxiety can take many forms, from panic attacks, agoraphobia, to free-floating anxiety. Many menopausal women have a feeling of foreboding or dis-ease just before a hot flash. When we explain to our patients that this brief experience is a natural precursor to a flash, they feel a sense of relief. Other women have a panicky feeling, which, combined with the heart palpitations, seems a bit like a panic attack. If you are having these symptoms at times other than a flash, then you may be suffering from some type of anxiety disorder. Treatments for anxiety, like those for depression, have made great advances recently, and help is available.

There are many avenues for help. Stress-management programs are available in many facilities. Your employer may have an employee assistance program (EAP). These programs are confidential, and usually provide general stress-management programs on an individual or group basis. They are not seen as "psychological malfunctioning" and most enlightened employers now see that stress management can only improve an employee's work rather than detract from it. Health maintenance organizations (HMOs) often have stress-management programs as well. Many social service agencies and community centers offer programs for managing stress also. These usually are not expensive and reduce visits to the doctors by providing alternative forms for reducing stress and anxiety.

If you find that you are suffering from some of the symptoms of anxiety and depression that we outline, then it is helpful to get in touch with a mental health professional. We detail this process in the chapter on depression. Almost every form of health insurance provides some mental health coverage. Whether you have a depression, an anxiety problem, or feel a general sense of stress, you may well benefit from meeting with the mental health professional. Many times you will feel relief after only a few sessions.

← COMMUNICATION

GET HELP AT HOME, AS WELL

Many menopausal women are working too hard at home. The 1980 census found that the average number of hours that a man contributed to household chores and child-care in a given week was eight. Women working full-time also worked another twenty hours at home. Arlie Hochschild details this situation in her moving book *The Second Shift* (Hochschild, 1989). The facts are that most working women work a full shift at work and another shift at home. Menopausal women are no

exception. Although the caretaking demands for young children usually do not exist, the household duties remain. Some women have less
energy at menopause and others are justifiably fed up!

A first strategy in obtaining help around the house is to renegoti-
ate the household duties with your partner. Many women find this
difficult to do for several reasons. First, many of us have been brought
up to believe that the house is our territory. Hochschild describes one
couple, both of whom were professional, where the woman did the
inside chores while the man did the outside chores. The couple dis-
torted the division of responsibilities as an equal split, even though the
indoor chores involved vacuuming, cleaning, washing the dishes,
cleaning the bathrooms and food preparation. Her husband's chores,
on the other hand, involved mowing the lawn, doing the laundry and
taking out the trash (Hochschild, 1989). Not quite a fifty-fifty split.
Many women are afraid to address this issue with their husband for fear
of causing conflict. Some of them have tried to discuss these issues in
the past with little success. Many of them have difficulty confronting
the fact that their husband is quite unwilling to be cooperative.

We have seen many women, however, who learn to negotiate
more forcefully at midlife. Conflict need not be frightening, particularly if there are no children in the home. In addition, many women are
able to give up the notion that conflict is bad, especially when it can
lead to a more equitable division of labor and a more comfortable
partnership. Many women regain some power in the marriage at midlife primarily because they have stopped being afraid of conflict. If such
accommodations are not made, many women have been extremely creative in getting help in other ways. For example, some families form
meal cooperatives, when one family, instead of making one meal, will
make four and share with other families. Then on other nights of the
week, the same family has no cooking to do. Other women learn to
share cleaning and organizational resources as well.

Finally, it is important to remember that there are *many avenues
for help*. For a number of reasons, many women do not go to stress-
management or psychotherapy programs. We wish this were not true
because so many women could benefit from these programs. Often
women turn to their families and friends for support and this, too, is
beneficial.

It is also important to keep all of this stress business in perspective.
At the end of his midlife crisis article, Eliot Jaques reminds us of the
gains of midlife: "The gain is in the deepening of awareness, understanding, and self-realization. Genuine values can be cultivated—of
wisdom, fortitude and courage, deeper capacity for love and affection

and human insight and hopefulness and enjoyment" (Jaques, 1965, p. 513). Remember his words. So, the next time you're feeling stressed, also remember Lorraine fighting off that bear, and Samantha taking charge of her MS. Remember Gladys who managed to go on, despite the loss of her husband, and Robin who took charge of her family. And Gina and Richard, working together through unemployment and family illness. And remember Audre Lorde, looking death right in the eye and still rejoicing in each day. These women are in all of us.

RESOURCES

In addition to the books we mentioned so far, here are some excellent resources on stress.

BOOKS

Joan Borysenko's *Minding the Body, Mending the Mind* (New York: Bantam, 1988) is a book based on the psychologist's work at the Deaconess Hospital.

Mind/Body Medicine (Yonkers, NY: Consumer Reports Book, 1993) is edited by Daniel Goleman, Ph.D., a psychologist who is an editor of *Psychology Today,* and Joel Gurin, the science editor of *Consumer Reports*. This is a well-written and extremely informative book, with contributions from many of the leading authorities in health care.

Mastering Stress: A Lifestyle Approach, by David H. Barlow, Ph.D., and Ronald M. Rapee, Ph.D., is a manual on stress reduction, available from the Learn Education Center of Dallas, Texas. This a clear and concise book, written by two leading experts in the area of stress and anxiety.

Trusting Ourselves: The Complete Guide to Emotional Well-Being for Women (New York: Atlantic Monthly Press, 1991) is written by Karen Johnson, M.D., former women's health editor of *Medical Self-Care*. This book addresses the issues of stress, anxiety depression and relaxation, and is accessible and informative.

Beyond the Relaxation Response was published in 1984 (New York: New York Times Book Company). Written by Dr. Herbert Benson and William Proctor, it emphasizes the importance of personal commitment to the basic issue of attaining relaxation.

Women's Encyclopedia of Health and Emotional Healing (Emmaus, Pennsylvania: Rodale Press, 1993) is edited by Denise Foley, Eileen Nechas and the editors of *Prevention* magazine. Hundreds of women who are health care professionals and other experts collaborated to produce this book that covers everything from anger to wrinkles.

AUDIOTAPES

There are many commercially produced tapes on stress management available. You need to find the one that is most effective with your individual needs. Jon Kabat-Zinn, Ph.D., has led meditation groups at Massachusetts Medical Center's Stress Reduction Clinic. His tapes can be ordered from P.O. Box 547, Lexington, MA 02173.

VIDEOTAPES

Bill Moyers's series on PBS, *Healing and the Mind,* is available on videocassette.

PAMPHLETS

The National Institute of Mental Health publishes a booklet titled "Plain Talk About Handling Stress." It is available by writing to Information Resources Branch, Room 15C-05, Office of Scientific Information NIMH-5600 Fishers Lane, Rockville, MD 20857.

CHAPTER NINE

Hysterectomy

YOU MIGHT BE WONDERING WHY WE HAVE INCLUDED A CHAPTER ON hysterectomy. After all, this is a book on the natural process of menopause, not on women's surgery. Our reason is inescapable: by the age of sixty, one-third of American women will have had hysterectomies (Carlson, Nichols and Schiff, 1993, p. 856). Some studies even suggest that the lifetime rate is as high as 58 percent. The ovaries are often routinely removed at the time of hysterectomy in premenopausal women, which causes menopause and its associated symptoms to occur earlier than they would naturally. Hysterectomy is the second most common operation performed on women, the first being a Caesarean section (Carlson and others, 1993, p. 856). Given these statistics, we hope that you can see how important it is to become well informed on the conditions which may lead to a recommendation for hysterectomy and to understand fully what the procedure involves.

Hysterectomy is major surgery. It involves general anesthesia, an incision, and the surgical removal of the uterus and cervix. It is often combined with an oophorectomy, which involves the removal of the ovaries. Abdominal hysterectomy usually requires four to five days of inpatient hospitalization, followed by months of recovery. Vaginal hysterectomy often results in a one- or two-day hospital stay. This major surgery has associated biological, psychological and sexual changes. A decision of this magnitude should be made conservatively and with great attention to your own personal medical symptoms.

A recent major review in the prestigious *New England Journal of Medicine* documented that a tremendous number of physicians are unsure about appropriate indications for hysterectomy. Drs. Carlson, Schiff and Nichols of Massachusetts General Hospital conclude that there are difficulties in diagnosis of the conditions that lead to hysterectomy, as well as a lack of information on the probable outcomes. They add that more attention should be given to alternative treatments. Finally, they conclude that women's preferences are not always taken into account. You need to know all you can before choosing a hysterectomy because this is an area where medical practice is rapidly changing (Carlson and others, 1993, pp. 856–860).

There is tremendous variation in rates of hysterectomy within our country. Women in the South have more hysterectomies than women in the North. One study revealed that in Maine, 70 percent of women in one city had hysterectomies whereas another city had a figure of 20 percent! In addition, African-American women have hysterectomies more often than white women. Hysterectomy is so common among African-American women in the South that it has been referred to as "a Mississippi appendectomy" (Morgan, 1982). Although African-American women tend to have fibroids more often than white women, hysterectomy may not be the most appropriate treatment for fibroids that are not life-threatening. These economic, regional, and racial differences need to be researched further. It is also clear that physicians' and patients' individual beliefs about hysterectomy must be factors. All the more reason for you to be an educated consumer when it comes to gynecological problems.

In the state of Florida, the average cost of a hysterectomy is over $10,000 (Health Survey, 1993). In other parts of the country, the cost is considerably less. Given the fact that so many hysterectomies are unnecessary, the cost to health insurance carriers, and ultimately to all of us, is enormous. With hospital costs of over five billion dollars on a yearly basis, it is financially wise to reevaluate hysterectomy as a routine surgical procedure.

Your individual health insurance plan plays a large role in how you are treated and advised. Research has shown that women whose insurance companies reimburse on a fee-for-service basis, have hysterectomies more often than women who are in health-maintenance organizations. Among the Western countries, the United States has the highest rate of hysterectomy, with Norway, Sweden and the United Kingdom having the lowest rates. Interestingly, those European countries also have national health insurance that monitors rates of hysterectomies as well as appropriate indications before the surgery can be performed. Unfortunately, there is no evidence that women in the United States have any improved health benefits from the high rate of hysterectomy. So the decision to have a hysterectomy and oophorectomy should be individually based on a woman's medical history, as well as her concerns.

We have provided Table 9-1 to help you understand the vocabulary that your doctor may use. Physicians use the term "total hysterectomy" to mean the removal of the uterus and cervix. If the hysterectomy is not total, it is called "subtotal" or "supercervical" and in that situation the uterus is removed and the cervix remains. The removal of the ovaries is called an oophorectomy. The removal of both the ovaries and the fallopian tubes is called a bilateral salpingo oophorectomy. Table 9-1 can clarify for you which organs have been left in and which organs come out in these various operations.

In our practice we have noticed a disturbing fact. Many women who have had a hysterectomy and/or an oophorectomy, do not know which type of surgery they have had. They may have heard the term

Table 9–1				
Medical Term	Uterus	Cervix	Fallopian Tubes	Ovaries
Subtotal, partial or supracervical hysterectomy	OUT	IN	IN	IN
Total hysterectomy	OUT	OUT	IN	IN
Oophorectomy	IN	IN	OUT	OUT
Total hysterectomy & bilateral salpingo oophorectomy	OUT	OUT	OUT	OUT

"total hysterectomy" and falsely believed that their ovaries have been removed as well. It is critically important for you to know whether the cervix or ovaries have been left intact. As you know from Chapter One, your ovaries produce not only the female hormones estrogen and progesterone, but also the male hormone testosterone, as well as other hormones. Unlike the gradual changes that are experienced during a natural menopause, oophorectomy leads to the abrupt cessation of hormone production. Women who have had this operation experience a sudden and dramatic drop in their hormones, which can cause hot flashes. The beneficial effects of the hormone estrogen in preventing osteoporosis and cardiovascular disease are therefore lost with surgical menopause, sometimes for no good reason. Then the question of whether or not to take hormone replacement therapy becomes crucial.

You may be surprised to discover that there are relatively few medical conditions for which elective hysterectomy is the only, or even the best option. There is no disagreement that hysterectomy is indicated in the following circumstances: invasive cervical or endometrial cancers, massive hemorrhage, uterine rupture, or severe uncontrollable infection (Cutler and Garcia, 1992). These clear indications for hysterectomy are listed in Table 9-2. Many of these cases are medical emergencies and will be done quickly, as well they should be.

Elective hysterectomy, which is surgery that is planned and not an emergency, may be offered for a variety of conditions. Other conditions for which hysterectomies have traditionally been performed are: fibroids, abnormal bleeding, endometriosis, chronic pelvic pain, en-

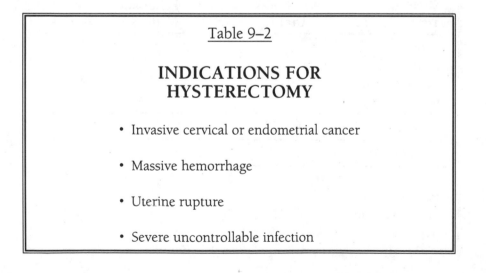

Table 9–2

INDICATIONS FOR HYSTERECTOMY

- Invasive cervical or endometrial cancer

- Massive hemorrhage

- Uterine rupture

- Severe uncontrollable infection

dometrial hyperplasia and genital prolapse. These indications are listed in Table 9-3 along with their alternative treatments. In each of these situations you need to discuss with your physician whether an alternative treatment is available. If it is available, you should consider it before deciding on a hysterectomy.

Of the hysterectomies performed in this country, 30 percent are for leiomyomas or fibroids. Fibroids are benign, not cancerous, overgrowth of smooth muscle tissue. Fibroids grow out of the wall of the uterus and can be as large as a football. There is a very small chance (less than 1 percent) of fibroids progressing to a type of cancer called leiomyosarcoma (Leibsohn and others, 1990). Some women may have multiple smaller fibroids in the uterine wall. Many women—in fact 30 percent of all women over forty years old—have fibroids, but have never experienced any symptoms. A smaller number of women will have symptoms such as bleeding, pelvic or back pain and later be told that they have fibroids. In most cases fibroids shrink at the time of menopause, because of the decreasing estrogen levels.

Not all bleeding is caused by fibroids alone. Other causes of bleeding include polyps, endometriosis, endometrial or cervical cancer and finally "dysfunctional uterine bleeding." We have always been troubled by this latter term because it seems like another harsh medical term that stigmatizes women's problems. Other similar terms include "incompetent cervix," "ovarian failure," and one of our own personal favorites "elderly first-time mothers" coined for pregnant women over the age of thirty-five. Dysfunctional uterine bleeding refers to excessive bleeding (either increased quantity, frequency or both) not related to fibroids, polyps, endometriosis, cancer, pregnancy, etc. This bleeding is presumed to be related to hormonal changes or imbalance and is actually more likely to occur in the perimenopausal period. Although it is often a reflection of changing menstrual cycles, it can also indicate something more serious like endometrial cancer. Therefore, abnormal bleeding needs to be fully evaluated by your doctor.

Another cause of hysterectomy (20 percent of all cases) is endometriosis. Symptoms of endometriosis (notably pelvic pain) are caused by the migration of tissue that normally lines the uterus to other organs in the pelvis. Although the number of hysterectomies for endometriosis is increasing, there are many new alternative treatments that are showing promise. Another bit of good news is that endometriosis is usually cured by menopause.

Genital prolapse (or pelvic relaxation), which is sagging of the rectum, urethra, or uterus through a weakened pelvic floor, is the reason given for about 15 percent of all hysterectomies. The two remaining reasons given for hysterectomy are chronic pelvic pain and endometrial hyperplasia. Chronic pelvic pain is one of the more complicated issues, and the underlying cause needs to be fully explored before hysterectomy should be recommended. Endometrial hyperplasia is the accumulation of the lining of the uterus, often related to a relative excess of estrogen. Although this condition accounts for almost 6 percent of hysterectomies, hysterectomy is not necessary in most of these cases (Carlson and others, 1993, p. 856).

Most women are unaware of the alternatives to hysterectomy. Medical technology has provided us with tremendous advances in the treatment of endometriosis and fibroids, conditions that have previously made up 50 percent of indications for the operation. If a hysterectomy is recommended to you, it is critically important that you get a second opinion. We will discuss this further in the communications section. Taking into consideration the inconsistent and often high rates of hysterectomy, it seems unlikely that women are participating enough in the informed consent process. Informed consent is an analysis with your physicians of the alternatives to hysterectomy, as well as the benefits and the risks involved. This should not be just signing a paper, but a lengthy discussion that allows you to see what your choices are and to talk over your concerns.

In addition to medical reasons, many experts believe that there are sexual and psychological reasons to avoid a hysterectomy if it is not truly necessary (Cutler, 1990). The wholesale removal of the uterus, as well as the resulting changes in the ligaments and the nerves in the area, can lead to changes in the sexual experience. The more we learn about sexual functioning, we know that the uterus, cervix and ovaries may be important sexual as well as reproductive organs. At one time, women were told what kind of orgasm to have, primarily by the orthodox psychoanalysts. The best orgasm, we were told, was the "mature vaginal" orgasm, in contrast to the "immature clitoral" orgasm. Now we know that women have a wide variety of sexual experiences (Masters and others, 1970). Linda Ellerbee once said that, "The best time to laugh is anytime you can" (ABC News, 1993). The same can be said for having any kind of orgasm. Many women experience some feeling of uterine contractions during orgasm and have had some cervical stimulation during intercourse. Thus, the removal of the uterus may have specific sexual implications.

Psychologically, hysterectomy is a major surgical procedure and can be very disruptive to a woman's life, involving several months of recovery. The literature on the association between hysterectomy and depression is complicated, as we will discuss. Although hysterectomy and oophorectomy do not necessarily cause depression in most women, they are major surgeries, with all that is involved. For some women, the loss of their reproductive organs may have a symbolic as well as a biological significance. In some cultures "no periods" implies "not feminine." One of our favorite gynecologists has even seen some patients whose husbands left them after a hysterectomy. Rather than experiencing a natural and gradual menopause, a woman literally wakes up to find that she can no longer choose to bear children. Overall, then, we do not view the reproductive organs as "not necessary anyway" as many of our menopausal patients have been told as a justification for a hysterectomy and oophorectomy.

OOPHORECTOMY TO PREVENT OVARIAN CANCER

Prevention of cancer is one of the common reasons for recommending oophorectomy. This may be an alternative for women who have strong family histories of ovarian cancer and who have completed their families. Doctors Winifred Cutler and Celso-Ramón García report that the recommendation of routinely removing the ovaries in the average woman was based on a false statistic that was reported in a medical journal. This statistic suggested that there would be a 5 percent chance that an ovary would become cancerous over a woman's lifetime. When Doctors Cutler and García checked this fact, they found that the true rate was only one tenth this amount. Thus, they have suggested that routine removal of ovaries in the average woman was unfounded (Cutler and García, 1992, p. 216).

Many women continue to be fearful of ovarian cancer specifically because it often lacks symptoms. Elizabeth, one of our patients, was told that the removal of her ovaries would alleviate her fear. Since she had no family history of ovarian cancer, the oophorectomy was being suggested to her for primarily psychological reasons. This suggestion was made without any psychological evaluation. The recommendation failed to consider the psychological impact of oophorectomy itself, and the fact that Elizabeth might certainly have gone on to worry about other forms of cancer, such as breast or colon cancer. These cancers are actually more common, but no reasonable person would suggest removing these organs ahead of time. In fact, removal of the ovaries does not absolutely guarantee the prevention of ovarian cancer if any bit of tissue remains.

One scenario for removing a woman's ovaries, or performing oophorectomy, occurs when the woman is having a hysterectomy for another reason. She then may decide or be advised that she may as well take out her ovaries to "prevent ovarian cancer." Women who are perimenopausal are sometimes told that "they don't need the organs anymore anyway." For women in general, a large number of healthy ovaries will be removed in order to prevent one case of ovarian cancer. Granted, ovarian cancer, a silent killer, is a truly terrifying fear. By now we all know the case of Gilda Radner, whose story exemplifies a woman's worst nightmare; a fear that a recurrent abdominal symptom, however vague, could actually be invasive cancer. But, the chances for the average woman who has no symptoms getting ovarian cancer are very small.

For women who do have strong family histories of ovarian cancer—that is, two first-degree relatives (mother, sisters) who have suffered from the disease—the situation is different. They face a more complicated decision involving whether or not to have the hysterectomy and oophorectomy to avoid cancer but risk the complications of the surgery. These women with strong family histories of ovarian cancer, who may have a risk of ovarian cancer up to 50 percent, are in a different situation than the thousands of American women who may undergo unnecessary oophorectomies.

What about women over the age of forty-five? There is some disagreement within the field about this. Drs. Cutler and García conclude that "the ovaries should not be removed unless they are diseased" (Cutler and García, 1992, p. 207). Doctors Carlson, Nichols and Schiff write that conserving the ovaries is "recommended for women under the age of forty-five and oophorectomy is recommended for women over the age of fifty. For women forty-five to fifty years of age, the decision should be individualized with consideration given to the patient's menopausal status, the risk of ovarian cancer and the ability to take estrogen replacement therapy" (Carlson and others, 1993, p. 859). So, the choice of surgically removing your ovaries depends on your age group and your individual medical situation, and should be discussed with your doctor.

✦ ALTERNATIVES TO HYSTERECTOMY

There is now a wide variety of alternative treatments for conditions that once led to hysterectomy. These treatments are summarized in Table 9-3. Fibroids, a common reason for hysterectomy, can sometimes be removed surgically without removing the entire uterus. This procedure is called myomectomy. It is technically more difficult, however, and has a higher risk for recurrence of fibroids. For these reasons, few people would consider this operation postmenopausally. If fibroids are big enough to obstruct bowel or urinary functioning, cause pain or persistent bleeding with anemia, and have not responded to other medical treatments, hysterectomy may well be the best alternative.

While a large percentage of white and African-American women approaching menopause may have fibroids, most have no symptoms. Since fibroids are stimulated by the hormone estrogen, they may subs-

---

Table 9–3

COMMON CONDITIONS ASSOCIATED WITH HYSTERECTOMY AND ALTERNATIVE TREATMENTS

Condition	Treatment
Fibroids (uterine leiomyomas)	Monitor During Menopausal Period Myomectomy
Dysfunctional Uterine Bleeding	Hormonal Treatment Endometrial Ablation
Endometrial Hyperplasia	Dilation and Curettage (D&C) Progestin Therapy and Monitoring
Endometriosis	Hormone Suppression Using Danazol
Genital Prolapse	Pessary, Topical Estrogen and Exercises
Chronic Pelvic Pain	Comprehensive Evaluation and Treatment, Including Psychological Nonsteroidal Anti-inflammatory Drugs

tantially decrease in size as estrogen declines during your natural menopause. So, one course of action, if your fibroids are not too troubling, is to monitor them over the perimenopausal period and to see if the situation improves. In addition, there are several drugs that can shrink fibroid tumors, a class of agents called gonadotropin-releasing hormone (GnRH) agonists. These drugs are known to decrease the size of fibroids, but in most cases they will grow back after the treatment is discontinued. In addition, there are side effects, including hot flashes and bone loss. However, the medication may be helpful in the short-term until the onset of menopause, or in cases to reduce the fibroids enough to enable a vaginal hysterectomy (Adamson, 1992). This medical treatment could avoid an unnecessary hysterectomy. However, this drug is very expensive—$375 per shot (monthly) and some insurance plans do not cover it.

A fibroid can be located by using a pelvic ultrasound or sonogram and it can be monitored to see how the treatment is proceeding. Gynecologists frequently express the size of a fibroid in terms of pregnancy, for example, ten weeks (odd but true). Laser surgery for fibroids causes less bleeding than traditional myomectomy and uses a device called a hysterascope, which allows the surgeon to look into the uterus itself. However, this procedure is indicated primarily for smaller fibroids, and only ones protruding substantially into the uterine cavity.

The first step in evaluating abnormal uterine bleeding is an endometrial biopsy. This involves taking a piece of the lining of the uterus. It is performed in a doctor's office and causes some minimal discomfort and bleeding. If an endometrial biopsy is normal, many women may choose to monitor the situation with the support of their primary professional. Some bleeding may be controlled by repeated short courses of progesterone treatment. A new technique has been developed that is called endometrial ablation, which shows increasing promise for perimenopausal women. This procedure uses either a high-frequency electrical current or a laser to destroy the endometrium or the lining of the uterus. To date, endometrial ablation is effective in its ability to stop unnecessary bleeding and preserve the uterus. There is limited experience with women in the perimenopausal years, but some studies suggest that this procedure can be used prior to taking HRT. Both myomectomies and endometrial ablation are new and very specialized techniques. So, you need to find surgeons who have performed many of these procedures. These gynecologic surgeons are often affiliated with medical schools.

Endometriosis is another condition that often improves at the time of menopause. This occurs because the monthly cycles of the building up of the endometrial lining begin to diminish and ultimately stop. So endometriosis may improve through your menopausal years. Endometrial ablation can also be used for endometriosis. In addition, medical alternatives include taking the medications Danazol or Lupron.

Genital prolapse occurs when the muscles of the pelvic floor are so weakened that they sag. Many women describe this as a feeling of heaviness or "drooping." This can occur in women who have had multiple pregnancies. One way to prevent prolapse is by taking care of ourselves during pregnancy and childbirth.

But for some of us, by now "the horse is out of the barn," since our childbearing years are long gone. So what can be done if there are symptoms of prolapse? First, it is never too late to try the Kegel's exercises. The Kegel's exercises we outlined in Chapter Three are a key part of maintaining our pelvic muscles. These are often used in combination with a vaginal pessary—a device that holds the uterus in place. Susanne Morgan in her book *Coping with a Hysterectomy*, also suggests certain yoga positions, or kneeling on the floor with your chest down to relieve discomfort (Morgan, 1982). Finally, there are surgical alternatives to hysterectomy. Gynecological surgeons can perform a suspension operation to lift and reattach the uterus.

Chronic pelvic pain is one of the most troubling reasons for hysterectomy. Chronic pelvic pain is defined as pain that has lasted at least six months. Chronic pelvic pain may have any number of gynecological causes or may be related to other medical problems, like irritable bowel syndrome or inflammatory bowel disease. Psychological factors may also play a role. One study found that almost 40 percent of women with chronic pelvic pain had experienced physical trauma as children (Rector, 1990, p. 117). Unless a precise cause for the pain has been found, such as an unusually large fibroid, it seems quite risky to have a hysterectomy. Chronic pelvic pain, like any aspect of sexuality, may involve more than the genital organs, including past history, attitudes and overall physical health. Unfortunately many women who have pelvic pain before hysterectomy, have pelvic pain after hysterectomy. One study found that 22 percent had persistent pelvic pain even after the surgery. Another found that a high percentage of women with pelvic pain had histories of sexual and/or physical abuse (Caldirola, 1983; Herman, 1986). It is tragic to think that these women may not have been evaluated thoroughly before experiencing a possibly unnecessary and ineffective operation for their presenting problem.

Chronic pelvic pain is sometimes linked to depression and depression has, in turn, been linked to hysterectomy. A study by the McKinlay group found that normal menopause is not associated with depression, but that hysterectomy is. This study found that 18 percent of women who had experienced hysterectomies were depressed. Since the McKinlays were able to follow these women before and after their hysterectomies, they were also able to pinpoint an additional concern. Many of the woman were depressed *prior* to their hysterectomies (McKinlay and others, 1987). Women who were depressed might have experienced more pains and gynecological problems. These chronic symptoms might have led them to visit numerous doctors, ultimately leading to the chain of events resulting in hysterectomy. The problem here is, of course, that the depression may be worsened by hysterectomy and oophorectomy. So it looks, once again, like depressed women may be especially prone to unnecessary medical procedures, including hysterectomies.

Given the fact that chronic pelvic pain and depression may ultimately lead to unnecessary hysterectomy, it is important that women be evaluated comprehensively. So, if your physician recommends a psychiatric evaluation as one part of a comprehensive evaluation for chronic pelvic pain, you should not be offended. Try to be open to it as part of a thorough assessment, because if there is a psychological component to chronic pelvic pain, it should be treated. If it is not treated, hysterectomy could make the problem worse. So, it is important to try to be open to psychological treatments as well as medical treatments. This is not to say that you should accept *only* a psychological evaluation for chronic pelvic pain. Too many women have experienced the "There, there dear, it's all in your head" approach and know that it is demeaning and often a manifestation of a physician's frustration.

← ALTERNATIVES TO OOPHORECTOMY TO PREVENT OVARIAN CANCER

This is an area in which more work is needed. Early detection of ovarian cancer is crucial. Some gynecologists now recommend a combination of ultrasound and a blood test called CA125 in order to monitor the possibility of ovarian cancer in high-risk patients. However, this technology is just developing. CA125 was actually developed in order to monitor the *progress* of treatment for ovarian cancer after it has been diagnosed, not to predict the development of it. An additional problem with this blood test is that it has a high degree of false positives, meaning that in many women, the blood level is elevated, even though there is no cancer present. Thus, sometimes the use of this blood test

can increase fear in women unnecessarily and may even lead to unnecessary oophorectomy. We hope there will soon be further development in the technology to detect ovarian cancer early.

Overall though, many hysterectomies and oophorectomies are
being performed for unclear reasons. We know, too, that there are
alternative treatments for many of the conditions that once automati-
cally led to hysterectomy. Many of you may feel that "just taking it all
out," especially during the menopausal years is a good idea. We believe
that you need to be aware of the advances in medical treatment and
that you should consider alternatives. Using this new information, you
will be better able to make your decision.

✦ COMMUNICATION

Hysterectomies are sometimes necessary. Alicia's story points out the
importance of doctor-patient communication, even when there is
agreement that a woman needs a hysterectomy.

Alicia, our fifty-one-year-old patient, first came to see us six
months after her hysterectomy. Her story reveals the importance of
communication, not only between doctor and patient, but between a
woman and her family. Alicia was "fed-up," to put it in her own words,
with her gynecologist and his office. For fifteen years she had gone to
see him, but been mildly irritated when he was more apt to talk about
books, or recent vacation plans, than to concentrate on Alicia's concerns about her health. She knew that her doctor was trying to build
rapport, but he was not meeting her needs, since she wanted to ask
more detailed questions about a variety of gynecological concerns. She
became somewhat resentful when she reached the menopausal years
and began to have questions about her hot flashes and, as time passed,
irregular bleeding.

Alicia had been married to Brian, her college sweetheart, for thirty
years and was content. Together they had raised three children. However, she did express concern about their communication. She was a bit
frustrated by always being the one to initiate conversations about feelings. He used "report talk," whereas Alicia needed "rapport talk."
Alicia did mention that if she and Brian were to enter a discussion
about politics, he would suddenly spend up to an hour exhausting
them both while expounding on his distrust and disgust of the system.
When it came to concerns about her health care, the only response
Alicia could get from Brian centered around whether or not the local
democratic representative in their district could be beaten.

When Alicia was about fifty she began to have irregular and heavy bleeding. She thought about reporting it to her doctor, but waited a few months because she thought it was just her menopause. When she finally did go to her doctor, he did a pelvic exam and then recommended that she have an endometrial biopsy. Alicia had no idea what an endometrial biopsy was. When she asked him if anything was seriously wrong he answered, "Don't worry about anything. In ninety-nine percent of these cases nothing is wrong." When she then asked about what an endometrial biopsy was, or what he was looking for, he told her again not to worry and left the office. Alicia then questioned the nurse in the office, hoping to get a little more information as she had in earlier years. This day, however, the nurse was too busy to answer her questions. As Alicia left the office, she looked back at the nurse and receptionist with a feeling of sadness and frustration.

Alicia came home in need of reassurance and comfort that Brian was unable to give. When Alicia told Brian of the endometrial biopsy, he replied by saying, "Don't get yourself worked up over nothing."

"But this is serious," she asserted.

"It'll be fine," Brian responded, feeling that he had adequately addressed his wife's fears. He was not aware, as many spouses are not, that his wife wanted to talk about this situation in some depth. Brian felt that if he did not have hard information about this medical condition, he could not talk to her about it. He was unfortunately not aware that just the process of sharing her fears would have made Alicia feel better.

Because she could not find comfort in Brian, Alicia chose to turn to a neighborhood friend whom she saw occasionally for coffee, or for dinner when their husbands were out of town. She felt supported as she shared her fears while her friend listened. She then turned to her daughter, Norma, but having been the mother for so many years, her long-distance phone call across country to her eldest daughter turned into a counseling session for Norma's failing marriage. But at least the conversation with Norma took Alicia's mind off the possibility of that dreaded word, cancer, for a moment. But on the whole, Alicia found little comfort from her friends and family, and spent a great deal of the following week anxious about what tomorrow would bring.

Because Alicia's doctor was off on the day that she was scheduled for her endometrial biopsy, one of his partners performed it. Alicia was on the examining table, nervous, waiting in her hospital johnny when the surgeon came in. This was their entire conversation: He walked in saying, "Endometrial biopsy. Please scoot down into the stirrups. Just relax. Okay. Bye."

At this point, Alicia felt a combination of such rage and fear that she was literally speechless. As much as she had had concerns about her regular physician, he did, at least, treat her as a person and tried his best to communicate. This person had literally spoken fewer than a dozen words to her in their entire encounter for a procedure that hurt a bit and could have meant a serious life-threatening condition.

Alicia's rage spilled over when the worst of her fears were validated and her gynecologist told her that the results of her pathology test indicated invasive uterine cancer, but that they should be able to "take care of it with a hysterectomy." She finally asserted herself and insisted that the gynecologist sit with her and Brian and spend some time going over her questions and concerns. Alicia was quick to point out that she felt that having Brian along during those consultations made the doctor more apt to take her requests seriously. When at home, Alicia addressed her fears and panic with Brian. When Brian started sounding "just like my doctor," Alicia told him that she needed his help and understanding now more than ever, and that he must give it his best shot. As the days passed, Brian learned to listen a bit more and tried his best to share feelings.

When the surgery was over, her gynecologist commented that he was "almost 99 percent certain" that he had gotten it all. Not realizing his earlier similar remark, suggesting that he was 99 percent certain that she did not have cancer. This response had a strong negative effect on Alicia. "What if he didn't get it all?" she thought. "Did he say that to everybody? What if I am in the one percent?" But her doctor was gone long before she could articulate any of these fears.

Alicia's recovery was long and tedious. It gave her enough time, however, to think about the fact that she wanted a new doctor. Having seen the movie *Network* when she first came to us she said, "I'm mad as hell and I'm not going to take it anymore!" By the time Alicia came to us, she and Brian had found a few more things to talk about. Because Alicia and Brian had always had an affectionate and sexual life together, they found ways to stay in touch while Alicia was recovering. Often that would mean sitting close together on the back porch and reading, while Brian gave his wife a shoulder massage. She was happy also that Norma came to visit from San Francisco, partly to get away from her marriage, and both Brian and Norma took care of the household chores and made sure that Alicia received a good amount of rest.

As part of Alicia's recovery, she was given a course of radiation therapy, and Brian was actively involved, helping her understand and deal with her concerns every step of the way. Because Alicia had been fifty-one, she accepted the recommendation that her ovaries also be removed. She was started on estrogen replacement therapy soon after the operation. Alicia chose the patch and has adjusted well to the therapy.

Now it is five years later and Alicia and Brian talk of all that had happened to her. They often speak of the hysterectomy and how it had saved Alicia's life. Brian, having witnessed an event that could have taken his wife away from him, grew to listen and appreciate the time that they had together even more. He completely understood Alicia's need to find a different doctor, listened and offered his opinion as she began to learn more about prevention and maintenance of her health.

Alicia learned to be more assertive in her health care. When she comes to Women's Health Associates, she often has a list of concerns written on a pad that she checks off one by one as they have been answered. She credits her hysterectomy with saving her life, and her previous gynecologist's attitude to making her the "demanding patient" she has become.

Alicia's case points out the different dynamics in doctor-patient relationships. Alicia's first gynecologist undoubtedly meant well in his rapport-building chats, but what this particular patient wanted was a slightly more detailed discussion of medical care. The second surgeon's attitude toward Alicia during the endometrial biopsy, however, left us speechless, as it did her. There is no justification for not discussing a procedure, no matter how hurried a physician might be. Even given these problems, Alicia had no doubt that her hysterectomy had been the right course of action.

It is a little more complicated when hysterectomy is an option, but not absolutely necessary. You can look at the list of medical reasons to consider hysterectomy and the alternative treatments on Table 9-3. This is just a beginning list and undoubtedly as treatments develop, you will be able to add to it. You can also investigate alternative treatments by contacting a women's health practice or a major university-affiliated hospital that deals in women's surgery.

After reviewing this chapter, if you do not find that you have enough information, you might seek additional resources to answer your specific questions. There are several excellent books addressing hysterectomy. *Hysterectomy, Before and After* was written by Dr. Winifred Cutler, a reproductive biologist who has written extensively on menopause and hysterectomy. She has been involved in independent research and is a faculty member of a medical school. Dr. Cutler's writing style on hysterectomy is both detailed and clear. The book will inform you as to every aspect of the changes that you will experience. Another book that focuses on alternatives to hysterectomy is *You Don't Need a Hysterectomy* by Ivan K. Strausz, M.D. (Reading, MA:

Addison-Wesley, 1993). *Ourselves Growing Older,* published by the Boston Women's Health Collective, is one of their most recent books to help educate women to be good health consumers. It summarizes much of the medical treatment but focuses more on alternatives to hysterectomy.

With these resources and others, you will get a wide range of information that can help you make an informed decision. After you have looked at the alternative treatments, if you are still considering a hysterectomy, you should get an independent second opinion. Your second opinion can come from another gynecologist who is certified by the American Board of Obstetrics and Gynecology. Another possibility is an internist, certified by the American Board of Internal Medicine. Many internists, especially those specializing in endocrinology, can suggest nonsurgical approaches to your problem. Most insurance companies now require this precaution, and this is good because women do not want to offend their doctors. This fear of giving offense is one of our worst enemies when it comes to getting good medical care. Alicia might well have been able to work things out with her first gynecologist if she had been able to talk about her concerns with him. Wanting a second opinion is a perfectly acceptable course of action and you should get another point of view before deciding upon hysterectomy. This means that you should not ask your doctor for the name of a close colleague. You might ask friends, or contact your local university hospital, in order to get a true independent second opinion.

Here is the problem in seeking a medical opinion, or any opinion regarding health care. If you go to a psychologist, she or he will probably recommend psychological treatment. As one of our colleagues put it, "If you go to Midas, you get a muffler." If you go to a surgeon, she or he may well recommend surgical treatment. For that reason, it might be best to talk to a primary care doctor or a gynecologist who does not perform hysterectomies, a general internist or family practitioner. By talking to one of these doctors about your condition, whether it is endometriosis, pelvic pain, or fibroids, you may get a true second point of view. A medical approach may be entirely different from a surgical approach. It is worth taking this additional time to think through your individual situation before making an important decision like this.

After obtaining a second opinion, and/or returning to your first physician, you might want to take a family member or friend with you. You need to know what specific condition you have, and can review alternatives to hysterectomy by asking what will happen if you do not have a hysterectomy. As we have discussed in earlier chapters, making serious decisions about your health care can increase your anxiety. Also, your anxiety can interfere with your ability to process information. That is what friends and family are for, to help you in this situation. Even though Brian was not a big talker, his mere presence signified to Alicia's doctor that this was an important situation. Also, Brian's support gave Alicia more confidence and a feeling that she was cared for. In addition, since hysterectomy requires an extensive recovery period, it is important for your family and friends to be informed so that they can be prepared to be supportive.

Talk to women who have had a hysterectomy. With the numbers we have discussed, it shouldn't be hard to find one. You will find a range of opinions about the procedure. Take Connie, for example, who after two years of completely unpredictable vaginal bleeding, was determined to have a hysterectomy. A busy, fifty-year-old educational administrator, Connie was fed up with the drug therapy and several dilation and curettage procedures that she had had in the last two years. When her gynecologist suggested that she should have a hysterectomy, she leapt at the chance and checked herself into a hospital three days before Christmas.

Unfortunately, the hospital was somewhat understaffed during the holidays, especially with respect to nurses. Connie was in a fair amount of pain after the operation, and found it difficult to get her nurses' attention during those moments when she needed assistance the most. Her friend Margaret, who was a particularly resourceful teacher on school break, moved into the adjacent bed in this two-bed room, put on a nightgown and pretended to be a patient so that she could take care of Connie twenty-four hours a day. Although Connie's nurses were aware that Margaret was only there to support her friend, they welcomed the intrusion. In addition to nursing Connie, Margaret brought in several magazines and favorite books, and when her friend was not resting, she would try to help her pass the time with inspiring stories and articles. Connie continued to improve and was able to leave the hospital several days after Christmas. She has had an excellent recovery and complains only of a little bit of weight gain. She is particularly grateful to Margaret for her supportive care.

This story points out the need for support from family and friends. Of course, it is not necessary to go to such lengths as Margaret did, but certainly your family and friends can pool together to support, encourage and listen to you during such an important time.

In addition, many hospitals have prehysterectomy groups that provide support and information that can help you make a decision.

✦ IF YOU DECIDE TO HAVE A HYSTERECTOMY

Our emphasis in this chapter has been prevention because of our strong feelings about the number of unnecessary hysterectomies. Nonetheless, we are aware that many times hysterectomy, even an elective hysterectomy, is indicated. Either medical treatments have failed, or you and your doctor have discussed it and opted for hysterectomy, knowing all the alternatives as well as the risks and benefits. Still, it's a good idea to prepare yourself for any surgery by understanding what will happen.

If you decide to have a hysterectomy, find a surgeon who is extremely experienced. You have the right to know how many procedures the surgeon has done. You have the right to know what hospital he or she uses, and you have the right to know what to expect. As a patient, remember that informed consent does not mean signing a piece of paper the day before surgery, as is usual procedure. It means having a full understanding of what the surgery involves and what the possible outcomes can be. Some hysterectomies are performed vaginally, but the majority are performed abdominally. In abdominal hysterectomy, the uterus is removed through an incision in the abdomen. In vaginal hysterectomy, an incision is made through the vagina and around the cervix. Although vaginal hysterectomy has a higher rate of infection, abdominal hysterectomy leaves an external scar. The type of surgery frequently is related to the reason for the hysterectomy. Some women choose to donate blood before their surgery. Both operations are major surgery, usually requiring general anesthesia and an inpatient hospitalization of one to two days for vaginal hysterectomy and four to five days for abdominal hysterectomy. Other forms of anesthesia, spinal or epidural can also be used.

You should know how much the hysterectomy will cost. In these days of cost containment, it is likely that your hysterectomy will need to be pre-authorized by any health plan. Nonetheless, even given this, there are often additional costs to a hospitalization that you should know about. This will help you do the appropriate financial planning.

The immediate surgical recovery period also means abstaining from sexual intercourse. You should not feel pressured to resume sexual activity until you feel comfortable. Preparation for surgery should involve your partner, so that there is an understanding of the sense of the delicate nature of hysterectomy. If a couple communicates well and shows consideration, then they are more likely to show a good adjustment after the operation. It is most important here that women not resume sexual activity until they feel comfortable and until their partner fully understands their physical and psychological needs related to the hysterectomy.

DEPRESSION AFTER HYSTERECTOMY

Although depression can occur in some women after a hysterectomy, you do not need to see it as inevitable. As we mentioned, the McKinlays found that many of the women who were depressed after a hysterectomy also had oophorectomies and may have been depressed before. Dr. Carlson and her colleague found no association in general between hysterectomy and depression.

There are several issues for you to consider. First, if you have an oophorectomy as well as a hysterectomy, your estrogen level will plummet. Thus, you will not experience a slow reduction as we have described in natural menopause; you will go cold turkey! So, the issue of hormone replacement therapy is quite different. So if you opt against hormone replacement therapy after an oophorectomy, you should try to use some of the alternative treatments for hot flashes in order to minimize your discomfort.

You will be less likely to become depressed if you plan your surgery carefully, provide yourself with ample social support, and allow yourself to explore any psychological issues that may arise.

✦ COMMUNICATING WITH YOUR FAMILY

It is important for your family to know that abdominal hysterectomy is a major operation. In addition to the recovery period, one study found that it took women a full thirteen months, on the average, to feel that they had gotten back to normal. This was in contrast to other operations, including gallbladder or appendectomy, where it only took 4.2 months, on average, to recover. The support of your family and friends is crucial in such a long recovery period.

We have found that many families have difficulty in reacting to the disability (even if temporary) of the mother, and even when the children are long since out of the house and grown with their own children. Sometimes denial sets in. The best way to cope with Mom's problem is to pretend that it doesn't exist. This might work well for everyone but Mom. Everyone goes back to business as usual, and unfortunately that often means that Mom is back to work at home entirely too soon. Don't do it! Household chores are often more strenuous than jobs outside the home. Everyone can learn to pitch in, and you need to take it slow after major surgery. Ask your family to treat you as you have treated them when they have been sick. Take it slow, and over time you will know how much you are capable of doing. It will not take thirteen months to make it back to your daily routine— most women can do so after two to three months, but your body will let you know when you've done too much. Talking to one of the nurses can be informative and supportive. This can be extremely helpful when you are planning your recovery period. Each woman is different, but you may begin to know what to expect in terms of when you would be able to get back to your daily routine, how you will feel and so on.

Again, it is a good idea to talk to a woman who has had a hysterectomy. You may be reluctant to do so. You may feel that you probably will not need it or that hysterectomy is a private matter. Nonetheless, talking with other women about a problem has a long history of serving women well. You will be relieved to know that your lack of sexual interest may be short-term, or that another woman has benefited from hormone replacement therapy. The reactions of other women's family members may be similar to yours. Women who have recovered from the hysterectomy often feel better by being able to share their knowledge with other women.

Try to become physically active as soon as you can after the procedure. This does not mean jumping on the StairMaster the day after surgery! By beginning to walk around your room as soon as you can, you will have a smoother recovery. Walking not only begins to help you regain use of your muscles, but will also help your gastrointestinal tract get moving, which can be a problem sometimes after surgery. As you feel better and can get more exercise on a daily basis, you will find that your mood will improve as well. This activity will also help you to firm muscles, and it can help in dealing with the mood changes that you may experience as a result of the operation.

If you have had an oophorectomy and you are perimenopausal, you need to consider the issue of hormone replacement therapy. You will probably have hot flashes, since they are reported by up to 70 percent of women after a hysterectomy. If, on the other hand, you are already postmenopausal and hot-flash free, you will not redevelop hot flashes because the reduction of hormones has already occurred. This is because the hot flashes associated with oophorectomy are triggered by the sudden reduction in estrogen from high premenopausal levels to low levels. The most important thing is to take care of yourself. This is major surgery, and you will recover. It will take time, and support will help. In the words of Alicia, "After all I've been through, I'm going to enjoy this recovery now."

◆ RESOURCES

"Come on up, I'll be your lifeline." This refrain from a poignant Holly Near song summarizes our feeling about social support for women who have had hysterectomies. We have identified other resources as well. You and your family, your relationship with your physician, and books can all help you not only decide whether to have a hysterectomy, but can help you plan ahead and minimize any disruption that the surgery might cause.

Through the hospital's social service or nursing department, you can often get in touch with a woman who has had a hysterectomy and is willing to volunteer her time to talk with you. Many communities have cancer support groups for women who have had breast or ovarian cancer. In some communities, specific hysterectomy support groups are also offered. Kara told us this story:

> The hysterectomy support group is small. Six women are sitting around a table drinking coffee and tea. Joanne, the social worker who leads the group, has sensitively put away the childbirth education materials used by another group that utilizes the same conference room. She usually begins the group with an open-ended question of how things have been going. This group has been together and meeting for six months. Two of the members have only been out of the hospital for several weeks. Two others have been out for several months and the "grandmothers" have been involved with numerous hysterectomy support groups over the years, having had their hysterectomies five years ago.

Kara is a forty-five-year-old African-American woman who had a hysterectomy because of recurrent fibroids that did not respond to medical treatment. Her surgery consisted of the removal of her uterus and her ovaries. The fibroids had been a problem all of her life, even preventing a normal pregnancy. Fortunately, she and her husband were able to adopt a healthy baby girl and Ruth was now a fun-loving ten-year-old who liked to rollerblade and play computer games.

Kara and her husband Roy have been having a difficult time more recently. Kara is having a slow recovery from her hysterectomy three months ago. She hasn't been able to pay as much attention to Ruth or Roy as she had in the past. She seems distracted and tired all of the time. As a self-employed business woman, she had lost a significant amount of money by taking two months off after the operation. Now that she was back to work, she felt a bit better but still hadn't regained her old passion for the "big sell." Roy, an insurance agent, always tried to be supportive of his wife, but he was having difficulty understanding her adjustment.

Sally, one of the older women in the group, asked her, "I'm wondering if this is raising old feelings of sadness for you?" Kara's eyes began to fill with tears. She hadn't realized that in addition to the normal adjustment after hysterectomy, she would be reliving some of her feelings of sadness over the infertility issue of earlier years. To be sure, she was a devoted and involved mother, and Ruthy was the center of her existence. Still, the hospital held for her many sad associations of feelings of loss, of anxiety and of tremendous disappointment.

The other women in the group were very protective of Kara. It was as if all their maternal feelings erupted at once and came to her aid. This feeling of connectedness and recognition that other women knew what she was going through helped Kara to sort out her feelings with the group over time. Some of the other members, those who had had children and those who hadn't, were able to share with her their feelings about the childbearing part of their life being over, and somewhat suddenly also.

One night the unthinkable happened. Some of the husbands of women in the group became interested enough to form a "men's group." These men decided to share their feeling of anxiety and concern for their wives when they did not know what to do. Many of these men had not been in a group with other men discussing anything related to their family since their childbirth education classes, which may have been anywhere from ten to twenty years ago, and some of them had never been in a group before. At the end of one of these evenings, the two groups and the couples were able to share their variety of experiences. It was somehow consoling to Roy to hear Jeff, the husband of another woman in the group, say that after a year his wife was back to her old self.

Kara's situation makes the point that although women don't tend to get depressed after a hysterectomy in general, the experience can bring out previous psychological issues. Undoubtedly, a woman having a hysterectomy at age forty-five is in a completely different category than a woman at the age of twenty-eight or thirty-eight. By forty-five she has either had her children or probably resolved the issue of childbearing in her life. But sometimes previous experiences with sexuality, infertility or hospitals themselves can lead to an awakening of old psychological pain. In such a case, the value of meeting with other women to discuss the situation is enormous. At other times, talking with an individual volunteer might also be helpful. If the pain becomes severe or if a symptom such as anxiety or depression occurs, then you can also discuss the situation with a mental health professional. But talking with other women is often the first step.

We have found that normal menopause also evokes these psychological issues in some women. This is especially true when there are unresolved issues concerning motherhood, abortion or infertility. Once again, sharing your concerns with a friend, participating in a support group or seeing a psychologist or other mental health professional will help.

CHAPTER TEN

Promoting a Healthy Lifestyle

PLEASE DON'T WORRY, THIS IS NOT A CHAPTER WHERE WE WILL INSIST that you eat huge quantities of oat bran and fish oil, work out with weights five times a week, jog three or four miles a day and abstain from all alcohol and sugar. Although, if you can do those things, by all means, carry on. However, most of our lives are full of responsibilities, time restrictions and old habits that make such a regimented diet and exercise program impractical. As you read on, keep in mind that our intention is not to burden you with unrealistic suggestions, but to give you a set of principles and ideas that, combined with your own good judgment, you can use to develop a plan that works for you.

Midlife is an ideal time for us to refocus on our health. Freed from some of the burdens of family responsibilities, we can now spend some of our time on planning for the future. We don't want to merely focus on longevity or the length of our life, but to improve the quality of our lives as well. None of us would look forward to living into her eighties if it means being severely crippled by osteoporosis or serious cardiovascular problems. Fortunately, with a careful assessment, and by setting some priorities, each of us can devise a plan that will improve and promote health throughout the next phase of our lives.

Prevention of illness is one of the most overlooked areas of medicine and all of health care. Unfortunately, only 1 to 3 percent of the American health care expenditures goes for preventive services. Given the clear link between such issues as smoking, substance abuse and lack of exercise to so many health problems, this small percentage reflects a problem in the priorities of the American health care system. By developing a good health-maintenance plan, you can do a lot to help prevent the development of serious illness. It's time to focus on healthy living.

There are six components of the Women's Health Promotion Plan. They are: routine health *Screening*, increased *Exercise*, *Relaxation*, *Eliminating* or reducing problematic behaviors, proper *Nutrition* and *Expanding* your social support system. We used the acronym SERENE, so that you can remember these five areas. We settled on "serene" for a very specific reason. One of the most important elements to a lifestyle focusing on health promotion is to remember to enjoy and accept life. As you will see, we believe that you should take control of your own health, especially in the area of promotion. But most importantly, we should all try to experience our middle years to the fullest, and take time to relax and enjoy our lives.

Before attending to any one of these six components, we need to look at some principles of change. You will have the best opportunity to change your life if you use these principles as a foundation. They are based on many years of psychological research investigating behavioral and cognitive factors in how people change. Each of these principles is well documented as having a positive effect on health promotion.

PRINCIPLE #1
Develop a realistic, specific and positive plan. At first, you might want to target only one or two behavior changes, like reducing the fat in your diet, for example. These targeted behaviors should have realistic goals. If, for example, you have always been overweight, do not try to lose forty pounds in two months. A realistic weight goal is especially important to women given our American socialization and emphasis on being too thin. In the areas of smoking cessation and alcohol treatment, most people feel that abstinence is the appropriate goal.

PRINCIPLE #2
Take small steps. Your changes can be small, but steady. You are not going to go from a diet of daily croissants to one of celery sticks. But, if you plan carefully and steadily, you will be able to make changes over the long run. Exercise plans, for example, have been found to fail

more often when they are overly heroic and intense. You need to walk before you can run, and so on.

PRINCIPLE #3
Think positive. This is not just some "don't worry, be happy" or Pollyanna approach, but once again is based on ample psychological research. We do not believe, though, that people who think certain ways or have certain personality styles are responsible for developing cancer. There is no evidence that this is true and this incorrect interpretation of the mind-body connection literature has been hurtful to many people with cancer. As we have discussed before, by trying to lower our stress levels, and maintaining an attitude of positive coping, we can improve our health. It is clear that as we age, we will encounter some health problems. With any luck, these health problems will be minor. But when coping with these problems, whether they are elevated blood pressure or increased stress, seeing them as a challenge and something that we can control is important. Stress is often a result of a lack of control in your life. By creating your own health-promotion plan with a positive attitude, you will be able to maintain control and feel better.

PRINCIPLE #4
Your commitment to change is key. After reviewing this chapter, you might choose only one or two categories to begin your health promotion plan. But make a firm commitment to do so. Many people find that, for example, choosing a quit date when they want to stop smoking is helpful if they do it long in advance and have a well-thought-out plan. This is also why so many smoking cessation programs are overwhelmed by new recruits shortly after the New Year. There is nothing wrong with New Year's resolutions, we just hope that you will be able to stick to them. By committing yourself to one or two areas for change, you are more likely to succeed.

PRINCIPLE #5
Restructure your environment to help you change. You can do this through small but steady changes. If you have targeted alcohol or smoking as your problem, you can limit your exposure by avoiding bars, restaurants and friends who continue to abuse those substances. If you are trying to cut back on fat, don't go to that Dunkin Donuts where you have always eaten a double-chocolate donut and assume that you will just buy coffee. In the area of exercise, find an exercise that is comfortable and easily available. By making these environmental

changes, you can help yourself follow through with your health-promotion plan.

PRINCIPLE #6
Provide yourself with ample reinforcement. Most of these behaviors have provided you with good feelings over the years. Food may have provided you with comfort, nicotine may have helped you feel more energetic, alcohol may have reduced anxiety. We understand this and know that this is why it is so difficult to give up so many of these behaviors. So, you need to fight fire with fire by developing a system of rewards. Try to structure the rewards frequently. For example, many women will buy themselves a new wardrobe once they have lost twenty or thirty pounds. But it is a long time between cutting down on some of those favorite foods and any significant weight change. A better strategy might be to buy yourself a new mystery novel on a weekly basis, or to go to a self-help group for support on a daily basis. So you can get rewards from yourself and from others.

PRINCIPLE #7
Try to avoid all-or-nothing thinking and other unhelpful cognitive styles. All-or-nothing thinking is perhaps the most destructive when it comes to changing difficult behaviors. Most of us know full well how it feels to have been successfully dieting for several days or weeks, or even months, only to experience a loss of control with resulting feelings of disappointment. Many women feel that they are either "on a diet" or "off a diet." It's important to rethink these changes as part of a new lifestyle. You are likely to slip up now and then. But by seeing the slipups as one bit of behavior and your next meal, or the next hour without cigarettes as one bit of behavior, you are less likely to be overwhelmed by your feelings and to go into an actual relapse. This is where the Alcoholics Anonymous motto of "One Day at a Time" got started and can be helpful to you when trying to conquer these difficult changes.

PRINCIPLE #8
Try to find a doctor who will help you in your efforts by focusing on prevention and support. Many doctors are less attentive to these issues than they should be. This is a result of a lack of training, as well as their need to attend to people who are suffering from acute illness. But with some care, you can find a doctor who will support your efforts. Many doctors at HMOs are more involved in preventive medicine. Yet you also need someone who can help you feel good and reinforce the

changes that need to be made. Your doctor can assist by helping you access self-help groups and university-affiliated behavioral medicine programs for your specific problem, and by just plain praising you when you have lost five pounds or abstained from alcohol or not smoked a cigarette for a month. Remember the other members of your health care team, including nurses, exercise physiologists, nutritionists and health psychologists, or other mental health professionals who can help you in this area.

James O. Prochaska, a clinical psychologist at the University of Rhode Island and his colleagues Drs. Carlo DiClemente and John Norcross have addressed the issue of relapse in their comprehensive analysis of how people change (Prochaska and others, 1992). Their stages of change model helps us to understand how to change some problematic behaviors like smoking and substance abuse. These researchers have studied thousands of people who are trying to change their problematic behaviors. They emphasize that people don't just change, but rather go through a set of predictable stages. The stages of change are: precontemplation, contemplation, preparation, action, maintenance and termination. Precontemplation is the stage where a person does not intend to change a behavior during the next six months. At this stage, many people do not have the problematic behavior identified as an issue. A women enters the contemplation stage when she has identified the problem and has begun to think about changing. Preparation involves planning to take action in the near future, like the next month, and may involve making some small changes already. The action stage is the time when a woman begins to change her problematic behavior. Maintenance involves maintaining the changed behavior. Most people feel that a behavior change should be maintained for six months before termination from a treatment program should be considered.

A major point of the stages of change model is that relapse is quite common. We do not emphasize this because we want to discourage you, but so you can understand that relapse is understandable. Most people, who relapse after trying to change their behavior, go back to an earlier stage of the model, but they don't go back to the precontemplation stage. In the area of smoking cessation, for example, people may make on the average between three or four attempts to change before attaining long-term maintenance. If you relapse, all that means is that you need to go over your plan and modify it. Try to identify what went wrong and plan your next attempt by addressing the problem. For example, you might find that you were able to maintain an exercise program during the summer, but as winter came, your exercise decreased. Your next exercise plan could include moving permanently to California or Florida, but that is probably not practical. So, you have to work harder on identifying an indoor exercise strategy that is affordable and comfortable for you.

By understanding the stages of change, you are more likely to find the appropriate treatment plan for you. For example, if you do not believe that you are drinking too much and your partner feels that you are, then an assessment of your drinking behavior by your primary care provider or a qualified substance abuse counselor may be helpful. If you identify where you are in the stages of change, you will be able to find the best target behaviors for you to change and to develop an appropriate treatment plan. You might be better off choosing a plan for which you are already prepared rather than a change about which you are ambivalent. For example, many people who are going from the contemplation to preparation stage go through a list of pros and cons. If, at the present time, your pros and cons are evenly balanced, then beginning a program based on behavior change may not be successful. This model shows great promise in helping us understand how people change.

Our work with Teresa exemplifies the attitudes of many midlife women when it comes to exercise and health promotion. Teresa has been our patient for many years. A sociologist, she appears on our public television and radio stations often as a consultant on sociological issues, especially the American family. At the age of fifty-one, Teresa feels that she has reached her prime. Teresa is witty, vivacious, committed to a number of feminist activities, and is particularly gifted at creating "sound bites" that are so valued by television.

Teresa grew up in a traditional Mexican/American family in Southern California. As one of three children, she was always very close to her siblings and her parents and committed to a family life. She came to the East coast after meeting her husband, Don, at UCLA. She moved to this area when Don was offered a professorship at a university. Teresa and Don have two children, Mark and Paula. As a young wife and mother, she opted to concentrate her energies on her family and home, taking graduate-level courses throughout their elementary school years and always maintaining that she would return to school full-time one day when her children were older. She was devoted to them, and she and her husband spent many hours following their sports, debates and other school activities.

When Mark and Paula reached high school, Teresa wanted to pursue her earlier interests. She kept that promise to herself and went back to school at the age of thirty-eight to obtain a doctorate in sociology.

She enjoyed graduate school, made many new friends, and finished her doctorate in four years. She states that she is fortunate to have a husband who has always been supportive of her aspirations, and admiring of her strong commitment to herself, her career and her family. Now, after almost ten years of publishing, she is in a tenured position at a local college. This tenure gives her the freedom to explore other professional activities like providing public information, a task that she always enjoyed tremendously. She is often called upon when some new study is released to explain the practical implications for American families.

Each time we meet with Teresa we are amazed at how well organized she is, planning her career and family-time down to the smallest detail. Although she credits this as the secret to her success, she recognizes that she has a tendency to be a little rigid. We discovered that Teresa has also been rigid in her diet. For the past twenty years, and perhaps most of her adult life, she has counted calories (Note: Technically a calorie is a unit of energy. What most of us refer to as a calorie is actually 1000 kilocalories, or a Calorie. Now that you know this bit of nutritional trivia, we will go back to using the word that you know best, calorie) and been careful to keep track of her daily intake of food. Teresa is a tall, large-boned woman. She comes to us normally for routine screening and health maintenance, rarely having any major medical complaints. But this past year was different for Teresa; she found that her normal dieting pattern was no longer working. For example, in the past, if she knew that she and her husband were going out to dinner on a Saturday night, she would be very careful to eat less during the week before and after. So, if she had gained a pound over the weekend, she could take it off within another week or so. This plan suddenly came to a screeching halt over the past year, and she gained five pounds. For a woman who was concerned about her weight and interested in her appearance because of her media exposure, this was a crushing blow.

When Teresa expressed her frustrations to us, we explained that over time the body's metabolism changes. The bad news is that not only does our metabolism slow down, and therefore we need fewer calories to maintain a certain weight, but in addition, if we do not exercise, our body weight will consist of a higher percentage of fat and a lower percentage of muscle, regardless of how muscular we may have been before. Teresa, never at a loss for words exclaimed, "Oh, wouldn't you just know it—all those cheesecakes I left by the side of the road and I'm still in trouble! Celery sticks and diet root beer for the rest of my life I suppose!"

We reassured Teresa that we were not going to suggest some rigid diet, where all she could have were vegetable sticks for snacks and a powdered shake in place of her morning muffin. We emphasized that although her diet was important, the role of exercise or physical activity could be a major player in her battle against the weight gain and in maintaining a good fat/muscle ratio. We recommended that Teresa work with an exercise physiologist to come up with an exercise program that would be suitable for her lifestyle. At first, she was extremely reluctant. She had never had the time for exercise and had functioned quite well with her previous plan. She was not particularly interested in becoming a "jock" at this point in her life. We reassured her that she need not resemble a woman in the "Just Do It!" sneaker commercial to reap the benefits of increased physical activity. After several conversations, she relented and met with an exercise physiologist and nutritionist; it was during that time that we discovered how Teresa's adolescence played a large part in her fear of exercise.

We also found out that Teresa's nutritional plan was quite sound. Fortunately, she had avoided the trap of so many women of alternating fasting with binging, or in depriving herself of calcium. She drank very little alcohol, consuming one to two glasses of wine on a weekly basis, if she and her husband went out to dinner. Although Teresa's calcium intake was more than the average American woman, she was still only consuming about 800 mg a day, and so we suggested that she use a calcium supplement. She decided to purchase large quantities of calcium carbonate–based antacids and would keep them in her purse so she could "pop one or two a day from time to time." We found that her diet was also high in fruits and vegetables, had an adequate amount of protein, and was overall a low-fat diet. Not that she didn't enjoy eating out and straying occasionally, but this was her general nutritional plan. Teresa, who likes to verbally spar with us, pointed out that she had an advantage growing up in California, where she developed an early appreciation of fruits and vegetables rather than the late conversions of so many people recently.

During those sessions, when we examined her attitude toward exercise, it became clear that she was similar to so many other women in the menopausal age group that we had known in our practice, having gone to junior and senior high school in the mid- to late fifties, when there was virtually no emphasis on women's health education in the schools. We laughed as Teresa shared with us her stories of the familiar dreaded gymsuit, a "tasteful" navy blue with capped sleeves and a built in belt that all the girls loathed. Besides feeling a bit silly in the exercise uniform, Teresa was never particularly coordinated and did her best just to get through the physical education class without too much embarrassment. She focused her skills and energies instead on academic events and the school chorus. Of course this was well before Title IX, the section of the Education Amendments of 1972 that outlawed sexual discrimination, so no attention was played to women's sports at all, and this was fine with Teresa. She preferred cheering in the stands and wearing her high school boyfriend's letter sweater on Fridays.

Further evaluation revealed that Teresa had also experienced what, for her, was a traumatic event in her early years. When Teresa was in the seventh grade, she and her family lived in a rural area where there were very few teachers. Therefore, her school system had hired two part-time physical education teachers from a local university. These were, unfortunately, attractive and flirtatious young men in their early twenties who had little or no experience teaching, but were physical education majors. The girls in the class, of course, developed mad crushes on these two young men. They were in a bind, wanting to do well in sports, but were afraid of looking silly during class. Teresa's fear and lack of coordination came out in an acrobatics class when she was awkwardly attempting a cartwheel which resulted in an embarrassing fall on the mat and a rip in the fashionable gymsuit. Although the teacher did, at first, rush to her side to make sure that she was not hurt, his response was to tease her, and even referred to the traumatic episode quite a few times throughout the semester. Teresa, of course, was mortified. She still could feel a slight twinge of embarrassment when she recounted the episode so many years later. She remembers her feelings more than the details of the event. She has wondered, over the years, whether the young men were engaged in good-natured teasing, or whether there was an element of prejudice involved, since she was one of the few Chicanas in a class dominated by Anglo girls. But overall, she still remembers her humiliation and this has carried over to her feelings about organized exercise.

Teresa had developed her tendency at that early age to compartmentalize things—to separate them into categories in order to cope. She quickly categorized physical education as a time where she could be humiliated and embarrassed. Physical education, as we have discussed in Chapter Four, "went off the list" for Teresa and many other women, never to return. Activity and physical education had a similar role in her life during college, where she was allowed to choose from several courses and thus chose shuffleboard, badminton and bowling. She preferred the games as they were less intimidating, shared activities that were already the source of humor among the other young women.

It took several sessions for Teresa to expand her view of physical education to include activities such as walking and swimming, as well as noncompetitive sports that she could share with other friends and her husband. After a careful analysis of her lifestyle, two things became clear. One was that now that she and her husband had more shared time, they were open to a joint activity. Don was a similarly intellectual and nonathletic man who maintained his health by walking to and from the university. He too knew he needed more physical activity, and over time, he and Teresa began to play tennis together on a weekly basis. One or two hours of tennis once a week is not enough to maintain bone mass or cardiovascular fitness, so we encouraged Teresa to find additional activities which she could add to her routine.

It was in fact a disagreement between Teresa and Don that finally helped her find her own exercise routine. Teresa was open to tennis as it would mean shared time with her husband, and now that Mark and Paula needed her less, she could relax and enjoy these activities. But, just as her career was taking off, Don insisted on getting a dog. Teresa knew this could mean trouble and her response was somewhat predictable: Although she had no interest in a dog, after a few months of heated debates on the issue, she realized that it was extremely important to her husband.

After extensive negotiations, Teresa agreed that she would try to be kind to the dog, but that she would not take major responsibility for feeding or other maintenance chores. Little did she know how attached she would become to the dog over time! Ultimately, Teresa's attachment to the new addition, a friendly copper-and-white Spaniel named Quayle, led her to begin walking their new pet. She not only walked Quayle, but she began to walk her a mile a day, twice a day, and was able to see the results of this added exercise within a few months. It is gratifying to us to see Teresa walking on a local bike-path trail, wearing her bulky parka and ski cap, with her dog in the midst of the harsh New England winters. Teresa found at this late date that walking was something that she could do not only to "help the damn dog," but to maintain her weight and her health as well.

After six months, not only was Teresa walking, but she was actually intermittently jogging a bit. After six months she came into see us once and exclaimed, "Not only am I developing muscles, but I think I may have felt one or two endorphins!"

✦ SCREENING

Although Teresa was a sedentary woman and needed to work on that area of her health, she represents the new breed of American women interested in health as she reaches her middle years. She knows it is very important to monitor health during the menopausal years in order to be screened for certain diseases and to maintain our present level of functioning. If you look at Table 10-1, you will find the screening plan that we recommend for the midlife woman.

One of the most critical screening procedures for women is the mammogram. There is some controversy, but the American Cancer Society recommends that women aged forty-five to fifty have mammograms every other year and that women after the age of fifty have annual mammograms (American Cancer Society, 1988). Unfortunately, despite these recommendations, it is clear that mammograms are underutilized. Only 25 percent of women above the age of fifty report having *ever had* a mammogram (Jacobs Institute, 1992). The rates of mammography in African-American and Hispanic women are even lower. In a recent review by the National Cancer Institute, less than 50 percent of white women had more than one mammogram (National Cancer Institute, 1990).

These low rates of screening reflect several problems. One study of women's decisions about mammograms suggested that women who had a positive orientation about mammograms and their value in health care were more likely to use mammography as part of their routine health screening (Rakowski and others, 1992). In the National Cancer Institute study, women who had not had a mammogram listed "not having thought about it" as their most common reason followed by "doctor never recommended it." This is a tragedy.

Some women falsely believe that having a mammogram will actually cause cancer and are afraid of mammograms. Although some women find them unpleasant, they are certainly not painful, especially when you go to a radiological facility that specializes in women. Some of these facilities offer reading materials and herbal tea while you wait for the results and the technicians are particularly sensitive to women.

The same NCI report found that women report that only 52 to 80 percent of them have had a breast exam by a health care provider in the last year (National Cancer Institute, 1990). We held a panel discussion recently of women medical students and physicians in training and they all commented that they had never been taught to examine the breast. As one recent editorial in the *Annals of Internal Medicine* put it: "Almost every internist, regardless of subspeciality, makes sure the patients blood pressure is taken routinely" with a resultant reduction in cardiovascular disease and death. "We can make similar strides in breast-cancer deaths if only we remember the breast is close to the heart" (Fletcher, 1992).

Table 10–1

HEALTH SCREENING FOR WOMEN AGES 45–55

	Appropriate Office Visit	Lab Test	Other
Yearly	Breast exam Pelvic exam Pap test Blood pressure	Stool for testing Occult blood (ages > 50)	Mammogram (ages 50–55 only)
	Dental prophylaxis		
Every other year			Mammogram (ages 45–50—only with no family history of breast cancer)
Every 5 years	Full physical exam	Serum cholesterol Glucose	
Every 5–10 years	Screening for vision/ Glaucoma		

Other areas of prevention should be part of regular health screening. You should have your blood pressure checked as part of your annual physical. Control of blood pressure is one of the major goals in preventing heart attacks and other cardiovascular problems. Your doctor will also order routine blood tests and screening for blood in the stool, a way to detect colorectal cancer. We also need to pay attention to regular dental and periodontal care. This involves checkups to see that your gums are not receding over time. Your dentist or periodontist may recommend X rays periodically.

Most of these screening procedures will be scheduled in your doctor's office, but it is possible that this will not happen. Offices are usually happy to remind you of your screening procedures, but, you may miss your physical or have to cancel an appointment. You can take charge of your own health by writing everything down on your calendar at the office or at home.

Self-awareness is useful in many areas, including early detection of possible malignancies. Remember to follow the American Cancer Society's acronym of CAUTION: The American Cancer Society's early warning sign of cancer.

C. *Change in bowel habits*
A. *A sore that does not heal*
U. *Unusual bleeding or discharge*
T. *Thickening or lump in the breast or elsewhere*
I. *Indigestion or difficulty in swallowing*
O. *Obvious change in a wart or mole*
N. *Nagging cough or hoarseness*

Any of the CAUTION acronym changes mean that you should contact your primary care physician right away to investigate them further. Self-awareness and monitoring really pays off. One of our patients, Elizabeth, saw a public service announcement about skin cancer. She then found a tiny malignancy—a melanoma on her leg—and proceeded to have it removed. That was five years ago. Elizabeth is doing fine and uses a #30 skin block, or wears long sleeves and a hat when she goes out into the sun.

❋ PHYSICAL ACTIVITY AND EXERCISE

Teresa is like so many of us: she's struggled with her weight for years mainly by restricting her food intake. Exercise was just never part of her life. Teresa is not alone. Only 22 percent of Americans engage in thirty or more minutes of light to moderate physical activity five or more times per week. And as we get older, we tend to exercise even less. We've been told to "take it easy" so often that many people falsely believe that we require less exercise as we age. The truth is just the opposite: most of us exercise less than we should. Physical activity is associated with increased life expectancy. It can also help prevent and manage some diseases, promote cardiovascular fitness, maintain muscle mass and strength, help control body weight and improve feelings of competence and reduce stress. A very impressive list of benefits! Overall, physical activity and exercise cannot only lengthen our lives, but can enhance the quality of life at every stage.

You might remember, from our chapter on healthy bones, that physical activity is any movement that uses energy. Exercise, on the other hand, is leisure-time physical activity that is structured and designed to improve physical fitness. Remember that even if you are not interested in exercise, that a physically active lifestyle can pay off. Figure 10-1 depicts the benefits of physical activity and exercise.

Regular physical activity can improve many aspects of our health. However, any physical activity is useful in maintaining a level of fitness

FIGURE 10-1
GENERAL BENEFITS OF PHYSICAL ACTIVITY/EXERCISE

Habitual Physical Activity/Exercise

⟶ **Physical/Physiological Benefits**

    ⟶ **Health Benefits**
        Health Maintenance
        Disease Prevention

        ⟶ **Daily Living Benefits**

            ⟶ **Emotional Benefits**

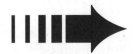 **IMPROVED QUALITY OF LIFE**

and can even improve our health to some extent. At any rate, a physically active lifestyle is associated with reduced morbidity and mortality. Dr. Steven Blair's research has followed more than ten thousand men and three thousand women over an eight-year period. The results were clear. People who had the lowest levels of physical fitness were more likely to die than those in the moderate or high-fitness categories. Small steps can be life-saving (Blair and others, 1989).

Women in the menopausal years have specific concerns. Table 10-2 is the exercise program for general fitness. You can use this as a basic plan. The specific plans for healthy hearts and healthy bones are included in chapters Four and Five. Many women in their fifties, sixties and seventies complete marathons and triathlons and compete in master's level competitions in swimming, tennis and other sports. Compared to sedentary people, these women almost always have a lower percentage of body fat, more energy, stronger muscles and less fatigue from normal daily activities.

One of the best examples of the value of consistent exercise is Tina Turner, who at the age of fifty-three is still a major force in rock and roll and is literally kicking up her heels. Despite her history of a hard life and a physically abusive marriage with Ike Turner, she is now thriving. When asked, Turner denies having any plastic surgery. She responds to the question with, "Look, this is me . . . I've been singing and dancing and that's exercise—thirty-five years, it's got to do something. I have muscle from control" (Orth, 1993)

Now we know that you are probably thinking, "Yeah, right. I'm really going to become a master swimmer or dancer like Tina Turner at this age." It is true that few of us will become master athletes or rock and roll stars. But, we can make some significant changes. First, you can work on increasing your daily physical activity. Here are the basics:

- Walk, don't drive, whenever you can.
- Use your lunch hour to walk.
- Take the stairs instead of the elevator.
- Don't stack things up at the foot of the stairs—take steps, don't "save steps."
- Take walking tours of cities where you live or travel.
- If you go to a shopping mall, don't waste time and emotional energy circling the parking lot for the ideal space. Use the physical energy and walk those extra yards.
- Consider walking when you visit a friend instead of, or in addition to, eating.
- Remember some of your high school dates? You didn't just go

Table 10–2

FIT PROGRAM FOR
GENERAL HEALTH
PHYSICAL ACTIVITY/EXERCISE PLANS

Purpose:	General health benefits
	Energy expenditure
	Enjoyment, feeling better
Frequency:	Start: 2–3 times per week
	Goal: 5 times per week
Intensity:	Light to Moderate
	(60% Max HR +)
Time:	Start: 10–20 minutes per session
	Goal: 30–60 minutes per session
Types:	Any physical activity
	Any recreational activity
	Walking, brisk walking, gardening

out to dinner or the movies or theater, you bowled, or went miniature-golfing. Try them again.

So physical activity can be part of your routine, and you will find that this change in your lifestyle can pay off. A second change is to do a *thorough* search for an enjoyable exercise. If this has been one of your areas for commitment, make a real attempt to find one that is fun for you and easily available. Many of us still have haunting memories of those navy blue gymsuits. In these days of the mirrored health clubs, we can be equally put off by overly thin young women in Spandex. But let's face it: most of us are not exercising now as a way to meet lovers. So we should try to attend to the exercise facilities and not be distracted by some of the other interpersonal games that are going on. The most important elements of success are to get comfortable and to get started! Be creative. You don't need to go to an aerobics class or jog, you can: go mall-walking, tap dance, swim, cross-country ski, the list is endless. Even a little change can help. Some studies find that the people who benefit the most from increased physical activity were those who went from being completely sedentary to being somewhat active. You do not need to be Jane Fonda or a marathon runner. Even Jane Fonda has reduced her number of workouts from five hours a day to a mere four hours per week (Boston Globe, 1993). Being a slightly more active you is a good start, and in many cases can have significant health benefits.

If you do begin an exercise plan, you need to consider your goals. Look at Table 10-3 for a reference. If you want some small benefit from increased activity, just get moving (walk, even garden) on a daily or at least every-other-day basis for thirty to sixty minutes. You can also take children to the park, play with them, push them on the swings. Do some errands by walking rather than driving, or use Don's example and get a dog that needs walking. Figure 10-2 illustrates a typical session. Remember, start slowly!

✦ RELAXATION

By now you are probably beginning to feel some stress. You may feel like we are pressuring you with all of these principles, and that you will not be able to change. You may even be discouraged. Let's take a break. Take heart, you are in control. You will be able to choose what and how much you want to change, and develop a reasonable plan. We are just covering all the bases. But, since you may be feeling a little stressed and burdened with information, now is a good time to remind you of the importance of relaxation.

The need for relaxation is universal. You don't need to be unusually stressed to have the need to relax. For most women in their midlife years, daily life alone has enough hassles to merit relaxation. We have discussed stress-management procedures in our chapter on stress, but we'll take the time to remind you again of our need for routine relaxation.

You need to find at least fifteen to thirty minutes a day where you can incorporate relaxation techniques into your life. It should be part of your daily routine. Many women incorporate relaxation into their lunch breaks. It doesn't matter when, as long as you use a consistent technique that you believe you will be able to stick to. Here are some key elements: Find a comfortable position and make sure that the temperature is suitable. Eliminate other possible distractions and responsi-

---

Table 10–3

DEVELOPING YOUR
PHYSICAL ACTIVITY/EXERCISE PLAN

Identify Your Reason to Exercise

•Optimal cardiovascular fitness and health benefits?
•Energy expenditure for weight control?
•Minimum activity for health benefits?
•Enjoyment, feeling better?
•Prevention of osteoporosis?

Considerations for a Physical Activity/Exercise Plan

•Frequency
•Intensity
•Time
•Type

Getting Ready—Check with Physician

•Obtain information about community programs and facilities; select location
•Get proper clothing (shoes, comfortable clothing)
•Identify convenient days and times
•Make arrangements with friend(s) if desired
•Determine a consistent time and days
•Set a starting date—mark it on calendar

Implement Plan

Use Friends and Family for Supports

---

bilities before you begin. Breathe slowly and deeply. Close your eyes for a few minutes. Be consistent; it may take time to remember how to relax! In *Mind-Body Medicine*, Dr. Herbert Benson, the developer of the Relaxation Response, points out that it is the end point of feeling

FIGURE 10-2

TYPICAL COMBINATION "EXERCISE" SESSION—FOR THE WOMAN WHO WANTS IT ALL
(60 min)

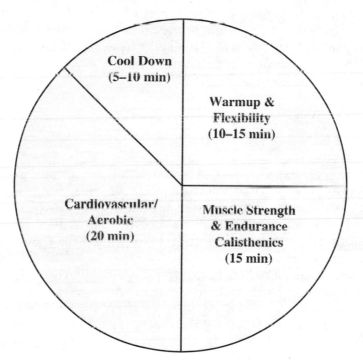

DEVELOPING A PLAN WITH VARIETY

Weekly Schedule for General Exercise & Fitness

- **Two days per week — Exercise session**
- **Two days per week — Physical activity (walking, jogging)**
- **One day per week — Special activity based on personal interests (swimming, golf, etc.)**

relaxed and calm that is the goal (Benson, 1993). How we get there can differ and you should explore the possibilities from transcendental meditation to Zen, to progressive relaxation, prayer or imagery in order to attain that state.

By incorporating relaxation into your daily life, you will be better able to face some of the tasks of career and family life. You will also be better at maintaining an exercise or behavior change program. Dance, listen to music, meditate, enjoy sex, read a good book, or even a bad book. Do something that takes you away from the daily struggles that life can bring. We all tend to get so preoccupied with the tasks of the day, that we forget this important part of our health. Just remember that relaxation is as important as any other part of the health-management plan and it needs to have high priority in structuring your life and incorporating it into a daily routine.

◆ Eliminating or Reducing Problematic Behaviors

Smoking, substance abuse and binge-eating are the three problematic behaviors which have particular implications for women. All three of these behaviors are difficult to change because they involve properties of addiction. All three can feel good because they provide relaxation or distraction from stress quickly. But, in the long-term, these quick fixes from problematic behaviors have negative health consequences. Women often begin these behaviors for specific psychological reasons, such as reducing anxiety or fighting off depression. Over time, the behaviors become reinforcing in themselves. We know full well how difficult it is to change any of these behaviors, but the health benefits and psychological benefits are so strong that we hope you will try.

Smoking

Teresa was fortunate in that she had not developed the habit of smoking, and therefore, did not have to worry about smoking cessation. She describes a humorous episode from her first year of college that illustrates the power of reinforcement and punishment. It was quite common at her college for the women in her dormitory to relax after dinner with a cigarette, over coffee. Teresa, like many women in their first year of college, longed to be included and to be sophisticated. In addition, smoking was becoming associated with the pleasure of good conversation, and an excellent cup of coffee. Teresa began to see smoking as part of the sophisticated style and so one night after dinner, she joined the other young women by lighting up. However, just as she did so, someone called her to the phone. She exited the dining hall, holding her cigarette and opening the heavy fire door. While doing so, she managed to smash one of her fingers on the other hand at the same time. ("Let's face it," she said. "Coordination is not one of my strong suits!") This led to an emergency visit to the infirmary, where a physician actually had to drill a small hole in her fingernail to release the pressure from the blood that was rushing to her finger. Teresa, knowing the principles of behavior modification, laughed as she shared this story with us saying, "Talk about major punishment. I never lit up again."

But for many women, smoking continues to be a major health hazard. Although the overall prevalence of smoking has declined in the United States since 1965, 26 percent of all Americans continue to smoke. It is predicted that by the mid 1990s, there will be as many women as men smoking (Burmen and Gritz, 1990).

The hazards of smoking are numerous and frightening. It is lung cancer, not breast cancer, that is the major cause of death by cancer among women. Smoking also increases your risk of cardiovascular disease (the major cause of death in women over the age of forty), oral cancers, and other related lung cancers (American Cancer Society, 1988). If you combined deaths due to alcohol, AIDS, fire, suicide, homicide, automobile accidents, as well as cocaine and heroin, you would still not reach the number of deaths that are attributable to cigarette smoking. That figure is now one in seven (Warner, 1991). Smoking also increases the aging process and brings on an earlier menopause. Women who smoke reach menopause, on the average, one to two years earlier than women who have never smoked. Smoking is also associated with an increased risk for osteoporosis. Finally there is good evidence that smoking causes wrinkles.

Since women's risk of heart disease increases after menopause, the interaction between smoking and cardiovascular reactivity to stress is important. The connections here are unclear for menopausal women, but it is quite possible that smoking increases reactivity to stress (Dembroski and others, 1985).

Second-hand smoke is an additional health problem. By smoking, you are exposing the people who live with you to an elevated risk of lung cancer (Brownson and others, 1992). Second-hand smoke has been identified as a major public health problem. Restaurants and corporations are making every effort to limit smoking as much as possible.

We know that for those of you who do smoke, you are well aware of the hazards and health problems related to smoking. Some of you have been smoking for years and are heavy smokers. Smoking is an extremely difficult behavior to change. Women continue to smoke for a variety of reasons, including nicotine addiction, weight control, psychological dependence, positive associations with smoking, as well as using smoking as a coping mechanism (Rigotti, 1992). So we understand the many reasons for your smoking. We just want you to consider quitting.

One of the primary concerns for women is that they are afraid they will gain weight if they stop smoking. We have listened to women worry about this many times, and there is good reason. Many women actually endorse smoking as a weight-loss strategy (Klesges and Klesges, 1988). Weight gain is, indeed, a legitimate concern since there is evidence that smokers who quit gain an average of five pounds (Rigotti, 1992). One of the Surgeon General's reports found that 75 percent of people who quit smoking did, indeed, gain weight (U.S. Surgeon General, 1990). The reasons for this are not completely clear, but may involve a reduced metabolic rate after withdrawal from nicotine, as well as eating more sweets during withdrawal.

The fear of weight gain is intense for many women. But you have to remember that there are things you can do within a smoking-cessation program to address this issue. Probably the most beneficial strategy would be to incorporate exercise into your smoking-cessation program. Exercise can use more calories and provide you with another stress-reducing mechanism. This is significant, since women also use smoking to cope with stress, and therefore may show more stress if they withdraw. Women who experience time pressure, whether they are working at home or outside of the home, are most likely to be smokers (Chesney, 1991). A final problem is that women have difficulty giving up smoking because they feel less confident that they will succeed.

It is clear then that women who smoke have special needs. We know that nicotine is one of the most difficult drugs to conquer. But we also know that many women manage to successfully quit smoking. Remember that there are many people who quit smoking on their own. We read less about these women because most researchers deal with people who come to formal smoking programs for guidance, and these people are usually those who have had more difficulty. So there are many success stories.

Dr. David Abrams and his associates have also conceptualized smoking as part of the way people try to cope with stress (Abrams and others, 1987). If you are one of the women who is concerned about her weight, as well as stress management, then you should know that there are many advances in smoking programs that can be helpful to you. Remember that you are not alone, and that many women need several attempts before they can finally quit smoking. Behavioral programs that combine stress management and weight-control procedures are offered at many university-affiliated hospitals. These programs are usually run by health psychologists and help you construct a careful analysis of the circumstances under which you smoke, the reasons for smoking and any past attempts at ending smoking that have not worked. The needs of women smokers are now finally being addressed in these assessments. By participating in such a program, you will be able to find other coping mechanisms for dealing with stress and weight control. If you have had problems with depression, smoking cessation may be extremely difficult for you. Some women who smoke and have a history of depression may experience symptoms of depression when they quit. This is all the more reason to be involved in a comprehensive smoking-cessation program.

One component of a smoking-cessation program that many women find helpful is nicotine replacement. This is especially helpful for women who are heavy smokers and who have smoked for many years. Many midlife women are in this category. The two methods of nicotine replacement are nicotine gum and the transdermal nicotine patch. It is best, however, to combine the gum or the patch with a multifaceted behavioral program as we have described. Your primary care physician can help you with the use of nicotine gum or the nicotine patch. It is important to set a quit date and to then be sure you have stopped smoking before adding nicotine to your system. The advantage of the gum is that it is a habit that can replace lighting up during the situations when you have smoked before. The patch, on the other hand, is applied on a daily basis and provides continuous absorption to keep the blood level of nicotine at a consistent level.

Over time, you do want to withdraw from nicotine as well, and therefore you can use the patch or the gum to gradually withdraw from nicotine, after you have broken the habit of smoking itself. You can try to structure your environment to avoid cigarettes by avoiding places where other people smoke, by informing your friends of your quit date, and by developing alternative behaviors, whether it is the gum, sipping herbal tea, or leaving situations with which you have associated smoking in the past.

If your first attempt to quit smoking is not a complete success, remember that you are not alone. Many women and men who try to stop smoking need several attempts to finally quit. If you go back to the stages of change model, you will see that this is part of the relapse that is quite possible during the change of any addictive behavior. This does not mean that you are lazy, stupid or have poor willpower, many of the unhelpful labels that we apply to ourselves when trying to change an addictive behavior. It means that you are making an extremely important but difficult change in order to improve your health and the health of those around you.

ALCOHOL

Eileen has been our patient for three years. When she first came to us, she did not perceive her drinking patterns as a problem. She and her husband would have a drink when they came home from work and one with dinner. It was only occasionally, on special holidays or weekends, that she might have an additional glass of wine, but never more than four on any particular evening.

When we discussed her family history, Eileen readily acknowledged that her father had had a problem with alcohol. She described him as a "functional alcoholic who went to work every day and rarely became truly drunk until his later years." It was in these later years that alcohol became more of a problem. Eileen's mother, who she describes as "a woman whose home could pass the old-fashioned white-glove test," drank much less and managed to keep the home together, despite her husband's frequent drunken episodes.

Eileen is now fifty, has two children ages nineteen and seventeen and is happily married to Roger, her second husband, who is an accountant. She is a buyer for a chain of women's clothing stores and describes herself as fairly stressed by the pressures at work and at home. She and Roger very much enjoy their evening drink together and see it as a time to relax and discuss the events of the day. Eileen is in very good health, although she acknowledges that she could certainly exercise more and be more careful in her diet. She comes to our Women's Health Associates for her yearly exam and a discussion regarding mammography for women fifty years old. Eileen has learned that she needs an annual mammogram now that she is fifty years old, but she is surprised when we discuss alcohol with her.

Eileen is fairly typical of American women, many of whom drink one to two alcoholic beverages a day. What Eileen did not know before she came to our practice was that for women drinking in this range, there are some well-established health risks. First, let's start with the basics. A drink is a drink is a drink. That is, one drink is equivalent to five ounces of wine, twelve ounces of beer, or a cocktail mixed with a shot or one and a half ounces of hard liquor. Many people assume that wine and beer, because of their lower alcohol content are less of a problem than hard liquor, but the lower alcohol content is usually offset by drinking a larger quantity. Any drink that is concocted with more than the standard quantity of alcohol is obviously comparable to more than one alcoholic beverage.

Eileen could not understand how drinking one or two drinks an evening could possibly be dangerous, particularly when she had seen her father drink for years in the range of six to ten cocktails an evening. This exemplifies one of the many inequities between the genders. While men can consume up to four drinks a day without experiencing long-term health consequences, women run the risk of experiencing the complications of alcohol by drinking over one and a half to two drinks a day. We now know that women absorb alcohol to a greater extent than men and have higher blood levels of alcohol even when differences in body weight are considered. So for any equivalent amount of alcohol consumed, a woman is going to experience the immediate effects to a much greater extent than a man. This becomes particularly important when considering the immediate consequences of driving while intoxicated.

The differences in the immediate effects carry over to differences in long-term effects. Women develop health complications of alcohol use after drinking for a much shorter time and at a much lower level than men. This is true for liver disease, ulcer disease, gastrointestinal bleeding and the neurologic effects of alcohol. Women who drink more than the equivalent of one and half to two drinks a day, increase their risk of developing alcohol liver damage after ten years. Eileen found this a shocking statistic, especially since Roger had been told by his physician to drink two drinks a day to elevate his HDL, the good part of his cholesterol. This is another area where the advice given to men may have one risk-benefit analysis, whereas the risks and benefits for women are quite different. Though it is true that alcohol has been shown to have some beneficial effect on cholesterol, the amount of alcohol that is recommended to achieve this benefit may put women at risk for a number of other complications. In the larger picture, the risk-benefit analysis of drinking for women makes it unwise to recommend this approach.

There are also a number of complications of alcohol use which are specifically problematic for women. Even at what some women see as low levels of alcohol consumption, women may increase their risk of developing breast cancer. This was demonstrated in several studies where women who drank in the range of even one drink per day were shown to increase their risk of breast cancer, up to one and a half times the rate of nondrinkers or moderate drinkers. For women who may already have an increased risk of breast cancer because of a family history, this is particularly important. The increased risk of breast cancer from hormone replacement is approximately equivalent to that which is conferred by drinking four or more drinks per week. Somehow, the information about estrogen and breast cancer has received much more attention than the information about alcohol and its link to breast cancer.

Osteoporosis is another condition related to alcohol consumption. Alcohol abuse increases the chance that a woman will develop osteoporosis as well as hip fractures in her lifetime. Coupled with cigarette smoking, these are two very preventable risk factors for osteoporosis. We may not be able to change our family history, but we certainly can try to change the behaviors which put us at an increased risk for this debilitating disease.

There are also a number of gynecologic problems associated with alcohol consumption. Many of these may have particular importance at the time of menopause. For example, irregular or heavy menstrual bleeding has been associated with heavy drinking. Many perimenopausal women have these symptoms anyway and it is likely that alcohol could worsen them. Although the obstetrical complications of alcohol are unlikely to be your primary concern during the perimenopausal period, they are well documented also.

Eileen was concerned about the health risks of drinking at her current level, but was reluctant to agree to give up her nightly two drinks. She saw these drinks as her reward at the end of what were often very hectic and stressful days. We discussed with her at some length the dangers of using alcohol as a relaxant medication. The dependence on alcohol for relaxation was already beginning to disrupt Eileen's sleep, but she did not understand this until we explained it to her. She would indeed feel relaxed right before going to bed, after drinking with Roger, but she was beginning to wake up in the middle of the night and did not understand that this could be a result of the alcohol. When alcohol enters the bloodstream, it does cause relaxation. However, approximately four hours later, when the alcohol level goes down, one becomes dehydrated and is often awakened.

In addition, Eileen was already at significant high risk of developing true alcohol dependence because of her father's history of alcoholism. Alcoholism is an inheritable disease, and it is particularly true that women who have alcoholic fathers are very much at risk of developing alcoholism. Women who use alcohol to improve their daily function-ing, seem to be at more of a risk of developing problems. Women who use alcohol to relax, to get to sleep, or to be more sociable have been shown to have higher rates of alcoholism than women who do not use alcohol in these ways. Although Eileen was controlling her alcohol consumption at that point in time, she did run significant risk of having future problems. It was also striking that she was so reluctant to con-sider giving up her nightly drinks. This reaction in and of itself indi-cated a potential dependence on alcohol that was more significant than she had ever realized. When we last talked with Eileen, she had reached the planning stage of her behavior change and was going to an Al-coholics Anonymous meeting with Roger. They were both consider-ing abstaining from alcohol, and Eileen wanted to learn more about the impact of her father on her own drinking and family life.

In addition to family history and the use of alcohol as a medica-tion, there are other factors which put women at an increased risk for developing alcoholism. Women who are married to or living with an alcoholic are at increased risk of developing problems with alcohol. Although there is some conflicting evidence, lesbian women may be at a higher risk of developing alcoholism than are heterosexual women. Some have suggested that this is a result of the discrimination and social stress of being in a minority group. There is considerable con-cern that the rates of alcoholism among African-American and His-panic women are increasing in the United States, and the tragic high rate of alcohol abuse among Native Americans is well documented. There is, in general, a higher rate of alcoholism among people from Eileen's Irish background, as well as French and German backgrounds.

For any particular woman, it is important to make a very detailed assessment of these risk factors. Although drinking may not be a signif-icant problem now, it may become one in the future. There have been a number of questionnaires which have been developed to assess whether a woman has a problem with alcohol. Most of these question-naires rely on information pertaining to problems with relationships that have developed, rather than the health problems that tend to occur late in the course of alcoholism. One questionnaire, which many physicians find useful, is called the CAGE Questionnaire and consists of four questions (Ewing, 1984). The questions are:

1. Have you ever tried to *Cut down* on your drinking?

2. Have you ever been *Annoyed by* criticism about your drinking?

3. Have you ever felt *Guilty* about your drinking?

4. Have you ever had an *Eye-opener* or an early-morning drink to treat a hangover?

Any positive response to these questions requires careful consideration of your drinking patterns. If you previously cut down on your alcohol consumption because of pregnancy, this may or may not represent a cause for concern. On the other hand, if you have tried to cut down on your alcohol consumption because you perceive that it was causing some problems in your life, this may be more significant. If you have two or more positive responses to these questions, you may have a problem with drinking, and you should consider getting an evaluation from a substance-abuse counselor or a mental health professional specializing in substance abuse.

If you suspect you have a problem with alcohol, or others are concerned about your drinking, it is important that you seek help. Although not all physicians are equipped to treat alcohol-related problems, they should be aware of resources within your community. There are a number of different types of treatment for alcohol abuse, including the self-help groups which rely on group process. The most familiar of the self-help groups is Alcoholics Anonymous, and it has been extremely helpful for many people dealing with alcohol problems. There are literally hundreds of meetings in any geographic area every week. There are meetings for women only, meetings which provide child-care, meetings for lesbians, and nonsmoking meetings, to name a few. Studies have shown that women do respond better to self-help programs and to all female groups (Jarvis, 1992). There is also a specific self-help group for women only called Women for Sobriety, which may meet in your area as well.

Many women also choose to see an alcohol counselor alone, in addition to self-help groups. The counselor can help to establish a treatment plan and monitor and support you through the recovery process. Alcohol counselors usually work closely with self-help groups and other resources in the community.

For some women, it is important that they be out of their usual situation in order to gain the most from treatment. Inpatient or residential treatment programs have been designed specifically for this purpose. Most of these programs involve hospitalization that is devoted to therapy and education about alcohol and its effects. Families and significant others are usually encouraged to participate in the program because long-term recovery depends not only on the individual with a drinking problem but also on their family and friends. Most residential programs also arrange for continued treatment after discharge in an outpatient setting.

Relapse may occur, of course, but treatment for alcoholism can be remarkably successful, and most people can look forward to happier and healthier lives in recovery.

SUBSTANCE ABUSE

Just as women are not immune to alcoholism neither are they immune to problems with other drugs which have the potential to be addictive. While only 5 percent of all women compared to 8 percent of all men reported using illegal drugs according to one survey, it is true that women abuse prescription drugs at a higher rate than men (National Institute on Drug Abuse, 1990). It is estimated that nearly half of women alcoholics are also dependent on other drugs, most commonly, sleeping pills or tranquilizers used for anxiety.

Not surprisingly, the factors which put women at risk for drug abuse include a family history of drug abuse, early age of onset of alcohol or other drug use, having a significant other who abuses drugs, and having been prescribed a mood-altering drug. We certainly can't do anything about our family history nor can we do anything about the age at which we might have begun drinking or using other drugs, but we do have some control over our significant others and our use of prescription drugs. Certainly no one begins taking a medication with the intention of becoming addicted to it. However, the path to addiction can be very insidious. There are extremely few women who do not have a complaint which could warrant the use of an addictive medication. Anxiety, insomnia, weight problems and chronic pain are all conditions that could be treated with medications which have addictive potential. Everyone is now aware of the dangers of Valium, which was prescribed too often to women with anxiety and stress. Only after a number of years of experience with the drug did it become clear that it was highly addictive for those who took it on a long-term basis.

Amphetamines were also used extensively in the past to treat weight problems, and many women became hooked on these uppers which gave them seemingly boundless energy and birdlike appetites. Narcotic pain medications used over the long-term can be addictive as well. This is not to say that pain medicine should be avoided altogether, but rather that any pain which has a potential to be chronic, such as long-standing lower-back pain or osteoarthritis, should be treated with medications that are nonaddictive, when possible. Although most health care providers are now aware of the addictive potential of many drugs, it is important that you question your physician and/or pharmacist when you are prescribed a new medication. If you do discover that there is the potential for addiction, you may ask for an alternative treatment, or reassurance that your treatment will be short-term and will not pose any long-term problems.

If you are worried that you may have developed an addiction to a particular medication, or to a nonprescription drug, it is absolutely important that you share this concern with your clinician. As in the case of alcoholism, physicians and other health care professionals may or may not be knowledgeable enough to establish a treatment plan with you, but they should be able to refer you to the appropriate resources. In the case of some drugs, it is important that the dose be gradually tapered rather than abruptly stopped in order to avoid symptoms of drug withdrawal. This can usually be done with the advice of your physician, counselor or in an inpatient setting designed for drug detoxification. The principles of drug treatment are similar to those of alcohol treatment and include self-help programs, including Narcotics Anonymous, drug counselors for outpatient treatment and residential programs for inpatient treatment. There is help available if you need it and want it. Remember the stages of change presented earlier in this chapter. The key is to move from precontemplation to action. Relapses may occur but should not be seen as signs of failure or reasons to lose hope.

← OVEREATING AND WEIGHT-LOSS PROGRAMS

American society, in general, and the medical profession, in particular, have been especially critical of overweight women. In fact, we find that most women are uncomfortable with their bodies. Most of us believe that we are too heavy or too thin, too flat-chested, or too full-figured. The pages of most women's magazines are filled with photographs of models who resemble boys or waifs, a completely unrealistic "look" for the majority of women. We only know a few women who have somehow escaped from the anxiety about body image.

Overweight people are one of the few remaining categories where prejudice is socially acceptable. You need only to look at any television program to see that overweight women and men take the brunt of numerous jokes. Midlife women, already subjected to discrimination, can be especially targeted for hurtful remarks when they are overweight. We are reminded of a visiting dignitary who came to one of our graduate programs in the early seventies and informed us that the women's movement would never take off because "after forty, women's hips spread." We knew even back then that this made no sense, particularly coming from a man who, although quite accomplished in his career, was not exactly Robert Redford.

Being overweight also continues to be seen as a character flaw, rather than a problem. This prejudice continues, even after progress has been made in other addictive behaviors, like alcohol abuse. This bias goes on despite the fact that it is clear that genetics play an important role in the determination of body weight and shape. In addition, little thought is sometimes given to the fact that treatment for obesity has usually not been very successful and has involved high rates of relapse. Treatment for overweight women is now somewhat controversial. Several psychologists who pioneered research on the efficacy of weight-loss treatments are now recommending caution in dieting. Drs. Susan and Orville Wooley believe that obesity alone should not be targeted for change. They recommend changes in eating behaviors like lowering cholesterol as a target behavior, rather than weight loss per se (Wooley and Wooley, 1979).

There are many hazards to being significantly overweight, as we have discussed in earlier chapters. Being moderately or severely overweight is associated with hazardous hypertension, cardiovascular disease, gallbladder disease, diabetes, musculoskeletal problems and certain types of cancer. These associations have not been found for slightly overweight people. So in many cases, weight loss is a good idea. However, overweight women have special concerns, including the hazards of weight cycling, or what is known as "yo-yo dieting" (Ernsberger and Nelson, 1988). By the time they reach midlife, many women have gained and lost weight a number of times, and these failures themselves have certain psychological hazards (Wadden and others, 1988). Many of these women, rather than understanding that being overweight is a complex and difficult set of behaviors to change, believe that *they* are failures and have resulting feelings of sadness and discouragement.

Nonetheless, many midlife women continue to try to lose weight. Others are trying to avoid the weight gain that is often associated with menopause. We believe that the first step should be to use the stages of change model that we have discussed. If there are other parts of our health-promotion plan where you have already begun to take action, it might make sense to follow through with those first. It doesn't make sense to tackle the weight problem again if you are not convinced and committed at this time.

What if you reach the preparation stage and you are only mildly overweight? You may be interested in losing weight primarily because of concerns about your appearance; then, you might consider an exercise program. One of our patients, Jeanette, is a fifty-four-year-old women who had a long history of being overweight and made multiple attempts to diet. She had previously lost between five and ten pounds, only to regain them over the last five years. She was frustrated because, as she got older, she noted it was even more difficult to lose weight than before. Jeanette decided that rather than change her diet, she would make a concerted and consistent effort to increase her physical activity level. Specifically, she had read that if she walked three miles a day, four or five times a week, she could lose ten pounds in a year. When we saw Jeanette for the first time she had been on her exercise program for less than a month. However, now a year has passed and Jeanette has indeed lost nine pounds without making any changes in her eating behavior. Jeanette has had great difficulty in sticking to her exercise plan but has managed to do so. She now wants to continue to exercise to maintain her weight loss.

Dr. Kelly Brownell of Yale University recommends that the key to successful treatment is a careful assessment in matching the patient to the treatment plan (Brownell and Wadden, 1991). The best place to have your weight-loss plan assessed is a comprehensive program, usually in departments of behavioral medicine in university-affiliated hospitals. These programs ensure that you will be able to be evaluated comprehensively, where the biological, psychological and social issues can all be considered in your treatment. Dr. Matthew Clark and associates at Brown University Medical School completed a review of all the literature on treatment of obesity and suggest that the following factors should be considered: First, it is important to have a psychological assessment. Two of the most important psychological issues are binge eating and a history of physical and sexual abuse. Some women who struggle with their weight are binge eaters and may require treatment for depression, not just another diet. Binge eating involves eating large quantities of food at a sitting and feeling out of control. This is now seen as a separate type of eating disorder that requires specific treatment. Some studies have found that up to 30 percent of women in weight-control programs have true eating disorders or another psychological problem (Clark and others, 1993). In addition, some women use food to treat their depressions. They may have had depressive episodes in response to dieting in the past. Finally, many women who have histories of sexual abuse, substance-abuse problems or anxiety, also need comprehensive psychological care. Additional parts of an evaluation should include a physical examination, laboratory tests and a nutritional and exercise assessment. Such an assessment will help you identify what your target behaviors are in order to provide an effective treatment program.

Components of a weight-reduction program usually involve behavior therapy, nutritional counseling and an increased exercise and physical activity program. Some recommend the use of a very low-calorie diet for people who have a lot of weight to lose. It should be noted that these programs need to be combined with a comprehensive treatment approach to maximize the possibility of long-term maintenance. Most experts, at this time, do not recommend surgery for obesity. The use of medications depends on the extent of weight loss necessary and should be carefully monitored. You should be especially wary of medications that can be addictive and affect the central nervous system.

Suppose you live in an area without a comprehensive weight-loss program? Remember, let the buyer beware, and use your own good common sense. Few weight-reduction programs have been evaluated scientifically and many of them spend a fortune on advertising, often using celebrities. Yet, do you really want to go on a liquid protein diet, and follow in the footsteps of Oprah Winfrey and proudly show off weight loss in a pair of tight black jeans, only to gain it all back in a few months time? Every weight expert we know shuddered and was concerned for Oprah when she announced her supposedly permanent new shape. You should be especially cautious about crash diets and programs that ask for a lot of money at the beginning of the plan. Some of these programs will give you a rationale that large amounts of money are needed "up front," in order to prevent you from dropping out easily. Although there is some truth to that, many programs for losing weight are quite similar and large amounts of money do not guarantee a good program. You want a program to focus on gradual nutritional planning, behavior modification and increased physical activity and exercise.

Consumer Reports analyzed the responses of 95,000 of their readers in order to evaluate commercial diet programs. Their results were sobering: Most of the people regained their lost weight within a year (Losing Weight, 1993). Among the top diet programs, there were no differences in helping people lose weight or keep it off. Members of Weight Watchers, however, reported the greatest level of satisfaction with the program. Although only 6 percent of the readers had been to hospital-based weight-reduction programs, these programs did as well as the others and received fewer complaints than other programs.

There were two particularly interesting results of this study. First, more than 25 percent of the people did not even meet the criteria for being overweight. More evidence that many of us are dieting unnecessarily. In addition, another 25 percent of the group did maintain weight loss, but the study could not determine what led to these successes.

In our experience, there are two key elements to keeping weight off. The first is as you know by now, a physically active lifestyle. The second is to identify and act on your need for social support, one of our favorite topics, which is more complicated when it comes to losing weight and maintaining weight loss. Although having a weight-loss or maintenance partner is usually helpful, a woman needs to decide if she prefers what Drs. Brownell and Rodin call a solo or a social plan (Brownell and Rodin, 1990). They found that some individuals do better with a buddy, whereas others preferred to lose weight alone. So look for support if you need it.

If, after an assessment, you are still unsure about the pros and cons of losing weight and are still in the contemplation stage, and if you have made multiple attempts to lose weight by dieting, you might consider an exercise/physical activity program. Some women break out of the diet habit by beginning a low-fat, rather than a low-calorie diet. The fact is that there are no easy answers to losing weight. One of the problems in losing weight is that the goal cannot be abstinence, as it can be in smoking cessation or substance-abuse programs. We cannot eliminate food from our environment. Thus, the exposure to temptation is frequent. In addition, gaining some weight as we age is to be expected. Thus, we should try to break out of the "you can never be too thin" mentality.

What if you are only ten pounds overweight and your physician is pushing you to lose weight? We have had many women come to us with this concern recently. Many of them have no other health-risk factors and are in good shape, but just tend to be heavier, as do many members of their family. Given the fact that we now know there is some genetic basis to being overweight and the fact that treatment for obesity is usually not successful for long-term maintenance, it seems that these women are being unfairly pressured. As much as we hope that you will be able to lose weight if you decide to do so, the fact is that this is still an area with a lot of relapse. Finally, some of the most recent research suggests that gaining a little weight as we get older may have protective health benefits like fewer hot flashes (Erlik and others, 1982). So this may be an opportunity for you to be assertive with your physician by suggesting that you do not feel this is a problem that you want to work on at this time and stressing your reasons for your beliefs.

Unfortunately, some health care providers are not as sensitive in this area as they could be. They may be unaware of the number of times you have tried to lose weight and your feelings about it. Your feelings are an important part of your health. It is appropriate and even necessary for you to share any feelings you may have with regard to your weight and past attempts at dieting. Remember that a healthy lifestyle overall is more important than the numbers on the scale.

✦ NUTRITION

As we have discussed in the previous section about overeating, all too many menopausal women have been prisoners of the calorie count for decades. By the time we reach midlife, many women have been dieting for a full thirty years. Most menopausal women are therefore experts in calories and calorie counting. This preoccupation tends to be destructive rather than beneficial. So we are not going to deal with calories. A better approach is to look at the components of nutrition that are necessary for good health during the menopausal years and to target problem areas. The components of good nutrition for midlife women are: a balanced diet, adequate calcium, lower fat consumption, avoidance of alcohol and caffeine and simple sugar, and adequate water intake.

Remember the four basic food groups that we learned in elementary school? Well you can forget them now, because the U.S. Department of Agriculture has launched a new food guide referred to as the new food pyramid. The pyramid (Figure 10-3) emphasizes for us, once again, that Americans have been eating too much meat. The foundation of our diet should be in the complex carbohydrates—the bread, rice, cereal and pasta group. Complex carbohydrates should compose from 55 to 60 percent of our diet. The next level of our diet should be composed of three to five daily servings of vegetables and two to four servings of fruit. We should be eating less of the proteins such as meat, poultry, fish and beans. Finally, we should eat very few fats, oils and sweets.

When the food pyramid was first released, Teresa laughed and mentioned that if she ate all of the servings of those foods, even as they were described, she would end up "looking like a pyramid." She has described her own dietary needs as "the shrinking pyramid." But the pyramid is a definite improvement over the old four food groups in that it emphasizes an increased intake of fiber and carbohydrates as an important component.

The American Dietetic Association has also suggested that within

Figure 10–3

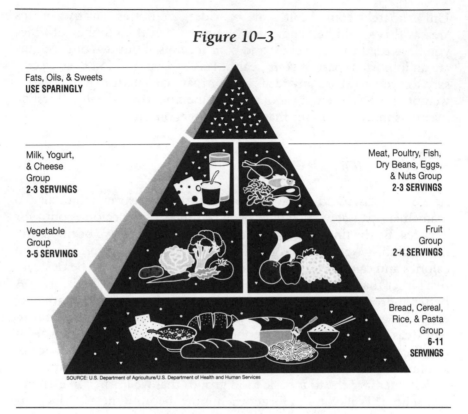

Fats, Oils, & Sweets
USE SPARINGLY

Milk, Yogurt,
& Cheese
Group
2-3 SERVINGS

Meat, Poultry, Fish,
Dry Beans, Eggs,
& Nuts Group
2-3 SERVINGS

Vegetable
Group
3-5 SERVINGS

Fruit
Group
2-4 SERVINGS

Bread, Cereal,
Rice, & Pasta
Group
**6-11
SERVINGS**

SOURCE: U.S. Department of Agriculture/U.S. Department of Health and Human Services

each of these groups, there are also variations in the amount of fats. Many sauces and additives contain lots of fat, and we should focus on keeping fat and cholesterol low, limiting excessive sodium and simple sugar and eating a broad variety of fruits and vegetables (1992a).

THE FAT QUESTION

Reducing fat is one of the most important changes for general health benefits and specifically for cardiovascular health. Two of the most important changes that we can make are to reduce the amount of red meat and to avoid high-fat dairy products. Many women have given up red meat entirely, but we must also be careful of high-fat dairy foods. In some gourmet ice cream, for example, 50 percent of the total calories is from fat, whereas in low-fat frozen yogurts only 6 percent of the calories comes from fat. So yes, you might want to give up chocolate-chip cookie dough ice cream and replace it with low-fat chocolate yogurt.

It is important to be careful about hidden fats. Fast-food and prepared foods are often extremely high in their fat and salt content. We should be eating no more than 30 percent of fat in our diet, and many nutritionists suggest that this figure should be closer to 25 percent for better health promotion. You can actually calculate the percentage of your calories that are fat, relatively easily. One gram of fat has nine calories. Most prepared foods now include a nutritional analysis that will list this figure. For example, one serving of a flavored cracker may have 50 calories. If the cracker serving has 2 grams of fat, then 2 (grams) × 9 (calories per gram of fat) = 18, or 18 of those 50 calories consists of fat. This is 36 percent of the total serving. This is actually a high figure for a cracker, especially when you compare it to a saltine, which has zero grams of fat. It is important then to read the label and not just assume that crackers, as a general rule, are all low-fat.

Another approach is to add up your grams of fat for the day. A 1,500 daily calorie diet could have about 40 grams of fat per day if you are aiming for the 25-percent figure. These quick calculations can help you make significant and consistent changes in your nutritional planning.

Beware of food labeling. The Food and Drug Administration has been mandated to develop a system of food labeling. This legislation is aimed at promoting consistency in labeling. In addition, the FDA will be cracking down on the terms that are vastly overused like "low-fat," and "light." They are in the process of providing definitions so that a company cannot slap a new label on an old product. We have all also seen the labeling that suggests that one serving of a coffee cake will have only 100 calories, only to find that that particular serving may be one-twentieth of a small cake (a tiny bite!). Another example is that a "light" hot dog may have a full two-thirds of its calories derived from fat. That may be "light" compared to other hot dogs that have 95 percent fat, but remember that we are aiming for less than 30 percent of our total daily calories to be derived from fat. You can accomplish a lot just by selecting low-fat foods. For example, one ounce of potato chips can have 10 grams (25 percent of your daily "fat allowance") of fat (Friedman, 1993, p. 1). Low-fat and no-fat muffins can replace the greasy ones. Frozen pizzas can vary from 5 grams of fat per slice (tofu or vegetarian), to about 13 to 14 grams (extra cheese or many "deluxe" toppings) (Friedman, 1993, p. 3). You can substitute a cup of unbuttered popcorn and eliminate fat.

The question of omega-3 fatty acid that is found in fish oils received attention when it was found that heart disease is quite rare among the Greenland Eskimos. Several studies suggested that these omega-3 fatty acids reduce the level of triglycerides which contribute to heart disease. In addition, there is some evidence that they reduce the tendency to form blood clots as well. Yet, most nutritionists agree that fish oil supplements are not necessary, but that eating fish two or three times a week is a good idea. This is true because fish is a good source of protein and also a natural source of the omega-3 fatty acids.

Adequate Calcium

Don't forget your calcium. As a result of inadequate calcium intake in youth and young adulthood, most of us reach the menopausal years with a low peak bone mass. In addition, as we age, our ability to absorb calcium decreases, especially at the time of menopause. This is particularly true for women after the age of fifty, but begins during the menopausal years. Remember, the calcium needs for perimenopausal women are somewhere about 1,200 mg per day. For the post-menopausal women, the suggestion is 1,500 mg per day.

One of the problems here is that women have long avoided dairy products because of a concern about gaining weight. As we discussed in our chapter on healthy bones, we can get enough calcium by replacing milk with skim milk, ice cream with low-fat yogurt, by eating a calcium-rich diet and by taking calcium supplements. Other vitamins and minerals can also be taken in a one-a-day supplement. This may be necessary because in our quest to cut calories, many women do not eat enough fruits and vegetables which greatly limits intake of vitamins and minerals (Winick, 1992).

The Iron Question

Sometimes women who are chronically dieting have an inadequate vitamin and mineral intake, especially iron. For perimenopausal women who are still menstruating, the recommended daily allowance of iron is 18 mg per day. Unfortunately, this would require an average caloric intake of 3,000 calories a day of a mixed, well-balanced diet! Obviously, this caloric requirement would lead to obesity over time, given the average activity level of most American women.

Until recently, it was believed that women who are premenopausal should be taking iron supplements. However, recent studies suggested that high iron stores have been associated with increased risk of heart attacks. Women's low stores of iron might protect us from heart disease before menopause. For that reason, women who have lower than the recommended intake of iron, but are not having any symptoms, may not benefit from iron supplements. This is clearly an area to watch for future developments.

H_2O

One of the healthiest choices that we can all make is to drink more water. Water makes up about 60 percent of our body and is needed for our body to function properly. The rule is that we should be drinking about four eight-ounce cups of water for every 1,000 calories we consume. For most women, that would be between six to eight glasses of water per day. This is particularly important because we tend to get dehydrated as we get older. Adequate intake of water can improve our skin, and can also keep us from overeating. Yet most of us have difficulty drinking this much water. Here are a few suggestions to make it easier: First, try replacing some of your caffeinated beverages with ice water. Because some of our tap water may contain contaminates, or may just "taste funny," using bottled water can help us feel more like drinking the water we need. It is as easy to order ice water when you are out to eat at a restaurant as it is to order a soda, and it is almost always free! Second, think about adding a water cooler to the office coffee room. We did this in both of our offices and it has had great results. You might also try drinking small amounts of water at a time. A three-and-a-half-ounce paper cup, for example, does not seem as overwhelming as an eight- or ten-ounce glass. Finally, you can follow the model of the character Susan Silverman in the Robert Parker novels about Spencer. Susan is prone to sipping warm water, perhaps with a bit of lemon or honey, while she is having those long intimate conversations with Spencer. You will be surprised how easy a habit that is to develop (the water, not the relationship with Spencer), especially during the winter.

CUT DOWN ON CAFFEINE AND ALCOHOL

With any luck, while you are drinking more water, you will be drinking less caffeine. Caffeine should really be limited to a maximum of two to three cups per day. Too much caffeine can inhibit the absorption of certain foods and can make us anxious and edgy. One study found that even people who drank between two and three cups of coffee per day experienced some symptoms of withdrawal when the caffeine was taken away. The symptoms included moderate to severe headaches, feeling depressed and feeling fatigued. This does not mean that caffeine should be avoided at all costs, but that we should be careful. In addition, the use of caffeine should be evaluated if you have a problem like headaches, anxiety or depression. It is often present in pain relievers and some other medications. Many over-the-counter weight-loss drugs are composed of high amounts of caffeine. Not only is caffeine a stimulant, it is also a diuretic. Therefore, all the good you do by drinking water can be undone if you match it with an amount of caffeine that depletes your system of water. Many women use both coffee and caffeinated diet sodas to get going during the day. Although we can certainly understand the need for coffee first thing in the morning, perhaps after one or two cups, you can stop. Diet sodas have recently become available in decaffeinated varieties so you can enjoy the taste without the caffeine or calories.

Alcohol abuse is associated with undernutrition. This is true because alcohol consumption affects the stomach, small intestine, pancreas, as well as the liver. It can also cause diarrhea which can result in the loss of nutrients. In addition to these problems, many women who drink too much are not eating a balanced diet. So we need to look at alcohol consumption when we are evaluating our overall nutritional status.

If you make up a new nutritional plan, try to remember our general rules. Try to make moderate rather than severe changes. You are unlikely to go from a diet that is composed of too much fat and simple sugar to an intense low-fat high-fiber diet. But, if you move toward lower-fat and higher-carbohydrate foods, you are more likely to succeed. You may make different choices over a given week. If you know that you are going to a party and it is likely that you will eat a favorite problematic food, it is okay to eat some as long as you try to balance out your diet at another time during the week. You can try to balance your diet over the course of any given week. You don't have to give up favorite problematic foods forever. If you limit your portions and only eat high-fat foods or sweets now and then, you can still continue to maintain a balanced diet.

◆ EXPANDING YOUR SOCIAL NETWORK

Social support is one of the most clearly beneficial factors in all health research. Expanding a social network can take many other forms. Many women have a strong network within their nuclear or extended family. Others have long-term friendships. Social support has been positively associated with everything from maintaining exercise programs to coping with chronic illness. In almost every area that we have described so far, you can find a social support system, whether it is working with a friend who has a similar problem, or participating in a formal self-help group. In the United States more than fifteen million people attend about 500,000 different self-help groups each week. In California alone, 4,600 self-help groups are listed (de Turenne, 1993). Most local newspapers devote a page to self-help groups on a daily or weekly basis. Self-help groups are now part of our culture and also part of a long tradition. We have, therefore, included self-help groups related to health promotion at the end of this chapter. We will discuss more general self-help groups and social-support groups in the next chapter. It is clear that despite the diversity of social networks, these links have been a particularly powerful source of strength for women.

Another way to expand our social network is by giving something back to the larger community. Erik Erikson suggests that the task of midlife is to struggle with the issues of self-absorption as opposed to generativity. Self-absorption can develop out of isolation. Without meaningful relationships, we can begin to turn inward and brood about the narcissistic losses of middle age. The growth-promoting aspect of generativity is the sharing with a younger generation the knowledge that comes with age. In this way, a woman in midlife can connect with others. Many women do so, through their paid employment, volunteer work, mentoring or grandparenting. So much for Helene Deutsch's nonsense that we have ended our service to the species. A study of menopausal women validated the importance of generativity, finding that when women had a commitment, whether it was paid employment or not, they reported fewer menopausal symptoms.

Hortence Powdermaker was an anthropologist who wrote about the importance of connection. In her description of life as an anthropologist, she too described her fear about doing field work in the Pacific. Her feelings of panic finally dissipated when she began to talk with one of the islanders. Her words can help all of us: "I was no longer alone. I had friends and went to bed and fell asleep almost immediately. No more thoughts of madness or leaving entered my mind. Several years later, I learned that a definition of panic is a state of unrelatedness" (Conway, 1992, p. 247). By remaining connected to others and expanding our social support, health promotion can become a new lifestyle.

You have now read about six components of the Women's Health Promotion Plan. But if your New Year's resolution was to attempt all six at once, it would be difficult to follow through. If, on the other hand, you use your own good common sense and identify one or two of these components with your primary care clinician, you are more likely to succeed. Please don't view us as the health police patrol, whose purpose is to remove all happiness and pleasure from your life. Use stress management, relaxation and pleasurable activities as the foundation. We don't want you to view the menopausal years as restriction and suffering, but we do want you to incorporate some of these changes into your lifestyle.

Keep in mind that no matter what changes or lifestyle we adopt, it is most important to enjoy life. Dr. Teresa Bernardez, a psychiatrist, gave a fascinating lecture to the Menninger's Institute on "Women and Self-Esteem" in 1989. She points out that we have enough struggles in midlife, and that to completely restrict our food intake and to make food a constant preoccupation is a tremendous loss for many women. She describes coming to the United States from her native Argentina in the 1950s and expecting to see a lot of free, comfortable, Katharine Hepburn-like women in comfortable slacks. In contrast, she found women whom she described as trapped in girdles, with hair that was controlled by lacquered layers of hair spray and a life of constant preoccupation with eating and not eating. Dr. Bernardez reminds all of us that food is extremely enjoyable for women, and that we can combine some good health habits with periodic relaxation and enjoyment (Bernardez, 1990).

RESOURCES

GENERAL RESOURCES

Melpomene
Melpomene Institute
1010 University Ave.
St. Paul, MN 55104
(612) 642-1951

Journal on women's health research; 3 journals a year with a membership to the Institute for $32. It includes profiles of older women, information on health, research and aging.

Prevention
Box 181
Emmaus, PA 18099-0181

A monthly magazine for $19.97 a year. Easy reading on nutrition, exercise, health-screening and maintenance.

Radiance Magazine
PO Box 31703
Oakland, CA 94604
(415) 482-0680

A quarterly magazine for large women, giving resources and information on health, including older women's health, fashion, politics, entertainment. $15 a year.

University of California at Berkeley Wellness Letter
PO Box 420148
Palm Coast, FL 32142
(904) 445-6414

Newsletter on nutrition, fitness, stress management and health. Somewhat technical and very informative. 12 issues for $24 a year.

HEALTH-SCREENING

Dial a Hearing Screening Test
(800) 222-EARS

This number, open Monday to Friday 9–6, EST, will connect you to an operator who will give you a local number to call. This number is a recorded hearing test consisting of 8 tones, with instructions. Operators also provide referrals.

EXERCISE

Living with Exercise, by Steven N. Blair. Dr. Blair is a major researcher in the area of physical fitness at the Institute for Aerobics Research in Dallas, Texas. Dr. Blair writes, "You don't have to be an Olympic champion to receive health benefits from physical fitness." His book is extremely valuable because of its approach. He emphasizes physical activities that are moderate, stressing that you do not need to begin to train for the Olympics, even though you have been a couch potato for most of your life. He takes a behavioral approach, helping you outline the rewards of exercise while eliminating the barriers. Finally, he focuses on increasing your physical activity as part of your daily lifestyle.

The American Volkksport is an association committed to promoting health and fitness through noncompetitive, safe sporting activities. They publish the *American Wanderer,* a bimonthly newspaper for $12 a year, with news on their groups and events. They can also send you a list of local walking clubs. An individual yearly membership is $20.

Rockport's Complete Book of Fitness Walking by Dr. James M. Rippe and Ann Ward, Ph.D. (New York: Prentice Hall Press, 1989).

Prevention Walking Club
Rodale Press
Box 6099
Emmaus, PA 18099
(800) 441-7761

A $9.97 membership includes a quarterly newsletter and annual magazine, both about various aspects of walking.

RELAXATION

There are many books dealing with the issue of relaxation. Some of the better ones include:

Beyond the Relaxation Response by Herbert Benson with William Proctor (New York: New York Times Book Company, 1984).

Mind/Body Medicine is an edited book, published by *Consumer Reports.* Some of the leading experts on psychoneuroimmunolgy present their views on how stress affects our health

Healthy Pleasures by Robert Ornstein and David Sobel presents a comfortable nonthreatening approach to lifestyle change. The upbeat tone helps us avoid the feelings at being trapped by the "health police" (Reading, MA: Addison-Wesley Publishing Co., Inc., 1989).

ELIMINATING OR REDUCING PROBLEMATIC BEHAVIORS—OVEREATING

Dr. Kelly Brownell and Dr. Judith Rodin have participated in research on obesity for many years. Two of the books that we have found helpful are: *The LEARN Program for Weight Control* by Dr. Brownell and *The Weight Maintenance Survival Guide* by Drs. Brownell and Rodin. The value of these books is that they are based on behavioral research and take a safe and gradual approach to weight loss. In addition, they are extremely sensitive to women's issues and to the concerns about weight-cycling that can also be hazardous.

ALCOHOL ABUSE

Alcoholics Anonymous or AA, the grandparent of self-help groups, is usually listed in the front of the telephone book and often on the pages of local newspapers. If, however, you cannot find a group in your area, you can check with the General Service Office at P.O. Box 459, Grand Central Station, New York, NY 10016—(212)-686-1100. Some women find AA to be too male-dominated and are more comfortable in groups where there are more women. This varies on a group by group basis.

Another group that works with women alone is called Women For Sobriety, P.O. Box 618, Quaker Town Pennsylvania, 18951—(800) 333-1606.

SMOKING

The American Lung Association provides pamphlets about quitting smoking. Your local affiliate can also send you a list of smoke-free restaurants in your area.

NUTRITION

Jane Brody is one of the best health writers around. Her articles in the *New York Times* are always balanced and practical. One of her books that is extremely helpful is called *Jane Brody's Nutrition Book* (New York: Bantam Books, 1987).

For women interested in vegetarianism, an interesting magazine is *Vegetarian Times,* published in Mount Morris, Illinois. This old guard vegetarian monthly magazine includes health topics, humane issues, vegetarian product information and recipes, but also covers educational articles promoting healthy lifestyles.

Fast Vegetarian Feasts, by Martha Rose Shulman (New York: Dial Press, 1982). This book proves that vegetarian cooking can be quick. It also includes menus.

Moosewood Cookbook, this meatless cookbook is one of the oldest and most popular, and has been recently revised to reflect the lower calorie approach. Written by Mollie Katzen (The Ten Speed Press, Berkeley California, 1993).

Tufts University Diet and Nutrition Letter
203 Harrison Ave.
Boston, MA 02111
(800) 274-7581

Newsletter that reviews studies, and gives the latest information on nutrition and health in a rather off-the-cuff, skeptical style. $20 a year for 12 issues.

← *CHAPTER ELEVEN*

Resources

So THERE IT IS. NOW YOU KNOW ALMOST EVERYTHING WE KNOW ABOUT menopause. You know that menopause does not need to be a time of multiple symptoms and deteriorating health. Menopause is not necessarily a time of significant losses. Menopause does not need to be a time when we retreat from society and withdraw into invisibility. Menopause is a time of new freedom from concerns about birth control, freedom from fulfilling but often draining family responsibilities, freedom to have more power to choose everything from our friends to our health care providers, and freedom to explore new ways of living.

Menopause is not merely a hormonal event, nor is it a negative event. Women need to be viewed as whole people, affected by our biology, yes, but by psychology, sociology and the political environment as well. As health care professionals we do see some women who are suffering from troubling symptoms at menopause. We know from our work with patients and our review of the research that problems associated with menopause can be treated effectively, and therefore that menopause is not a particularly troubling time for most women.

This chapter will help you get the most out of your own resources.

When it comes to coping with issues around menopause and dealing with other problems, women have long turned to one another for strength and guidance. We can turn inward to trust our own feelings, and we can turn outward to other women and resources that can be extremely beneficial. Intuitively you will know how to approach certain problems. If you trust your feelings, you will know what your needs are, and your emotional response to many suggestions or ideas about solutions can tell you a lot. This chapter will provide you with resources, but remember that you are your own best health expert.

Two of the most important resources in dealing with the menopausal years are maintenance of good health and focusing on relationships. By maintaining good health, we can promote a lifestyle that prevents as much disease as possible. Focusing on health, rather than illness, also helps us keep an optimistic and coping attitude, instead of focusing on the next phase of life as a series of losses and symptoms. By using the preventive strategies we detailed in the previous chapter, we can continue to lead, not only long, but active and healthy lives. Part of that lifestyle involves developing a women's health team, which we will describe shortly. By maximizing our choices and obtaining as much information as possible, women can work with a primary care provider to develop a healthy lifestyle and flourish during the menopausal years.

Whatever problems we face in life, our relationships and social connections can help us. In every area of women's health from depression to maintenance of exercise routines to dealing with the issue of hormone replacement therapy, women have received support from their relationships with others. These relationships can consist of our family, our friends, our health care providers and self-help groups. If you combine the information that you have taken away from this book, with an assertive attitude toward your own health care and an openness to relationships that can provide you with a feeling of support, you will be well able to cope with whatever life brings. These principles can continue to guide you long after you finish reading this book.

✦ CREATING YOUR OWN WOMEN'S HEALTH TEAM

One of the most significant, positive changes you can make is to take charge of your own health care. You can do this by creating your own women's health team, maintaining a healthy attitude, becoming an educated health consumer and accessing resources.

As we write this book, the health care system in the United States is under intense scrutiny and in the midst of revolutionary change. This change is necessary because of the escalating health care costs that threaten our economic livelihood. We know all too many women who have been shut out of good health care because they lack health insurance. This may be due to poverty, unemployment, inadequate health benefits or the results of a divorce. We should all recognize the impact of the "feminization of poverty"—that is, the fact that most of the people on welfare in the United States are women and their children, and older women as well. As women entering the menopausal years, we must remember that we are the largest segment of the American population and that as we age, we must continue to develop political power so that no woman or man is shut out of the health care system.

We hope that any changes in the health care system will support an effort to emphasize the role of primary care providers. Primary care professionals are the key to women's health during the menopausal years. A primary care provider can help us process the explosion of new information and access appropriate resources when necessary. By creating a partnership in which a woman makes her own health care decision with her primary care provider, health care costs can be maintained, with the best possible health resulting.

Given the changes in the health care system, there is tremendous uncertainty about what types of health insurance will be available, and what will be included in health care coverage. Nonetheless, whether your health insurance is provided on a fee-for-service basis, or in a health-maintenance organization, or in a primary care clinic, you can use certain principles to guide you.

The first principle is to develop a good relationship or partnership with your health care professional. This significant relationship must be based on mutual respect and the ability to talk over the rapidly developing information regarding choices and health care for women in today's changing world. All too often, we have heard our patients say, "I can't really talk with my doctor, but I don't want to hurt his or her feelings" or "My doctor really doesn't have the time to talk to me much." Although we understand the stresses in being a doctor, we know that it is not a woman's job to take care of her doctor, or to worry about taking up too much time. We see many confident and successful women who may be assertive in their everyday lives, but who are still anxious when they need a few moments time from their physicians. It is imperative that we stop feeling like we are "wasting the doctor's time" or that "the doctor has more important things to do than listen to me complain." Spending productive time with our doctor is a meaningful activity, since communication is the key to understanding and the road to prevention and healing. You need to be able to feel free to share your feelings with your physician and to feel comfortable asking questions. Your doctor does not need to be your best friend, but there should be a minimal amount of tension and an attitude of mutual respect, and the ability to share feelings as well as information.

Remember to focus on your own communication skills. The more prepared you are for the office visit, the more you will get out of it. This means first thinking through what your goals are. If there is information that you want to explore during an office visit, you can state that as soon as possible. If, on the other hand, you have several symptoms or problems that are of concern, try to emphasize the ones that are most bothersome or cause you the most anxiety. You might want to review some of the interactions we describe in other chapters of this book to help you along.

Your primary care professional should coordinate your health care. This means providing referrals to appropriate subspecialties and helping you understand their role in your health care. Too many of our patients who have had extensive medical evaluations for infertility, cancer or cardiac problems have stated that the most troubling part of these experiences was dealing with the health care system in general. Trying to coordinate these various specialists is a difficult proposition and your primary care provider should be able to do it for you.

It is important that your health care focus on health, not on illness alone. You probably knew this by now, since in every chapter we have emphasized the issue of prevention. The lifestyle changes that we have outlined are sometimes difficult. But, once they have been established as part of your daily routine, they can make all the difference in your menopausal years. We know that we can reduce the risk of heart disease in women if we begin early. We know that exercise and the appropriate calcium intake, as well as hormone replacement therapy, can reduce the risk of osteoporosis. We know that exercising and eliminating substance abuse can make us all feel better. This emphasis on a healthy lifestyle should be one of your health care provider's values as well.

Do not hesitate to involve a health psychologist or mental health professional. Women tend to use the mental health care system more than men. This is not evidence of some growing mental illness in women, but is a strength. We can conclude from these numbers that most women know when they need help, and we should all trust our instincts and access the mental health system when necessary. Counseling or psychotherapy can make all the difference when coping with stress, family problems or depression. Still, national estimates are that only 8 percent of people with psychological problems receive the appropriate care. Your primary care provider should have a positive attitude toward psychological care as well. Usually, he or she can help you find a competent psychotherapist when necessary. If not, you can refer to our chapter on depression for other ways to access the system of psychological care.

You should be able to have some choice in selecting your primary care provider. This includes choosing a female clinician. Medicine has long been dominated by male physicians. For too many years, women did not have access to female psychologists or physicians. Fortunately, the situation changed rapidly in the last twenty years, with 30 percent of the graduates of medical schools and more than half of the graduate schools of doctoral programs in psychology being female. But female gender alone does not guarantee either an attitude of mutual respect or necessarily an expertise or interest in women's health. This was summed up to us once when one of our patients who was thinking of going to a female gynecologist was told by a close friend, "If you are the type of woman who wants a woman doctor, that woman doctor is not the right one for you!" Complicated, but we knew what she meant.

A significant part of the women's health approach involves a woman's family. Whether your family includes a spouse, partner, children, or a close friend, these people are important resources, not a burden to your health care. Your family should feel comfortable, accompanying you to appointments and even meeting with the doctor when you are either feeling anxious or perhaps facing a major crisis. Most primary care providers are eager to include your family, so you should not hesitate to do so.

✦ THE ROLE OF MENOPAUSE CLINICS

Menopause clinics are springing up everywhere, and we are somewhat concerned about this popular trend. If a menopause clinic involves the comprehensive and interdisciplinary approach we have described, with attention to doctor-patient communication, then it is likely to be an excellent facility for you. However, some menopause clinics focus exclusively on the issue of hormone replacement therapy, and may even involve unnecessary testing (for example, bone densitometry for every woman). Other such clinics are primarily screening centers, but do not offer continuing primary care for women. Your best bet for finding comprehensive care, is to look for a women's health associates practice, using the same principles that we have described above. In addition, the North American Menopause Society (NAMS) can provide you with a resources list for your area. These resources provide the type of professional services available from NAMS members. NAMS is composed of professionals from many disciplines and has national as well as regional meetings to disseminate new treatments and advances in research.

Whether you choose a menopause clinic or a women's health practice, a primary care provider or an individual in an HMO, you should consider scheduling a first meeting essentially as a consultation. This may not always be feasible, depending on your health insurance plan or financial situation. If you can, use that meeting to get a feeling for your comfort level with the provider and to share expectations of what the relationship will be. Ultimately, you are the best judge of your relationship with your primary care provider. If, after two visits you are uncomfortable, be sure to seek out another health care provider or facility.

Be sure to avail yourself of the resources in your community. Although many of the resources such as health education and behavioral medicine programs may be out there, you may not know about them if you do not seek them out.

Above all, do not let yourself become invisible. Most health care providers respect their patients and know that good communication with an actively involved patient may require extra time, but ultimately is worthwhile. If you are treated without respect, you should work with a patient advocate if you are in an HMO or clinic, or find another primary care doctor if your insurance is fee for service. In most cases you will be able to work things out by taking an informed and assertive approach to your own health care. If all else fails, you may need to risk being labeled cranky, or even a "bitch," when your health is at stake. As U.S. Supreme Court Justice Ruth Ginsburg has been quoted, "Better bitch than mouse" (Rosen, 1993).

◆ BECOMING AN EDUCATED CONSUMER

Every Thursday morning on the morning news programs and radio shows, we learn the results of the most recent medical breakthroughs, possible cures and hazards. Often, a doctor of one sort or another is brought on the program for approximately three to four minutes to explain an article published in a medical journal. At times, this overload of information can become unbelievably confusing—do this, don't do that, take this, stay away from that. A prime example was described by

Dr. James Muller, a cardiologist at Harvard Medical School. He was listening to a talk show in which a caller drew a conclusion from two separate studies that had been reported. One study had suggested that heart attacks tended to occur in the morning, another that eating grapes could reduce the risk of heart attacks. Conclusion? "The best way to stay healthy was to stay in bed, eating grapes, until noon" (Rosenthal, 1993). Although such a lifestyle has a certain appeal, this example illustrates how we can make false conclusions when we receive just a little information!

But how can we make sense of these new articles, facts and findings? The best advice is "Do not panic!" over tomorrow's miracle cure or killer. It is rare that the results of one study alone are enough to necessitate a major change in your lifestyle. It is also true that sometimes the media picks up studies that are more sensational than they are reputable. However, if you begin to hear the same results over and over again, then it is time to take notice. Talk all of this new information over with your clinician. In addition, there are several good health magazines that can help you process the information. We list some of them in the back of this chapter, but one of the best is *Prevention*. It tends to review current and reputable articles, rather than the most sensational ones.

We appreciate and respect your interest in understanding the literature. We know that the traditional medical establishment has not paid enough attention to women's health until recently, and so women have needed to be active consumers of information. We do *not* think that you should take a passive view, but should remember to try not to be frightened based on one study. There are several questions you can ask when trying to understand the results of medical literature. One issue involved in understanding the study includes methodology, or how the study was conducted. You need to know if the study is a new study, or has it been done before with other people? The most notorious examples here were many of the cardiovascular studies that were done only on men, ignoring the issue of women's health. Another example is the exaggeration of a study that commented on women's declining fertility in their thirties. The original overly dramatized study was actually based on a small group of French women whose chief complaint was the couple's infertility—hardly a group from which to generalize to the larger American society.

Remember also that association does not mean causation. If we see that, for example, baldness is *associated* with heart disease, that does not mean that baldness causes heart disease in general. Nor does it mean that if someone you know is bald, he will suffer a heart attack.

It may be, for example, some underlying factor that affects most bald men that may also be associated with heart disease. There are a few factors that we know are directly causal. (One thing we do know for sure, however, is that smoking causes lung cancer, the cancer most likely to kill women. So we will take this opportunity to ask you again to quit smoking if you are a smoker.) But in general, Dr. Muller rightly cautions us that we shouldn't "live off tidbits of epidemiological data." Epidemiological studies merely point in certain directions. It takes much more careful study to understand how and why certain medical problems occur.

Risk factors can help us make general decisions, but do not completely protect us from illness, nor do they always apply to any individual woman. For example, let's say that your risk of getting bitten by a mosquito was .0001. If a new study came out and found that women who wore perfume increased their risk tenfold, this could be met with quite a bit of excitement. But that still only increases the risk of that individual to .001, that is, only one out of a thousand women would still be bitten by the mosquito. So, in this situation, the numbers can tell you a lot. Scientists, like other people, have points of view, and so they can use numbers in many ways. You can use your own common sense to help you decide how much or how little the risk factors or numbers involved in a study apply to you.

Note who paid for the study. The publicized study linking baldness to heart attacks was funded by the UpJohn Corporation, which wanted to prove that it was the baldness and not minoxidil, the drug produced by UpJohn to treat baldness, that was associated with heart attacks. More importantly, studies that have been funded by pharmaceutical companies that produce hormone replacement drugs, or institutes which rely on these companies for a large proportion of their income, should also be viewed accordingly.

Remember again to think over your concerns and bring them up with your primary care provider. Some women prefer not to follow the psychological and medical literature and prefer to let their primary care provider let them know appropriate new information. But most of our patients are avid consumers of health news. Most physicians and psychologists enjoy talking over these findings with their patients and are usually prepared to do so.

✦ ACCESSING RESOURCES

There are a number of general resources for the menopausal woman. These resources have been included at the end of this chapter.

There are two resources that we find are vastly underutilizied. Both of them are good examples of taxpayers' dollars at work, something we do not hear much about these days. Both of them are practically free, and readily available. First, on the local level, ask your librarian. Some of you may remember how exciting it was to walk into a library when you were ten or eleven years old and suddenly realized the amount of information that could be found there. If you were very lucky, you met a friendly, rather than intimidating librarian, who could show you available resources and answer your questions. Guess what? She (or he) is still around! You just need to find the library where she works. This is, after all, what reference librarians do best. For you, it costs nothing. It is easy, and there is usually a public library nearby.

On the federal level, one of our exciting discoveries was the Bureau of Public Documents (U.S. Government Printing Office, Superintendent of Documents, Mail Stop: SSOP, Washington, D.C. 20402-9328). You can obtain a monthly list of documents that are published. They are quite wide ranging and informative, from growing lima beans to an excellent review of the hormone replacement therapy literature. So you can keep up with what the government is publishing on a regular basis and order these documents for a minimal cost.

✦ RESOURCES

We have selected several resources for you in a number of categories. This list is not meant to be exhaustive, but rather is included to give you an idea of some of the best resources available.

BOOKS

The Columbia University 40+ Guide to Good Health (Fairfield, OH: Consumer Reports Books, 1993). This book is published by the Columbia University School of Public Health faculty. It debunks many of the myths of aging and provides coping strategies, biological and psychological problems.

ASSOCIATIONS

AARP—American Association of Retired People
601 E St., NW
Washington DC 20049
(202) 434-2277

We know that you are probably not retired yet, but the AARP works to enhance the quality of life for older people through education and policy change and has more than 33 million members over 50. One program within the Association is the Women's Initiative, which focuses specifically on older women's issues. Members receive a bimonthly magazine, Modern Maturity, *and a newspaper with information about the AARP's activities and achievements,* The AARP Bulletin, *eleven times a year. Other free publications are available on a variety of topics, including exercise, diet, older women's health concerns, mental health, and the health needs of various ethnic groups.*

American Board of Medical Specialties
1007 Church Street, Suite 404
Evanston, IL 60201-5913
1-800-776-CERT—certification line
(708) 491-9091—number for the Board

Call or write to find out if a doctor is board-certified. The board also offers a pamphlet, "Which Medical Specialist for You?," describing medical specialties, for $1.50.

American Board of Obstetrics and Gynecology
4225 Roosevelt Way NE, Suite 305
Seattle, WA 98105
(206) 547-4884

This is a certifying board: call or write to find out if a gynecologist is certified.

American Cancer Society
1599 Clifton Rd., NE
Atlanta, GA 30329
(800) ACS-2345—This number connects you to your state office.

Check your white pages for the nearest local office.
The ACS provides information, guidance, support groups, and referrals to other community resources. They can send you free pamphlets and factsheets on mammograms, breast self-exams, Pap smears, reproductive cancer, and general cancer information.

American College of Obstetricians and Gynecologists (ACOG)
409 12th St, SW
Washington, DC 20024
(202) 638-5577

The ACOG can give you a listing of board-certified physicians in your area. They also offer a number of free patient-education pamphlets on menopause and related issues, osteoporosis, hysterectomy, and fitness and exercise.

American Dental Association
211 E. Chicago Ave.
Chicago, IL 60611
(312) 440-2500

The ADA can give you a listing of dentists in your area. They also publish free pamphlets on dentures, diet and dental health, and dental tips for older adults.

American Dietetic Association
216 W Jackson Blvd, Suite 800
Chicago, IL 60606

This association and its newsletter are geared toward dieticians, but brochures on dietetics and nutrition are also available for consumers.

Gray Panthers
1424 16th St, NW, Suite 602
Washington DC 20036
(202) 347-6471

A coalition of activists that promotes the concerns of older people. The group has a newsletter and other publications on a variety of issues.

Health/PAC (Policy Advisory Center)
853 Broadway, Suite 1607
NY, NY 10003
(212) 614-1660

The Center is a nonprofit advocate for progressive health policy. They publish a quarterly journal on health care policy, HealthPAC Bulletin, for $35 a year, $22.50 for people with low income. The group also sponsors seminars on health care and policy.

National Senior Citizens' Law Center
1815 H Street, NW, Suite 700
Washington, DC 20006
(202) 887-5280

This is a legal-service support center which advocates for low-income older clients and offers referrals.

North American Menopause Society
University Hospitals of Cleveland
2074 Abington Rd.
Cleveland, OH 44106
(216) 844-3334

The NAMS has publications on menopause, a listing of literature about menopause, and lists of menopause clinics across the country.

Older Women's League (OWL)
666 11th St, NW, Suite 700
Washington, DC 20001
(202) 783-6686

OWL lobbies for the needs of older women. They have a referral resource file for support groups, and will answer your letters and questions. They sponsor the Campaign for Women's Health, which lobbies and publishes the newsletter "Women's Health," and also put out a bimonthly newspaper, The Owl Observer. *They are in the process of publishing a brochure on menopause.*

Women's Action Alliance
370 Lexington Ave, Suite 603
NY, NY 10017
(212) 532-8330

A nonprofit group working for positive change and self-determination for girls and women. Women's health is one of their focuses but nothing on menopause has been published. The Alliance has a publication catalog.

FEDERAL GOVERNMENT

National Cancer Institute
9000 Rockville Pike
Building 31, Room 10A24
Bethesda, MD 20892
(800) 4-CANCER—number answered regionally

The NCI has a listing of free publications which you can order, in English or Spanish, on smoking, nutrition, breast cancer, cancer tests

*for those over 65, and mammograms. It also sponsors the Cancer
Information Service: free cancer information and support from trained
counselors, referrals to physicians, quit smoking counseling, and
resources for medical care and counseling.*

The Cancer Information Service
Office of Cancer Communications
333 Cedar Street, LEPH 139
PO Box 3333
New Haven, CT 06510

National Heart, Lung, and Blood Institute
9000 Rockville Pike
Building 31, Room 4A 21
Bethesda, MD 20892
(301) 951-3260

*The institute publishes a directory of resources for relevant health
concerns, including somewhat technical-free pamphlets and factsheets
on healthy eating, weight loss and exercise.*

National Institute on Aging
Information Center
PO Box 8057
Gaithersburg, MD 20898-8057
(800) 222-2225

*The institute publishes a very complete resource directory for Women's
Health and Aging, the pamphlet "The Menopause Time of Life," and a
series of factsheets or Age Pages on menopause and other aspects of
aging, exercise, and nutrition. They also sponsor workshops on
menopause.*

INFORMATION CENTERS/CLEARINGHOUSES

Boston Women's Health Book Collective
240A M Street
Davis Square
Somerville, MA 02114
(617) 625-0271

*A medical consumer organization that publishes books and brochures on
women's health issues. They have available a listing of their publications*

and services and literature packets on a variety of women's health topics, including HRT and menopause.

Center for Medical Consumers
237 Thompson St
NY, NY 10012
(212) 674-7105

The center has a library and a monthly newsletter, "Health Facts," which includes information for menopausal women. A pamphlet on the benefits and risks of mammography screening, "Mammography Screening: A Decision-Making Guide," is available for $5.

Consumer Information Center
PO Box 100
Pueblo, CO 81002
(719) 948-3334

They have a listing of publications, the Consumer Information Catalog of government publications, covering a lot of topics, including health, aging, exercise, and nutrition.

National Council on Patient Information and Education
666 11th St, NW #810
Washington, DC 20001

The council publishes "Medicines: What Every Woman Should Know," a pamphlet on proper use and behavior related to medicines.

National Institute on Drug Abuse
Prepares the brochure "Elder-Ed: Using Your Medicines Wisely." To receive it, write to:

Government Printing Office
710 N Capitol St, NW
Washington, DC 20402
(Stock No 00017002400969—$4.75)

National Self-Help Clearinghouse
25 W 43rd St, Room 620
NY, NY 10036
(212) 642-2944

*The clearinghouse is a databank and "switchboard" for information
and referrals to self-help groups. It publishes manuals, training
materials and group-starting materials, as well as a quarterly
newsletter, "Self-Help Reporter," for $10.*

National Women's Health Network
1325 G Street, NW, Lower Level
Washington, DC 20077-2052
(202) 293-6045

*A member-based educational organization and clearinghouse for
information on women's health. They have a database of current
resources, 56 literature packets available for $8 each on women's health
issues, a free directory of publications, pamphlets, and factsheets
available, and can provide referrals. A $25 membership includes the
"National Women's Health Report," a bimonthly newsletter. They also
publish "The Network News," a newsletter on women's health and
resources.*

National Women's Health Resource Center
2440 M St, NW, Suite 325
Washington, DC 20037
(202) 293-6045

*An information clearinghouse on women's health, focusing on public
education, clinical services, and research. The Center publishes a
newsletter, "National Women's Health Report." They publish a
brochure on HRT and sponsor conferences and seminars on menopause.*

Santa Fe Health Education Project
PO Box 577
Santa Fe, NM 87502
(505) 982-3236 or 982-9520

*They publish a newsletter, "Healthletters," with bilingual health
information for women. "Menopause—a Self-Care Manual" is also
available for $3.85.*

Vintage 45 Press
PO Box 266
Orinda, CA 94563-0266

*Publishes a Selected Booklist catalog, with books on all aspects of being
an older woman, including one on menopause.*

SELF-HELP GROUPS

Red Hot Mamas
Connecticut Center for Menopause Management
Ridgefield, CT
(203) 431-3902

The Red Hot Mamas was founded by Karen Giblin. They offer support groups in Connecticut and can help women establish new chapters.

Supportive Older Women's Network (SOWN)
2805 N 47th Street
Philadelphia, PA 19131
(215) 477-6000

Helps women over 60 with aging-related concerns through support groups, consultation, and outreach programs. The Network also puts out a newsletter, "The Sounding Board," and publishes guidelines for developing a group.

PHARMACEUTICAL COMPANY PUBLICATIONS

US Pharmacopeial Convention, Inc.
Drug Information Division
12601 Twinbrook Parkway
Rockville, MD 20852

Publishes the USP Catalog of patient education materials, such as "About Your Medicines," a book on common prescription drugs, patient education leaflets, and computer products.

Bristol-Myers Squibb
PO Box 907
Spring House, PA 19477-9945
(800) 937-4025

Offers a free newsletter on aging, menopause and HRT, "Transitions," put out by company that makes ESTRACE, a brand of estradiol.

NEWSLETTERS

Consumer Reports Health Letter
Consumer Union of US, Inc.
101 Truman Avenue
Yonkers, NY 10703-1057

Information on prevention, risks, treatment of various health issues with a focus on keeping the consumer informed.

Johns Hopkins Medical Letter: Health After 50
PO Box 420176
Palm Coast, FL 32142

12 issues of medical information on women's health and older people's medical concerns for $24.

Network
National Gray Panther Newsletter
3635 Chestnut St.
Philadelphia, PA 19104

Bimonthly newsletter on aging, health care, political action, and local chapter activities.

Magazines/Periodicals

Lear's
PO Box 420353
Palm Coast, FL 32142-9648

Monthly magazine geared toward older women with articles on entertainment, health, fashion, politics, money. $18 a year.

Hippocrates
301 Howard Street, Suite 1800
San Francisco, CA 94105

Monthly magazine of health information.

Menopause Management
9 Mt. Pleasant Turnpike
Denville, NJ 07834
(201) 361-1280

Magazine endorsed by the North American Menopause Society with articles on all aspects of menopause: symptoms, prevention, treatment, lifestyle. Primarily oriented to health care professionals. Published bimonthly for $25 a year.

Midlife Wellness Center for Climacteric Studies
University of Florida
901 NW 8th Ave, Suite B1
Gainesville, FL 32601

Quarterly journal on menopause and aging for health professionals and the general public.

CHAPTER TWELVE

Moving On

AS YOU KNOW BY NOW, WE SEE THE MENOPAUSAL YEARS AS EXCITING AND full of a new sense of freedom. Yet, the negative views of the menopausal years persist in medical literature, in the popular media and within all of us. There is, of course, a long history of bashing the menopausal woman, and older women. But the combination of the negative attitude with medicalization of women's lives has a particularly destructive effect. This combination can be traced back many centuries. Our job, as women today, is to fight it every step of the way, in every form we see it.

In 1816, French physician C.P.L. de Gardanne described a syndrome called "De la ménépausie ou de l'age critique des femmes" (Gardanne, 1821). Over one hundred pages of the manuscript is dedicated to a myriad of illnesses that may accompany menopause, including hemorrhoids, rebellion and severe mental illness. If we were to read *La Ménépausie* today, and take it to heart, we would conclude that menopause was merely a batch of horrifying symptoms that would make us deteriorate over time, filling the remainder portion of our lives with misery.

Our experience has provided us with a much more optimistic outlook. We know that women are strong, and that they have most likely survived many life crises by the time they reach menopause. But if you are still a nonbeliever, consider the following women. Many of these women's stories have been collected and edited in an excellent book by Jill Ker Conway, the first woman president of Smith College and a professor at the Massachusetts Institute of Technology. In *Written by Herself*, we can learn about the stories of women of all ages (Conway, 1992).

• Marian Anderson, who died while we were working on this book, was the first black person to sing at the Metropolitan Opera Company on January 7, 1955. She describes her anxiety and excitement over this accomplishment.

> ". . . Mother arrived, and she threw her arms around me and whispered in my ear, 'We thank the Lord.' Her only words before the performance had been, 'Mother is praying for you,' and after it she just stood there, and though she is not outwardly demonstrative, I could see that there was a light around her face. She did not know much about opera, but she knew the significance of what was going on that night and she was profoundly moved by it. If she had said more she would have said, 'My cup runneth over' " (Anderson, 1992, p. 97).

Marian Anderson was fifty-three on that exciting night.

• Ruth Bader Ginsburg was one of ten women in her law school class of five hundred from the late 1950s. She was elected to the law reviews of both Harvard and Columbia University. Proposed by one of her Harvard Law School professors as a potential clerk to Justice Felix Frankfurter, the justice told Professor Albert Sacks that "while the candidate was impressive, he was not ready to hire a woman" (Lewis, 1993). Ruth Bader Ginsburg became the first tenured female law professor at Columbia. Judge Ginsburg credits her mother as "the bravest and strongest person I have known, who was taken from me much too soon. I pray that I may be all that she would have been, had she lived in an age when women could inspire and achieve, and daughters are cherished as much as sons. I look forward to working to the best of my ability for the advancement of the law in the service of society" (Lewis, 1993). You know where Ruth Bader Ginsburg, now in her sixties, is today.

• Cecilia Payne Gaposchkin became the professor and chairman of the Department of Anthropology at Harvard University at the age of fifty-six. She had a loving family life, and had worked at Harvard for many decades. Perhaps some of her energy was fueled by the discrimination she faced. Despite the fact that she was an accomplished woman who had received her Ph.D. from Radcliffe in 1925 and had written extensively, her salary from the Harvard Observatory had to be paid directly from her mentor, Harlow Cheply. For twenty years she was not paid a fair salary and her courses were not even listed in the catalogue. Cecilia, too, has words of wisdom, "On the material side, being a woman has been a great disadvantage. It is a tale of low salary, lack of status, and slow advancement . . . it is a case of survival, not of the fittest, but of the most doggedly persistent. I was not consciously aiming at the point I finally reached. I simply went on plotting, rewarded by the beauty of the scenery, toward an unexpected goal. . . . Your reward will be the widening of the horizon as you climb. And if you achieve that reward, you will ask no other" (Gaposchkin, 1992, p. 282).

• Vida Dutton Scudder challenged the conventions of society when she opposed Wellesley College's accepting money from the Rockefeller family because she felt it was tainted, and when she addressed workers who were on strike in Lawrence, Massachusetts. All this occurred in 1912, when Scudder was fifty one years old (Scudder, 1992, p. 333).

• In July 1966, Nien Cheng survived the loss of her husband and the prejudices of Chinese society. Nien Cheng saw her house ransacked and lived more than six years in solitary confinement because she refused to confess that she was an enemy of the state. She was fifty-one when she was arrested. Her imprisonment was followed by the tragic discovery of the death of her daughter. Nien Cheng pursued the mysterious details of her daughter's death for over a decade, until she discovered that her daughter had been murdered. She, like the mothers of the Plaza de Mayo in Argentina, would not let the matter drop. She came to the United States and wrote the book *Life and Death in Shanghai,* as a testament to her daughter. She writes, "I live a full and busy life. Only sometimes I feel a haunting sadness. At dusk, when the day is fading away and the level of my physical energy is at a low ebb, I may find myself depressed and nostalgic. But the next morning I invariably wake up with a renewed optimism to welcome the day as another opportunity given me by God for enlightenment and experience. . . . I feel a compulsion to speak out and let those who have the good fortune to live in freedom know what my life was like during those dark days in Maoist China" (Cheng, 1988, p. 538).

• The photographer and writer Margaret Bourke-White was in her late forties when she was an official army and air force photographer during World War II, and much of her work was published by *Life* magazine. She was at the peak of her career when she reached her mid-fifties, and even when she was diagnosed with Parkinson's disease, fought against it by using photographs of people during rehabilitation to encourage others. Bourke-White chose never to marry and wrote this, "Mine is a life into which marriage doesn't fit very well. If I had children, I would have chartered a widely different life, drawn creative inspiration from them and shaped my work to them. Perhaps I would have worked on children's books rather than going to wars. It must be a fascinating thing to watch a growing child absorb his expanding world. One life is not better than the other, it is just a different life. . . . There is a richness in a life where you stand on your own feet, although it imposes a certain creed. There must be no demands, others have the right to be as free as you are. You must be able to take disappointments gallantly. You set your own ground rules, and if you follow them, there are great rewards" (Bourke-White, 1992, p. 453).

• Frances Sherwood is a fifty-three-year-old woman who is a professor, and mother of three grown children. She wrote a brilliant novel based on the life of eighteenth-century feminist Mary Wollstonecraft. The novel was rejected by four agents. Frances Sherwood then sent her manuscript directly to a publisher and her novel was published in 1993. The title of her novel? *Vindication* (Olshan, 1993).

• Maya Angelou was named one of the one hundred most influential American women in 1983 when she was fifty-five. Author of *I Know Why the Caged Bird Sings,* this gifted poet and writer was asked to create a poem especially for the inauguration of President Clinton when she was sixty-five years old.

We read frequently that women used to die in their forties and fifties, and that perhaps we were never meant to live another forty years without estrogen. But these statistics have an artificially low average age of death because they include many women who died during childbirth. Although our life spans are increasing, there have always been thriving older women around, if only we would pay attention to them, and heed their words. Like Ellen Glasgow: "Yes, I have had my life, I have known ecstasy, I have known anguish, I have loved, and I have been loved. With one I loved, I have watched the light breaking over the Alps. If I pass through, 'the dark night of the soul,' I have had a far off glimpse of the illumination beyond. For an infinitesimal point of time, or eternity, I have caught a gleam, or imagined I caught a gleam, of the mystic vision. It was enough, and now it is over. Not for everything that the world could give me would I consent to live over my life unchanged, or to bring back unchanged my youth" (Glasgow, 1992, p. 400).

Did these women have hot flashes? Probably. Did some of them have headaches or other difficulties? Maybe. Did they survive and flourish? Most definitely, and we are the better for it. Knowing now what we know about menopause, perhaps it is time to treat our symptoms seriously when we should, and then to move ahead with the strength that women share.

APPENDIX A
MISCELLANEOUS PROBLEMS
AND SYMPTOMS

In this appendix we have included a variety of symptoms and problems that have been reported by our menopausal patients and in the medical literature. If a symptom has not been covered in a previous chapter, you will be able to find a description of it here. We have titled this appendix "Miscellaneous Problems and Symptoms" because these are less frequently reported. However, we know that any symptom that is *yours* is extremely important. "Miscellaneous" certainly does not imply minor. Some of the symptoms listed below may be your only, or most troubling, symptom of menopause.

There is a danger, however, in listing every problem that has ever been reported by menopausal women. Many women do not have regular health care prior to menopause. We go to the obstetrician when we are pregnant, we may go to a gynecologist for routine pelvic exams and Pap smears, but often we do not obtain ongoing health care. It is often during the menopausal years that some women will visit a physician regularly for the first time in their lives. This is good for any individual woman's health, but it leads to certain problems in research and misrepresenting the "typical menopausal woman." There have been too few studies of the menopausal women who choose not to visit physicians, so it is difficult to obtain the "normal picture." One study of Swedish women found that a full 35 percent of menopausal women did not experience any changes other than cessation of the menstrual cycle. The remaining 65 percent reported changes in weight gain and redistribution of body fat, some changes in skin or hair and stiffness of the joints. But, the vast majority of these women did not see that these symptoms had any negative effect on their life (Collins, 1992).

We should not generalize to all women from the small groups of women who begin to visit doctors at the time of menopause, or from other women who may be visiting doctors very frequently.

There are some difficulties with the symptoms mentioned in this chapter as well. Because of the lack of research on women's health issues, we do not know which problems are common to all women, which are a function of aging, and which are associated specifically with menopause. This appendix will try to sort through these factors. Still, there has been so little research on women, that we will not be able to give you all the answers at this point in time.

What we can give you is an assurance that any discomfort from these miscellaneous symptoms can, for the most part, be treated effectively. Part of our major motivation for writing this book was our emotional reaction to other books about menopause that literally listed dozens of problems potentially associated with menopause, without listing their relative frequency. Many of the problems that were listed were equally common to aging men, but were presented as menopausal problems. We ask one favor of you. *Do not* read this appendix and believe that you *will necessarily* experience any or all of these problems and symptoms. Be reassured that it is extremely unlikely that you would experience more than one or two of them, and even if you do, most women have found that these problems are not severe and can be managed quite well. Rather, use this appendix as a reference point for miscellaneous symptoms that you did not find in other chapters.

A good reference is the *Johns Hopkins Medical Handbook: One Hundred Major Medical Disorders* of people over the age of fifty. This is a detailed and accessible book that is an excellent reference. It provides discussions of the major problems of midlife people and also provides an additional section on resources for treatment.

✦ BACK PAIN

Fifty to eighty percent of Americans complain of back pain at some time. Back pain actually represents a large category of problems. We found that for most women chronic back pain can occur at any time. Low back pain can also be aggravated by osteoarthritis or rheumatoid arthritis. It is important to read the chapter on osteoporosis to understand the necessity for trying to maintain our bone mass as much as possible. Chronic back pain can be improved by weight loss, as well as by exercise.

Acute back pain, which may be mild or severe, is usually the result of an injury, an accident or a ruptured disc. It is important to consult your physician as soon as possible when experiencing acute back pain. The most likely treatment for acute back pain is actual bed rest for several days. We don't know many women who follow these instructions, given their multiple roles and the demands of daily household responsibilities; however, it is extremely important to treat acute back pain with care. Heat treatments are often recommended. We find that many people misunderstand the use of heat treatments. Do not use heat for more than fifteen minutes at a time. Alternate heat treatment with rest in order to benefit from it.

Exercise can prevent chronic back pain. By exercising, we strengthen our back and abdominal muscles. It is also important to maintain good posture and to be cautious in lifting heavy objects. Bending the knees instead of the back and holding an object close to the body is the most important precaution to take. We find that many women, believing that they are immune from heart disease, will shovel snow on a regular basis. They do this to prevent their husbands from experiencing a sudden heart attack. But shoveling snow is one of the most dangerous exercises with respect to back pain. If it is not possible to get help in shoveling snow, it is important for women to use as much caution as men in approaching the task, to use good posture and to do small amounts of lifting at any one time.

✦ Breast Changes

Our breasts are composed of glandular tissue and fat. Glandular tissue reacts to the presence or absence of hormones. This is one of the reasons that hormone replacement therapy is not indicated for women who have breast cancer. Estrogen can stimulate the growth of cancer in these glands.

Just as our breasts can become swollen and retain water prior to our menstrual period, hormones can affect the breasts at menopause as well. After the production of estrogen slows, the glandular tissue in the breasts shrinks. At the same time there are ligaments, Cooper's ligaments, that continue to support the breast tissue. Over time, they lose some of their elasticity and begin to lengthen, thus our breasts tend to become somewhat smaller and sag. Although estrogen replacement therapy may reverse this situation somewhat, this cosmetic concern should not be a major factor in making the decision whether or not to begin hormone replacement therapy.

✦ Chest Pain

See Chapter Five, on healthy hearts.

✦ CHOLESTEROL

Cholesterol is one of the fats found in all of the body's cells. Elevated cholesterol is associated with the development of atherosclerosis. Since an elevated cholesterol is associated with a higher risk of cardiovascular disease, it is important to maintain a low-fat diet and to exercise. We discuss the cardiovascular risks in Chapter Five, our chapter on healthy hearts, and the importance of diet and exercise more in our chapter on prevention, Chapter Ten.

✦ FATIGUE

Fatigue is one of the most common complaints of not only menopausal women but of all women. Fatigue can be the result of any number of conditions, including depression and stress. It is clear that women who suffer from hot flashes may have their sleep disturbed and that insomnia leads to fatigue. A woman who had been functioning quite well may now need more sleep or feel overwhelmed at times during the day. Thus, the treatment of hot flashes may effectively treat the insomnia and the resulting fatigue. Menopause can be a time of increased vulnerability. Women who are entering the perimenopausal period seem to develop and report more symptoms than women either before menopause or after menopause. For some women, fatigue is just the natural response to unrealistic responsibilities in and out of the home, combined with emotional burdens.

✦ FOOT PROBLEMS

There are some changes in the structure of our feet that are associated with aging, unrelated to menopause. The skin becomes more easily dehydrated and less elastic over time. Our feet become more susceptible to infections from bacteria or fungus. At the same time, the soles and heels of our feet lose some of their padding fat and calluses can develop on these weight-bearing points. These changes can actually lead to change in shoe size. This should not be a cause for concern. Walking, foot massage and a consultation with a podiatrist might be helpful.

A persistent complaint of having cold feet may be due to poor circulation. This may be a result of artherosclerosis or also could be a sign of diabetes. Any consistent complaints of feelings of coldness or numbness of the extremities should be a cause for concern.

✦ HAIR CHANGES

Most of the changes in our hair over time are due to the natural aging process. After approximately age forty, our hair tends to become dryer and often begins to turn gray. There is a tremendous amount of variability in this process. We all know people who begin to turn gray in their twenties, and others who have only a few gray hairs into their sixties. But eventually we all become gray, men and women alike. Poor nutrition can lead to brittle hair, and this is a separate problem not associated with aging. Sometimes thyroid conditions can affect hair and cause noticeable changes. The concerns with hair changes are primarily cosmetic and we are concerned that some of our patients worry excessively about these changes. They are not indicating any medical problem.

Hirsutism is the growth of excessive dark hair. As the female hormone estrogen decreases, the relative amount of testosterone, the male hormone, increases. Some hair is responsive to hormonal changes and will therefore become excessive and thicker. Our patients complain when they develop excessive hair on their faces. This can usually be managed though, with hair removal or bleaching techniques, and tends not to be a major problem for most women. Hirsutism is also sometimes associated with obesity. The interaction between obesity and the related hormonal changes in menopause can worsen this situation.

✦ HEADACHES

Headaches are one of the most common problems of Americans. There are several categories of headaches, including migraines and tension. In addition, substance abuse can be a factor here, as a possible cause or when a woman may turn to pain killers for relief. Headaches are described in greater detail in Chapter Eight, our chapter on stress.

✦ INSOMNIA

Insomnia is one of life's most frustrating problems. All of us have trouble falling asleep from time to time, and as we age our sleep becomes more disrupted. One study by the National Institute of Health found that more than half of the people over the age of sixty-five experienced some sleep disturbance (Foley and Nechas, 1993). We find that many menopausal women who complain of insomnia are having problems with night sweats. A night sweat is a hot flash that occurs at night and often awakens a woman. In a study of normal menopause, the McKinlay group found that women who experienced hot flashes were twice as likely to report insomnia as women who did not. This can be an extremely disruptive experience and some women have tremendous difficulty getting back to sleep. Estrogen replacement therapy is an effective treatment for hot flashes and will reduce night sweats and the resulting insomnia. Vitamin E and other treatments have not been thoroughly evaluated, but can provide some relief for many women. Wearing cotton bedclothes can also help.

However, since some insomnia and sleep disruption are also associated with the aging process, it is important to take other precautions as well. There are several behavioral techniques we can use. First, get up at the same time every day regardless of what time you went to sleep. Try not to go to bed unless you are sleepy. Exercise regularly and avoid caffeine within six hours of bedtime. Try an hour of relaxation before getting into bed. Use your bed only for sleeping—not for reading or doing paperwork. You want to develop a strong association between the bed and sleeping. The only exception to the rule is sex.

The elimination of naps is needed in order to reestablish a consistent sleep cycle. It is extremely important to avoid using alcohol or sleeping medications to treat this problem. Although both may seem to work, they are associated with significant problems if used consistently. Most physicians will not prescribe sleep preparations for more than several nights and of course it is extremely important never to mix a sleeping pill with alcohol.

✦ JOINT PAIN

Joint pain is often caused by an inflammation of the joints called arthritis. There are two major types of arthritis, rheumatoid and osteoarthritis. Arthritis can occur in any joint but is commonly found in the hips, feet, spine and knees. Many women also complain of arthritis in their finger joints. *Osteoarthritis* is associated with the aging process and is common to most people over the age of sixty. In a normal joint, the ends of bones are covered by cartilage, a rubbery, protective coating. This cartilage cushions the area between the bones. The bones are held together by ligaments and tendons. Over time, the joint tissue breaks down, the cartilage can soften and become frayed and loses its elasticity. In some cases, sections of the cartilage actually wear away. This leads the unprotected bones to rub together with any movement and cause pain. When the cartilage deteriorates, a joint may change its shape, with the bone ends thickening. These changes cause pain.

There is no evidence that osteoarthritis is associated with menopause. It is associated with the aging process in that it is rarely reported by people under the age of forty unless the joints have had overuse or injuries. There is also some evidence that people who are overweight are more likely to have arthritis because of the extra pressure on the knees and the hips—the weight-bearing joints. When osteoarthritis is diagnosed in these joints, weight loss is often recommended to reduce the wear and tear on the joints and the resulting pain.

Rheumatoid arthritis is a different problem. It is a systemic disease and affects the entire body. Although rheumatoid arthritis tends to affect women more than men and begins in the forties and fifties, it is not specifically associated with menopause either. Rather than being caused by a breakdown of cartilage, in rheumatoid arthritis the lining or membrane between the joints becomes inflamed and the joints can appear to be swollen. Rheumatoid arthritis often causes redness and warmth whereas osteoarthritis does not cause redness. Osteoarthritis is usually limited to specific joints whereas rheumatoid arthritis affects many joints. Rheumatoid arthritis causes a more general feeling of sickness and fatigue. Your doctor can make the distinction between rheumatoid and osteoarthritis by testing your sedimentation rate, using a simple blood test. In addition, the morning pain associated with osteoarthritis tends not to last more than thirty minutes, whereas with rheumatoid arthritis it lasts much longer. Osteoarthritis is less common in the wrist, elbow, shoulder and ankle joints. The pain associated with osteoarthritis gets better with time and hand functioning is maintained. In rheumatoid arthritis there is a loss of grip strength. Osteoarthritis can also be confirmed by X-ray findings that show bone and cartilage overgrowth and narrowing of joint spaces.

Treatment of arthritis begins with the appropriate diagnosis. It is important to seek treatment because arthritis can be one of the most chronic and crippling diseases. Arthritis responds to several forms of treatment. Both types of arthritis respond to the nonsteroidal, anti-inflammatory drugs which are known by the acronym NSAID. Ibuprofen is the most common of the NSAIDs, but your doctor can help you choose one of the others as well. One of the problems with the NSAIDs is that they have many side effects that affect the gastrointestinal system. These include mild stomach pain, as well as nausea and vomiting. The chronic use of the NSAIDs can sometimes lead to ulcers. It is important to take them with a full meal and to drink plenty of liquids.

Aspirin is actually the oldest and most common NSAID. Like other NSAIDs it can cause gastrointestinal side effects which may be partially avoided with the buffered form. One problem with aspirin, however, is that the dose required is somewhere between 3 and 6 grams or nine to eighteen pills per day. Many women who may be dieting or concerned about their weight, do not have the regular eating habits necessary to appropriately take this much aspirin. For many women, it is difficult to take medications more than three times a day, so that taking pills every four hours is unthinkable.

Although there is no treatment that can prevent or reverse osteoarthritis at this time, it is important that we try to keep up with our daily activities.

Exercise can be alternated with rest in order to maintain our level of functioning. Swimming is a particularly good exercise for women with arthritis, since it takes all of the weight off the joints and allows movement and muscle development with less pain.

✦ MOOD CHANGES

Many women experience mood changes around the time of menopause. The perimenopausal period is often associated with feelings of emotional instability. Others believe that the hormonal factors themselves may lead to some emotional malaise, but this has not yet been documented. Some women feel irritable or describe themselves as nervous, as we have discussed in Chapter Seven, "Myths of Depression." Most of these changes are mild, time-linked, and do not affect women at menopause any more often than women at other ages. However, if changes in your mood are disruptive and long lasting, it is time to consult a mental health professional. Our chapter on depression discusses this in great detail.

✦ SKIN CHANGES

Some women complain of itchy or uncomfortable feelings of dry skin. This can be combated by using milder soaps and moisturizers. One of the most important changes we can make during the menopausal years is to drink large quantities of water.

There are also age-related changes in pigmentation such as liver spots and "ruby spots." These are groups of dilated capillaries that can appear on the face, neck, arms and legs. Environmental conditions can also lead to dry skin. The most obvious culprit here is sun, and if by now you haven't restricted your exposure to the sun, menopause is a good time to do so. Using a sunscreen and avoiding direct exposure to the sun by wearing protective clothing and sunglasses is wise. Even when swimming, it is important to use sunscreen.

With skin cancers accounting for more than half of the malignancies in the United States each year, it is important to learn to examine ourselves for moles that are asymmetrical, with irregular borders, with a color that is not uniform and with a diameter that is larger than the size of a pencil eraser. Any change in a wart or mole represents an early warning sign of skin cancer—the O in the American Cancer Society's CAUTION.

The American Cancer Society's early warning signs of cancer:

C. *Change in bowel habits.*
A. *A sore that does not heal.*

U. *Unusual bleeding or discharge.*
T. *Thickening or lump in the breast or elsewhere*
I. *Indigestion or difficulty in swallowing.*
O. *Obvious changes in a wart or mole.*
N. *Nagging cough or hoarseness.*

Some women describe a feeling of pins and needles or a sense of tingling. A small number of menopausal women report experiencing that insects are crawling on their skin. This is called formication. One study found that 20 percent of women experienced formication around the time of the their last period, but only 10 percent of them described the problem over time. Like many menopausal symptoms, the cause is unknown, but thankfully it tends to be a short-lived problem.

✦ PALPITATIONS

See the chapter on healthy hearts, Chapter Five.

✦ VISION CHANGES

Most of us will eventually need to use reading glasses, but menopause cannot be blamed for this. Men and women alike have changes in their vision, beginning approximately at age forty. This is because, as we age, the lens of our eye begins to lose some of its elasticity. We find it increasingly difficult to focus on objects that are near. This gradual farsightedness is known as presbyopia, the visual change associated with aging.

Although corrective reading glasses can be purchased over the counter at almost any pharmacy, it is important to begin to check in regularly with an ophthalmologist. An ophthalmologist can begin to screen for other eye problems associated with aging such as glaucoma and cataracts. In addition, the farsightedness does change over time and prescription lenses will need to be adjusted accordingly.

Some of us will experience a disruption in our vision. Behind the lens of our eye is a large compartment filled with a clear fluid called the *vitreous humor*. When tiny bits of material drift in this clear fluid, we may see spots or strings dropping down into our field of vision. These are called "floaters." These are usually harmless but should be discussed with an ophthalmologist. If you experience any sudden change in vision (including an increase in floaters) you should seek medical attention immediately.

◆ WEIGHT LOSS

If you have experienced a sudden or significant weight loss, and you have not been dieting or exercising more, then it is important to consult with a physician as this can be a symptom of a serious problem. Thyroid disease and diabetes can also cause unexpected weight loss.

◆ WEIGHT GAIN

At midlife our metabolism slows down, making it more likely for us to gain weight if we continue to eat as we have previously. Obesity can contribute to the development of diabetes, heart disease, high blood pressure and joint pain. However, many women diet unnecessarily because of unrealistic standards. Weight gain at midlife is expected and natural. If you are concerned about this, you are more likely to successfully maintain your weight with increased exercise than by rigid dieting. We discuss the possibilities of healthy eating behaviors and exercise in our chapter on prevention.

Gaining weight, of course, can lead to a thickening around our abdomens. It is important to note that abdominal and pelvic disorders (including ovarian cancer) sometimes manifest themselves by the sudden distention of the abdomen. If you have not been gaining weight because of lack of exercise or overeating, a sudden bloated feeling or change in your abdomen should prompt you to schedule a visit with your physician for a complete evaluation including a pelvic exam.

There are some reports of weight gain with hormone replacement therapy and this is a great concern to menopausal women. This may be caused by fluid retention and is believed to be associated with the hormone progesterone rather than estrogen. Some researchers have also suggested that hormones can also make a person hungrier and can lead to overeating if control is not maintained. Weight gain is discussed thoroughly in Chapter Five, "Healthy Hearts" and Chapter Ten, "Promoting a Healthy Lifestyle."

As we met with women in our "menopause town meetings," we began to compile the most common questions. Here they are, along with the corresponding page numbers.

◀ Town Meeting: Women's Health Questions

Hormone Replacement Therapy

Do I have to take progesterone with estrogen?   pp. 149, 160–161

Doesn't estrogen cause breast cancer?   pp. 149–153

Can I stop taking estrogen suddenly if I don't like it?   p. 144

What is the advantage of the estrogen patch?   pp. 140–141

Will estrogen prevent me from getting heart disease?   pp. 118–119, 128, 146

Will estrogen make me look younger?   p. 147

Sex

Symptoms

General Health

Do I need to eat a low-fat diet if I'm in good health?   pp. 124–127, 294–296

How much exercise do I really need?   pp. 56, 100–102, 123–125, 225, 271–276

I've been reading a lot about heart disease. What can I do to prevent it?
   pp. 121–127, 278–298

I've tried to stop smoking three times. I feel like giving up. Any ideas?
   pp. 121–122, 263–264, 278–282

If I swim three times a week, will that prevent osteoporosis?   pp. 100–102

If I take HRT, do I need to worry about osteoporosis?   pp. 95–104

Does everyone get osteoporosis?   pp. 88–90, 91–93, 98, 107

How much calcium should I be consuming?   pp. 95–97

Should I be taking vitamin D in addition to calcium?   pp. 96–98

I don't like dairy products. How else can I take in enough calcium?
   pp. 96–97

I went to a menopause clinic and they said I need to have the density of my
   bones measured. I'm in good health. Do I really need this?   pp. 93–94

Should I have my cholesterol checked?   pp. 115–116, 124–126, 270

PSYCHOLOGICAL ISSUES

Will I get depressed at menopause?   pp. 29–31, 168–170, 258

Don't most women have midlife crises?   pp. 201–203, 212–216

How can I handle family stress? I thought it would be over by now.
   pp. 184–185, 208–212, 231–233

Will estrogen help me if I'm depressed?   pp. 171, 178–179

What can I do about anxiety?   pp. 219–226, 230–231

I need some psychological help, but I don't have insurance coverage for it.
   What can I do?   pp. 188–189, 199, 232–233

What's all this I read about Prozac? Is it a wonder drug? Is it addictive?
   pp. 189–191

If I had PMS, should I expect the same at menopause?   pp. 30, 178

I have a lot of "down" days—is that depression or normal mood swings?
   pp. 173–179

HYSTERECTOMY

What is the difference between a hysterectomy and having my ovaries removed?   pp. 235–238

I had a hysterectomy five years ago. How will that affect my menopause? pp. 140, 158, 247–250

My doctor is suggesting that I have a hysterectomy because of my fibroids. I'm forty-three. Are there other treatments available?   pp. 239–241, 242–244

I'm almost fifty and I am having a hysterectomy. Should I have my ovaries removed too?   pp. 242, 250–252

My doctor says I should have a hysterectomy because of my pelvic pain. I want to get a second opinion, but I don't want to hurt his feelings.   pp. 16–17, 240–241, 245–246, 251–252

If I have had a hysterectomy, how will I know I'm going through menopause? pp. 27–28, 45, 140, 143–145

HEALTH-CARE AND DOCTOR-PATIENT COMMUNICATION

My doctor doesn't seem to listen to me. What can I do?   pp. 15–18, 36–38, 106, 111–112, 193–194, 307–309

I'm fifteen pounds overweight, and my doctor keeps telling me to lose weight. I've tried every diet there is. What should I say?   pp. 292–293

My doctor says I need to do "weight-bearing exercise." Isn't all exercise weight-bearing?   pp. 100, 102

I'm worried about heart disease, but my doctor thinks I'm silly to worry. pp. 111–112, 129–130

I can't understand my doctor's answers to my questions. What should I do? pp. 15–17, 37–38, 128–129, 193–194, 250, 307–309

GENERAL

Is there any way to predict when I will go through menopause?   pp. 24, 40, 142

Can a blood test predict when I'll go through menopause?   pp. 138, 142

When does menopause occur?   pp. 24–25, 27, 142

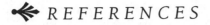 *REFERENCES*

ABC News. (1993). *Prime Time Live,* 6. Transcript #304. New York.

Abrams, D.B., Monti, P., Pinto, R., and Elder, J. (1987). Psychological stress and coping in smokers who relapse or quit. *Health Psychology, 6,* 289–303.

Adamson, G.D. (1992). Treatment of uterine fibroids: Current findings with gonadotropin-releasing hormone agonists. *Am J Obstet Gynecol, 166,* 746–51.

Albrecht, B.H., Schiff, I., Tulchinsky, D., and Ryan, K.J. (1980). Objective evidence that placebo and oral medroxyprogesterone acetate therapy diminish menopausal vasomotor flushes. *Am. J. Obstet. Gynecol. 139:* 631–635.

American Cancer Society. (1988). Summary of current guidelines for the cancer related checkup: recommendations. New York: American Cancer Society.

American Heart Association. (1989). Women and heart disease. Summary of proceedings. Meeting, Washington, D.C.

American Psychiatric Association. (1987). *Diagnostic and Statistical Manual of Mental Disorders.* Third Revised ed., Washington, D.C.: The American Psychiatric Associations.

Anderson, M. (1992). My Lord, what a morning. In J.K. Conway (Ed.), *Written by Herself*, pp. 55–97. New York: Vintage Books, A Division of Random House.

Andrasik, F., and Kabela, E. (1988). Headaches. In E.A. Blechman and K.D. Brownell (Eds.), *Handbook of Behavioral Medicine for Women*, pp. 206–221. New York: Pergamon Press.

Aneshensel, C. (1986). Marital and employment role-strain, social support and depression among adult women. In S. Hobfoll (Ed.), *Stress, Social Support, and Women*, pp. 99–114. Washington, D.C.: Hemisphere.

Are You Eating Right? *Consumer Reports*, October 1992a, 647.

Associated Press. (1993, March). U.S. health study to involve 160,000 women at 16 centers. *New York Times*, p. A21.

Avis, N.E., and McKinlay, S.M. (1990). Health care utilization among mid-aged women. In M. Flint, F. Kronenberg, and W. Utian (Eds.) *Multidisciplinary perspectives on menopause*, pp. 228–256. New York: New York Academy of Sciences.

Bachmann, G.A. and Leiblum, S.R. (1991). Sexuality in sexagenarian women. *Maturitas, 13,* 43–50.

Barnett, R., Biener, L. and G. Baruch. (1987). *Gender and Stress*. New York: The Free Press.

Barrett-Connor, E. and Bush, T.L. (1991). Estrogen and coronary heart disease in women. *JAMA, 265,* 14: 1861.

Beckman, H.B. and Frankel, R.M. (1984). The effect of physician behavior on the collection of data. *Annals of Internal Medicine, 101,* 692–697.

Bell, S.E. (1990). The medicalization of menopause. In Formanek, R. (Ed.), *The Meaning of Menopause: Historical, Medical and Clinical Perspectives.* Hillsdale, N.J.: The Analytic Press.

Benson, H. (1993). The relaxation response. In D. Goleman and J. Gurin (Eds.), *Mind/Body Medicine: How to Use Your Mind for Better Health.* Yonkers: Consumers Union of United States, Inc.

Bergkvist, L. (1989). The risk of breast cancer after estrogen and estrogen-progestin replacement. *NEJM, 321,* 293–297.

Bernardez, T. (1990). Older women: Inventing our lives. In *Seventh Annual Women in Context Conference in Topeka, Kansas,* The Menninger Foundation.

Blair, S.N., Kohl, H.W., and Paffenbarger, D.G. (1989). Physical fitness and all-cause mortality: a prospective study of healthy men and women. *JAMA, 262,* 2395–2401.

Blumstein, P. and Schwartz, P. (1983). *American Couples.* New York: William Morrow and Company.

Boston Globe, Quote unquote, p. 30, January 4, 1993.

Bourke-White, M. (1992). Portrait of myself. In J.K. Conway (Ed.), *Written By Herself,* pp. 423–453. New York: Vintage Books, A Division of Random House.

Brown, G.W., Bifulco, A., Harris, T.O., and Bridge, L. (1986). Life stress, chronic subclinical symptoms and vulnerability to clinical depression. *The Journal of Affective Disorders, 11,* 1–19.

Brownell, K.D. and Rodin, J. (1990). *The Weight Maintenance Survival Guide.* Dallas: Brownell & Hager.

Brownell, K.D. and Wadden, T.A. (1991). The heterogeneity of obesity: fitting treatments to individuals. *Behavior Therapy, 22,* 153–177.

Brownson, R.C., Alavanja, M.C.R., Hock, E.T., and Loy, T.S. (1992). Passive smoking and lung cancer in nonsmoking women. *American Journal of Public Health, 82* (11), 1525–1530.

Budoff, P.W. (1983). *No More Hot Flashes: And Other Good News.* New York: Warner Books.

Bullock, J.L. (1975). Use of medroxyprogesterone acetate to prevent menopausal symptoms. *Obstetrics and Gynecology, 46* (2), 165–68.

Burmen, B. and Gritz, E. (1990). Women and smoking: Current trends *Journal of Substance Abuse 3,* 221–238.

Burns, D.D. (1980). *Feeling Good: The New Mood Therapy.* New York: William Morrow & Company.

Bush, T.L. (1991). Epidemiology of cardiovascular disease in women. In G.P. Redmond (Ed.), *Lipids and Women's Health,* pp. 6–20. New York: Springer-Verlag.

Byyny, R. and Speroff, L. (1990). *A Clinical Guide for the Care of Older Women.* Baltimore: Williams & Wilkins.

Caldirola, D. (1983). Incest and pelvic pain. *Health and Social Work, 4,* 309.

Carlson, K.J., Nichols, D.H., and Schiff, I. (1993). Indications for hysterectomy. *New England Journal of Medicine,* 856–860.

Cheng, N. (1988). *Life and Death in Shanghai.* New York: Viking Penguin.

Chesney, M.A. (1991). Women, work-related stress and smoking. In M. Frankenhaeuser, U. Lundberg & M.A. Chesney (Eds.), *Women, Work and Health,* pp. 139–55. New York: Plenum Press.

Clark, M.M., Ruggiero, L., Pera, V., Goldstein, M.G., and Abrams, D.B. (1993). Assessment, classification, and treatment of obesity: a behavioral medicine perspective. In A. Stoudemire and B.S. Fogel (Eds.), *The Psychiatric Care of the Medical Patient,* New York: Oxford University Press.

Clayden, J.R., Bel, J.W. and Pollard. (1974). Menopausal flushing: Double blind trial of a non-hormonal medication. *British Medical Journal 1,* 409–412.

Collins, A. (1992). Emotional responses and symptomatic changes during transition to menopause. In K. Wijma and B. von Schoultz (Eds), *Advances in Psychosomatic Obstetrics and Gynecology.* Park Ridge, N.J.: Parthenon.

Conway, J.K. (Ed.) (1992). *Written By Herself.* New York: Vintage Books, A Division of Random House.

Cooper, Kenneth, H. (1989). *Preventing Osteoporosis.* New York: Bantam Books.

Cutler, W. and Garcia, C. (1992). *Menopause: A Guide for Women and the Men Who Love Them.* New York: W.W. Norton & Company.

Dembroski, T.M, MacDouguel, J.M., and Cardozo, S. (1985). Selective cardiovascular effects of stress and cigarette smoking in young females. *Health Psychology, 4,* 153–167.

de Turenne, Veronique. (1993, March 24). Support groups link people in similar situations. *Sarasota Herald-Tribune,* 1E, 4E.

Deutsch, H. (1945). *Psychology of women.* Vol. ii. New York: Grune & Stratton.

Deykin, E. (1966). The empty nest: Psychological aspects of conflict between depressed women and their grown children. *American Journal of Psychiatry,* 1422–1425.

Doress, P.B., Siegal, D.L., and The Midlife and Older Women Book Project. (1987). *Ourselves, Growing Older: Women, Aging with Knowledge and Power.* New York: Simon & Schuster/Touchstone Books.

Douglas, P., Clarkson, T.B., Flowers, N.C., and Hajjar, K.A. (1992). Exercise and atherosclerotic heart disease in women. *Medicine and Science in Sports and Exercise* 24 (6): S26.

Dukes, M.N.G. (Ed.) (1992). *Meyler's Side Effects of Drugs: An Encyclopedia of Adverse Reactions and Interactions.* Amsterdam: Elsevier.

Eaker, E.D. and Castelli, W.P. (1987). Coronary heart disease and its risk factors among women in the Framingham study. In E.D. Eaker, B. Packard, N.K. Wenger, T.B. Clarkson, and H.A. Tyroler (Eds.). *Coronary Heart Disease in Women: Proceedings of an N.I.H. Workshop,* pp.122–130. New York: Haymarket Doyma, Inc.

Ellis, A. and Harper, R.A. (1975). *A New Guide to Rational Living.* North Hollywood: Wilshire Book Company.

El-Mallakh, N. and Rif, S. (1987). Marijuana and migraine. *Headache,* 8, 442–444.

Erikson, E. (1950). *Childhood and Society.* New York: W.W. Norton.

Erikson, E. (1970). *Identity Through the Life Cycle.* 2nd ed. New York: W.W. Norton.

Erlik, Y., Meldrum, D.R., and Judd, H.L. (1982). Estrogen levels in postmenopausal women with hot flushes. *Obstetrics and Gynecology, 59:* 403.

Erlik, Y., Tatryn, I.V., Meldrum, D.R., Lomax, P., Bajorek, J.G., and Judd, H.L. (1981). Association of waking episodes with menopausal hot flushes. *JAMA, 245:* 1744.

Ernsberger, P. and Nelson, D.O. (1988). Refeeding hypertension and dietary obesity. *American Journal of Physiology, 254,* R47–55.

Ernster, V.L. (1988). Benefits and risks of menopausal estrogen and/or progestin use. *Preventative Medicine 17,* 301–323.

Ettinger, B., Genant, H.K., and Cann, C.E. (1987). Postmenopausal bone loss is prevented by treatment with low-dosage estrogen with calcium. *Annals of Int. Med., 106,* 40–45.

Ewing, J.A. (1984). Detecting alcoholism: The cage questionnaire. *JAMA, 252,* 1905–1907.

Faludi, S. (1991). *Backlash: The Undeclared War Against American Women.* New York: Crown.

Fleming, L.A. (1992). Osteoporosis: Clinical features, prevention and treatment. *J. Gen Int Med, 7,* 554–561.

Fletcher, S.W. (1992). The breast is close to the heart. *Annals of Internal Medicine, 117,* 969–971.

Foley, D. and Nechas, E. (Eds.) (1993). *Women's Encyclopedia of Health and Emotional Healing.* Emmaus, Pa.: Rodale Press.

Friedman, M. and Rosenman, R.H. (1974). *Type A Behavior and Your Heart.* New York: Knopf.

Friedman, R.M. (Ed.) Pizza: however you slice it. (1993, June). *University of California at Berkeley Wellness Letter,* 3.

Friedman, R.M. (Ed.) (1993, June). Fascinating facts. *University of California at Berkeley Wellness Letter,* 1.

Gaposchkin, C.P. (1992). An autobiography and other recollections. In J. K. Conway (Ed.), *Written By Herself,* pp. 248–282. New York: Vintage Books, A Division of Random House.

Gardanne, Ch.P.L de. (1821). *De la ménépausie ou de l'age critique des femmes.* Paris. Chez Mequignon, Marvis, Libraire.

Gershoff, S.N. (Ed.) (1992, July). How many calories? More than the label says. *Tufts University Diet & Nutrition Letter, 10* (7), 1–2.

Glasgow, E.A.G. (1992). The woman within. In J. K. Conway (Ed.), *Written By Herself,* pp.372–400. New York: Vintage Books, A Division of Random House.

Goldberg, R.J. (1988). Depression in primary care: DSM-III diagnoses and other depressive syndromes. *Clinical Reviews, 3,* 491–497.

Goleman, D. and Gurin, J. (1993). *Mind Body Medicine.* Yonkers: Consumers Union of United States, Inc.

Grady, D., Rubin, S., and Petitti, D. (1992). Hormone therapy to prevent disease and prolong life in postmenopausal women. *Annals of Internal Medicine, 117,* 1016–1037.

Greenwood, S. (1984). *Menopause Naturally: Preparing for the Second Half of Life.* Volcano, CA: Volcano Press.

Greer, G. (1970). *The Female Eunuch.*

Greer, G. (1992). *The Change: Women, Aging and the Menopause.* New York: Alfred A. Knopf.

Hallstrom, T. (1977). Sexuality in the climacteric. *Clinics in Obstetrics and Gynecology 4,* 227–239.

Harris, R.B., Laws, A., and Reddy, V. (1990). Are women using post-menopausal estrogen? A community survey. *American Journal of Public Health, 80* (1): 1266–1268.

Haynes, S.G., Feinleib, and Kannel, W.B. (1980). The relationship of psycho-social factors to coronary heart disease in the Framingham study. III. Eight-year incidence of coronary heart disease. *Am J Epidemiol, 111* (1): 37–58.

Health Survey. (1993, March 24). *Sarasota Herald Tribune,* 1.

Helson, R. and Wink, P. (1992). Personality change in women from the early 40s to the early 50s. *Psycholog-Aging, 7* (1): 46–55.

Henderson, I.C. and Wender, R.C. (1991). Breast cancer. *Am Cancer Soc Newsletter,* 2, 1.

Henrich, J.B. (1992). The postmenopausal estrogen/breast cancer contro-versy. *JAMA, 268* (14): 1900–1902.

Herman, J.L. (1986). Long-term effects of incestuous abuse in childhood. American Journal of Psychiatry, *143:* 1493.

Herman, J.L. (1992). *Trauma and Recovery.* Cambridge: Harvard University Press.

Hochschild, A. (1989). *The Second Shift: Working Parents and the Revolution at Home.* New York: Viking Penguin, Inc.

Hunter, M. (1990). Emotional well-being, sexual behaviour and hormone replacement therapy. *Maturitas, 12,* 299–314.

J.S. (1992). ERT: Helping Women Decide. *Journal Watch, 10* (5): 39–40.

Jacobs Institute of Women's Health. (1992). Mammography Attitudes and Usage. Washington, D.C.: Jacobs Institute of Women's Health.

Jaques, E. (1965). Death and the midlife crisis. *International Journal of Psy-choanalysis, 46,* (4): 502–513.

Jarvis, J. (1992). Gender of problem drinkers points to different treatment needs. *Br. J. Addiction, 87,* 1249.

Jones, B.M. and Jones, M.K. (1976). Male and female intoxication levels for three alcohol doses or do women really get higher than men? *Alcohol Technical Reports, 5,* 11.

Jones, K.P., Ravnikar, V., and Schiff, I. (1985). A preliminary evaluation of the effect of lofexitine on vasomotor flushes in postmenopausal women. *Maturitas, 7,* 135–139.

Kaplan, A. G. (1986). The "self-in-relation": Implications for depression in women. *Psychotherapy: Theory, Research, and Practice, 23,* 235–242.

Kaslow, F.W. (1981). Divorce and Divorce Therapy. In A. Gurman and D. Kniskern (Eds.), *Handbook of Family Therapy.* New York: Brunner/ Mazel.

Katz, L. (1992). Beyond the hot flash. *Seasons,* 4–7.

Kegel, A.M. (1951). Physiologic therapy for urinary stress incontinence. *Jour-nal of Am. Medical Assoc., 146,* 915–917.

Keeping your weight steady found better than "yo-yo" dieting. (1993, January 17). *Providence Journal.*

Klesges, R.C. and Klesges, L.M. (1988). Cigarette smoking as a dieting strategy in a university population. *International Journal of Eating Disorders, 7,* 413–419.

Kronenberg, F. (1990). Hot Flashes: Epidemiology and Physiology. In *Annals of New York Academy of Sciences* 56–86.

Kronenberg, F. (1993, May 21). Menopausal hot flashes. Paper presented at Menopause: The Background and Skills for Effective Therapy. Symposium of the North American Menopause Society.

Kübler-Ross, E. *Living with Death and Dying.* New York: Macmillan, 1982

LeGuin, U. (Summer 1976). The space crone. *The Co-Evolution Quarterly.*

Leibsohn, S., d'Ablaing, G., Mishell, D.R. and Schlaerth, J.B. (1990). Leiomyosarcoma in a series of hysterectomies performed for presumed uterine leiomyomas. *Am J Obstet Gynecol, 162,* 968–976.

Lewis, N.A. (1993, June 15). "Clinton Names Ruth Ginsburg, Advocate for Women, To Court." *New York Times,* A1, A23.

Lindsay, R. (1991). Estrogens, bone mass, and osteoporotic fracture. *Am. J. Medicine, 91,* 10S–12S.

Lipid Research Clinic Program. (1984). The lipid research clinics coronary primary prevention trial results. *JAMA, 251,* 351–364.

Lock, M. (1991). Contested meanings of the menopause. *The Lancet, 337,* 1270–1272.

Loo, C. (1988). Sociocultural barriers to the achievement of Asian American women. *Annual Meeting of the American Psychological Association.* Paper presented at the meeting of the American Psychological Association, Atlanta, GA.

Losing Weight: What Works. What doesn't. *Consumer Reports,* June 1993, 347–357.

Lutter, J. (1992). A question of age: similarities and differences of melpomene members across the lifespan. *Melpomene, 11* (1): 28–34.

Mahowald, M. (1992). Beyond Motherhood: Ethical Issues. In *3rd Annual Meeting of the North American Menopause Society* (p. 56). Cleveland, Ohio: Case Western Reserve University.

Manson, J., Stampfer, M., Colditz, G., Willett, W., Rosner, B., Speizer, F., and Hennekens, C. (1991). A prospective study of aspirin use and primary prevention of cardiovascular disease in women. *JAMA, 266* (4): 521–527.

Margolis, S., and Moses, H. (1992). Headaches. In *The Johns Hopkins Medical Handbook,* pp. 120–131. New York: Rebus, Inc.

Masters, W., and Johnson, V. (1970). *Human Sexual Inadequacy.* Boston: Little Brown & Co.

McCrady, B.S. (1988). Alcoholism. In E.A. Blechman and K.D. Brownell

(Eds.), *Handbook of Behavioral Medicine for Women,* pp. 356–368. New York: Pergamon.

McGill, H.C. (1989). Sex steroid hormone receptors in the cardiovascular system. *Postgrad Medicine,* 64–8.

McGrath, E., Keita, G.P., Strickland, B.R. and Russo, N.F. (1990). *Women and Depression.* Washington, D.C.: American Psychological Association.

McKinlay, J., McKinlay, S., & Brambilla, D. (1987). Health status and utilization behavior associated with menopause. *American Journal of Epidemiology, 125,* 110–121.

McKinlay, J., McKinlay, S., & Brambilla, D. (1987). The relative contributions of endocrine changes and social circumstances to depression in mid-aged women. *Journal of Health and Social Behavior, 28,* 345–363.

Miller, S. (1993). *For Love.* New York: HarperCollins.

Mills, P.K., Beeson, W.L., Phillips R.L., & Fraser, G.E. (1989). Prospective study of exogenous hormone use and breast cancer in seventh day adventists. *Cancer, 64,* 591–597.

Morgan R. (Ed.) (1993). Audre Lorde obituary. *Ms. 3* (5), 58.

Morgan, S. (1982). *Coping with a Hysterectomy.* New York: The Dial Press.

Moyers, B. (1993). *Healing and the Mind.* New York: Bantam Doubleday Dell.

Nabulsi, A.A., Folsom, A.R., White, A., & Patsch, W. (1993). Association of hormone replacement therapy with various cardiovascular risk factors in postmenopausal women. *The New England Journal of Medicine, 328,* 1069–75.

Nachtigall, L. & Heilman, J.R. (1991). *Estrogen: The Facts that Can Change Your Life.* New York: HarperCollins.

National Cancer Institute. (1990). The NCI breast cancer screening consortium screening mammography: A missed opportunity?: Results of the NCI Breast Cancer Screening Consortium and National Health Interview survey studies. *JAMA 264,* 54–58.

National Institute on Drug Abuse Sample Size and US Population Size Tables. (1990). National Household Survey on Drug Abuse: Population estimates, 17.

National Institute of Mental Health. (1987). National Lesbian Health Care Survey. Washington, D.C.: The U.S. Dept. of Health and Human Services, 1987.

National Osteoporosis Foundation. (1991). Boning up on osteoporosis: A guide to prevention and treatment. Washington, D.C.: National Osteoporosis Foundation.

Neaton, J.D., Lewis, H.K., Wentworth, D., & Borhani, N.O. (1984). Total and cardiovascular mortality in relation to cigarette smoking, serum cholesterol concentration, and diastolic blood pressure among black and white males followed up for five years. *Am Heart Journal, 108,* 759.

Nolen-Hoeksema, S. (1987). Sex differences in unipolar depression: Evidence and theory. *Psychological Bulletin, 101,* 259–282.

Olshan, J. (1993, June 28). Picks & Pans: Pages. *People,* p. 10.

Orlander, J., Jick, S., Dean, A., & Jick, H. (1992). Urinary tract infections and estrogen use in older women. *JAGS, 40* (8), 817–820.

Orlandi, M.A. (1987). Gender differences in smoking cessation. *Women's Health.*

Orth, M. (1993, May). The lady has legs. *Vanity Fair,* 171.

Otto, W. (1991). *How to Make an American Quilt.* New York: Ballantine Books.

Parke, E. (1991). A funny thing happened on my way to middle age. In D. Taylor and A.C. Sumrall (Eds.), *Women of the 14th Moon,* p. 7. Freedom: The Crossing Press.

Perspectives. (1993, July 12). *Newsweek.*

Petitti, D.B., Sydney, S., & Pearlman, J.A. (1988). Increased risk of cholecystectomy in users of supplemental estrogen. *Gastroenterology, 94,* 91–95.

Polivy, V. & Herman, C.P. (1985). Dieting and binging. *American Psychologist, 40,* 193–201.

Prochaska, J.P., Norcross, J.C. and DiClemente, C. (1992). In search of how people change: Applications to addictive behaviors. *American Psychologist, 47* (9), 1102–1114.

Quinn, J.B. (1993, April 5). What's for dinner, mom? *Newsweek,* p. 68.

Rakowski, W., Dube, C.E., Marcus, B.H., Prochaska, J.O. (1992). Assessing elements of women's decisions about mammography. *Health Psychology, 11,* 111–188.

Ravnikar, V.A. (1987). Compliance with hormonal therapy. *American Journal of Obstetrics and Gynecology, 156,* 1332–1334.

Ravnikar, V. (1990). Physiology and treatment of hot flushes. *Obstetrics & Gynecology, 75,* 3S–8S.

Rector, R.C. (Ed.) (1990). *Chronic Pelvic Pain Clinical OB:GYN.* Vol. 33. New York: Lippincott.

Rigotti, N. (1992). Smoking cessation strategies for women. Paper presented at *Harvard Medical School Continuing Education Course Primary Care of Women.* Boston, MA.

Rodin, J., Silberstein, L.R., & Striegel-Moore, R.H. (1985). Women and weight: A normative discontent. In T.B. Sonderegger (Ed.), *Nebraska Symposium on Motivation: Psychology and Gender, 32* (pp. 267–301). Lincoln: University of Nebraska Press, 1985.

Rosen, J. (1993, August 2). Book of Ruth. *The New Republic,* pp. 19–31.

Rosenthal, E. (1993, March 21). Conversations: James E. Muller. *New York Times.*

Rothert, M. (1991). Perspectives and issues in studying patients decision making. In M.L. Grady (Ed.), *Primary Care Research: Theory and*

Methods, (pp. 175–179). Rockville: Agency for Health Care Policy Research.

Rountree, C. (1993). *On Women Turning 50: Celebrating Mid Life Discoveries.* San Francisco: HarperSanFrancisco.

Russo, N.F. & Olmedo, E.L. (1983). Women's utilization of outpatient psychiatric services: Some emerging priorities for rehabilitation psychologists. *Rehabilitation Psychology, 28,* 141–155.

Sachs, J. (1991). *What Women Should Know About Menopause.* New York: Bantam Doubleday Dell Publishing Group, Inc.

Salonen, J.T., Nyyssonen, K., Korpela, H., Tuomilehto, J., Seppanen, R. & Salonen, R. (1992). High stored iron levels are associated with excess risk of myocardial infarction in eastern Finnish men. *Circulation, 86,* 803–811.

Schiff, I. and Walsh, B. (1989). Hot flashes. In C.B. Hammond, F. Haseltine, and I. Schiff (Eds.). *Menopause: Evaluation, Treatment and Health Concerns.* New York: Wiley, 1989

Schiff, I., Tulchinsky, D., Cramer, D., & Ryan, K. (1980). Oral medroxyprogesterone in the treatment of postmenopausal symptoms. *JAMA, 244,* 1443–1445.

Schmidt, P. & Rubinow, D. (1991). Menopause-related affective disorders: a justification for further study. *American Journal of Psychiatry, 148,* 844–852.

Scudder, V.D. (1992). Modeling my life. In J.K. Conway (Ed.), *Written by Herself,* pp. 333–371. New York: Vintage Books.

Sheehy, G. (1991). *The Silent Passage.* New York: Random House.

Sheehy, G. (1992, May 14). The silent passage: Menopause. *Vanity Fair,* p. 6.

Sherwin B. (Chair) (1993, September). Menopausal depression: Myth or realty? Symposium conducted at the Fourth Annual Meeting of the North American Menopause Society, San Diego.

Stampfer, M.J. (1991). Postmenopausal estrogen therapy and cardiovascular disease. *The New England Journal of Medicine, 325,* 756–62.

Stampfer, M.J., Graham, A.C., Willett, W.C., Rosner, B., Speizer, F.E., & Hennekens, C.H. (1987). Coronary heart disease risk factors in women: The Nurses' Health Study experience. In E.D. Eaker, B. Packard, B. Packard, N.K. Wenger, T.B. Clarkson, and H.A. Tyroler (Eds.), *Coronary Heart Disease in Women: Proceedings of an N.I.H. Workshop* (pp. 112–116). New York: Haymarket Doyma, Inc.

Stampfer, M.J., Hennekens, C.H., Manson, J.E., Colditz, G.A., Rosner, B., and Willett, W.C. (1993). Vitamin E. consumption and the risk of coronary disease in women. *The New England Journal of Medicine,* 1444–1449.

Stark, M. (November, 1992). Ask your doctor. *Boston Magazine, 84,* 11: 67–69.

Stunkard, A.J. and Rush, J. (1974). Dieting and depression reexamined: A critical review of untoward responses during weight reduction for obesity. *Annals of Internal Medicine, 81*, 526–533.

Sturdee, D.W., Wilson, K.A., Pipili, E., & Crocker, A.D. (1978). Physiological aspects of menopausal hot flush. *British Medical Journal, 2*, 79–80.

Swartzman, L., Edelberg, R., & Kemmann, E. (1990). Impact of stress on objectively recorded menopausal hot flushes and on flush report bias. *Health Psychology, 9*, 529–545.

Tamerin, J.S., Tolor, A., & Harrington, B. (1976). Sex differences in alcoholics: A comparison of male and female alcoholics and spouse perceptions. *American Journal of Drug and Alcohol Abuse, 3*, 457–472.

Tannen, D. (1990). *You Just Don't Understand.* New York: Ballantine Books.

Taylor, D. and Sumrall, A.C. (Eds.). (1991). *Women of the 14th Moon.* Freedom: The Crossing Press.

Todd, A.D. (1989). *Intimate Adversaries: Cultural Conflict Between Doctors and Women Patients.* Philadelphia: University of Pennsylvania Press.

Tuyns, A.J. & Pequinot, G. (1984). Greater risk of ascitic cirrhosis in females in relation to alcohol consumption. *International Journal of Epidemiology, 13*, 53.

United States Congress, Office of Technology Assessment. (1992). *The Menopause, Hormone Therapy, and Women's Health.* (OTA-BP-BA-88) Washington, D.C.: U.S. Government Printing Office.

United States Surgeon General. (1990). *The Health Consequences of Smoking Cessation.* U.S. Dept. of Health and Human Services: Public Health Service, Office on Smoking and Health.

U.S. Dept. of Health and Human Services. (1988). Indian Health Service: Chart Series Book. Washington, D.C.: The United States Government Printing Office.

Wadden, T.A., Stunkard, A.J., & Liebschutz, J. (1988). Three year follow-up of the treatment of obesity by very low calorie diet, behavior therapy and their combination. *Journal of Consulting and Clinical Psychology, 56*, 926–928.

Walling, M., Anderson, B., & Johnson, S. (1990). Hormonal replacement therapy for postmenopausal women: A review of sexual outcomes and related gynecologic effects. *Archives of Sexual Behavior, 19*, 135.

Warner, K.E. (1991). Health and economic implications of a tobacco free society. *Journal of the American Medical Association, 258* (15): 2080–2088.

Weissman, M.M. (1980). The treatment of depressed women: the efficacy of psychotherapy. In C.L. Heckerman (Ed.), *The Evolving Female: Women in a Psychosocial Context* (pp. 307–324). New York: Human Sciences Press.

Weissman, M.M. & Klerman, G. (1985). Sex differences and the epidemiology of depression. *Arch Gen Psychiatry, 34*, 98–111.

Wenger, N.K., Speroff, L., & Packard, B. (1993). Cardiovascular health and disease in women. *The New England Journal of Medicine, 329,* 247–256.

Wilson, R.A. (1966). *Feminine Forever.* New York: M. Evans.

Winick. (1992). Nutritional Needs of the Menopausal Woman. Paper Presented at the North American Menopause Association. Cleveland, Ohio.

Wolfe, L. (1992, October 12). New York Woman. *New York,* pp. 46–55.

Wooley, S.C. & Wooley, O.W. (1979). Obesity and Women: I. A Closer Look at the Facts. *Women's Studies International Quarterly, 2,* 69–79.

Ylikorkala, O., Kuusi, T., Tikkanen, M.J., and Vinikka, L. (1987). Desogestertrel- and levonorgestrel-containing oral contraceptives have different effects on urinary excretion of prostacyclin metabolites and serum high density lipoproteins. *J. Clin. Endocrinol. Metab., 65,* 1238–42.

Young, R.L., Kumar, N.S., & Goldzieher. (1990). Management of menopause when estrogen cannot be used. *Drugs, 40* (2), 220–230.

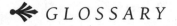

amenorrhea: Absence of the menses.

androgen: A class of male hormones including testosterone.

anemia: A condition in which the blood is deficient of red cells, hemoglobin or total volume.

artery: A vessel through which the blood passes away from the heart to the various parts of the body.

atherosclerosis: A condition characterized by thickening and loss of elasticity of the arterial walls.

atrophy: A wasting away; a diminution in the size of a cell, tissue, organ, or part.

beta-blockers: A class of drugs used for a variety of conditions including cardiovascular health.

bilateral oophorectomy: Surgical removal of both ovaries.

biopsychosocial: Pertaining to the interactions between mind, body and society in the formation and continuation of the personality.

cardiovascular disease: Diseases pertaining to the heart and blood vessels.

cervix: The lower and narrow end of the uterus which protrudes into the vagina.

chemotherapy: The use of chemical agents in the treatment of a disease, usually cancer.

cholesterol: A pearly fatlike steroid substance which circulates within the bloodstream and is found in foods.

conjugated estrogen: A form of estrogen therapy commonly derived from the urine of pregnant mares.

depression, major: A psychiatric disorder that includes depressed mood or markedly diminished interest and three of the following symptoms: The symptoms have occurred for two weeks and are a change from usual functioning. They include: changes in weight or sleep and agitation or retardation, fatigue or loss of energy, feelings of worthlessness, inability to concentrate and recurrent thoughts of death or suicide.

diabetes (diabetes mellitus): A disease that occurs when insulin is absent or ineffective. Insulin is the hormone that processes sugar.

diuretic: Tending to increase the flow of urine.

dyspareunia: Difficult or painful coitus/intercourse in women.

dysthymic disorder: A chronic condition that includes symptoms of sadness or irritability and at least two of the following symptoms: changes in appetite, sleep, energy level or concentration and low self-esteem and feelings of hopelessness.

endometriosis: The migration of tissue that normally lines the uterus to other organs.

endometrium: The lining of the uterus.

epidemiology: A branch of medical science that deals with the incidence, distribution and control of a disease in a population.

epithelium, vaginal: The tissue lining of the vagina.

estrogen: A female sex hormone. It is responsible for the development of the female secondary sex characteristics.

extrusion: A form that is pushed or pressed out.

fallopian tube: The pair of tubes through which eggs are transported from the ovary to the uterus.

fibroids: Benign, not cancerous, overgrowth of smooth muscle tissue in the uterine wall.

follicle: The structure on the ovary surface that nurtures a ripening oocyte. At ovulation the follicle ruptures and the oocyte is released.

FSH: Follicle-stimulating hormone. This hormone is produced in the pituitary gland and stimulates estrogen production in the ovary. A high level of FSH is associated with low levels of estrogen.

hot flash: Subjective experience of intense warmth throughout the upper body.

hot flush: The objective change during a hot flash that produces visable redness of the upper chest, neck and face followed by perspiration.

HRT (Hormone Replacement Therapy): Usually including both estrogen and progesterone.

hypertension: An elevation of the blood pressure.

hypothalamus: The portion of the diencephalon (part of the brain) that regulates many vital functions.

hysterectomy: Surgical removal of the uterus.

incontinence: Inability to control urination.

invasive: Tending to invade healthy tissue.

lactose: A type of sugar present in milk.

LH: Luteinizing hormone produced by the pituitary gland to act on the ovaries.

menarche: The establishment or beginning of menstruation.

menopause: The cessation of menstruation.

oocyte: Immature eggs produced by the ovaries.

osteoarthritis: A chronic process that wears away the cartilage between the bones, leading to joint stiffness and pain.

osteoporosis: A condition of bone thinning that can lead to fractures.

ovaries: The female reproductive organs that produce eggs and the female sex hormones.

perimenopausal: The time around the menopause when menstrual cycles begin to be irregular.

postmenopausal: Occurring after the menopause.

progesterone: One of the principal female hormones. Progesterone causes the lining of the uterus to shed in the absence of a fertilized egg.

regimen: A strictly regulated scheme of diet, exercise, or medication designed to achieve certain ends.

sonogram: See ultrasound.

stress: The sum of the biological reactions to any adverse stimulus, physical, mental, or emotional, internal or external, that tends to disturb the organism's equilibrium.

symptom: The subjective experience of a disease

syndrome: A group of symptoms that produce a pattern typical of a particular disease.

thyroid: The endocrine gland lying at the base of the neck that produces thyroid hormone. Thyroid hormone regulates metabolism.

ultrasound: Diagnostic technique for the examination of internal body structures that involves an image created by ultrasonic or echo waves.

urethra: The canal that carries urine from the bladder to the exterior of the body.

urinary stress incontinence: Involuntary escape of urine due to strain on the orifice of the bladder, as in coughing or sneezing.

uterus *pl. uteri:* The hollow muscular female organ located in the pelvis where a fetus can grow.

vasoconstriction: Reversible narrowing of blood vessels which decreases the blood delivered to an area.

vasodilation: Reversable expansion of a vessel that increases blood flow; **re-**

flex vasodilation, vasodilation occurring as a reflex to a stimulus, or after an initial vasoconstrictive response.

vasodilator: A medication that widens blood vessels and increases blood flow.

vertebra *pl. vertebrae:* Any of the thirty-three bones of the spine, including the seven cervical, twelve thoracic, five lumbar, five sacral, and four coccygeal vertebrae.

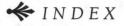# *INDEX*

104–5; osteoporosis, 96. *See also* Calcium, supplements; Hormone replacement therapy; *Vitamin headings; specific names and types*
Meditation, 55, 56, 219, 226
Medroxyprogesterone. *See* Progesterone
Men: alcohol effects, 127, 228, 283; heart disease/prevention, 111, 112, 114, 115, 128; hot flashes, 45; midlife problems, 213–15; sexuality changes, 31–32, 70, 73–74
Menopause: average age, 24, 142; changes with, 26–31; common complaints/symptoms, 17–29, 129, 329–38; common questions, 339–42; cross-cultural differences, 28; defined, 24, 357; diagnosis, 46, 138, 140; and fertility, 77–78, 142–43; negative views of, 33–35, 61, 64–65, 169–70, 323; phases, 23–24, *25;* popular culture depictions of, 33–34, 64, 169–79; surgical: *see* Hysterectomy; Oophorectomy; as transition, 23–24, *see also* Aging process; Perimenopausal; Postmenopausal; Premenopausal; *specific aspects*
Menopause clinics, 309–10
Menopause: Hormone Replacement and Women's Health (book), 166
Menopause Self-Help Book, The (Lark), 162
Menstrual periods: abnormal bleeding, 148–49, 154, 239, 244, 284; contraceptive use after last, 77, 142–43; cyclical biological changes, 27, 139, 149; ending suddenly, 24; estrogen therapy while having, 143; headaches and, 227; hot flashes while having, 46, 143; as HRT side effect, 155–56, *159,* 160, 161; normal premenopausal, 139; perimenopausal, 24, 142
Metabolism, 117, 265, 338
Midlife crises, 202, 212–15, 232–33
Migraine headaches, 154, 227–28
Milk. *See* Dairy products
Mind/body connection, 219–20, 228, 261, 276, 278, 302
Mood swings, 24, 30, 157, 165, 255, 336
Morgan, Susanne, 245
Movies, menopause depiction in, 169–70
Moyers, Bill, 219–20, 234
MR. FIT (Multiple Risk Factor Intervention Trial), 111, 117
Muller, James, 31, 312
Muscle-contraction headaches. *See* Tension headaches
Music, as stress reliever, 224–25
Myomectomy, 242, 244

Nachtigall, Lila, 143, 166
NAMS. *See* North American Menopause Society
Narcotics. *See* Substance abuse
National Association for Mental Health, 189

National Cancer Institute, 269, 316
National Lesbian Health Care Survey, 195
Native American women, 181, 285
Nausea, 157, 335
Newsletters. *See* Publications
New York magazine, 170–71
Nicotine gum/patch, 122, 281
Night sweats, 44–45, 46, 142, 178, 332, 333–34
Nolen-Hoeksema, Susan, 192
Nonsteroidal anti-inflammatory drugs (NSAIDs), 91, 103, 228, 335
Non-weight–bearing exercise, 100
Norcross, John, 263
North American Menopause Society, 310, 316
NSAIDs. *See* Nonsteroidal anti-inflammatory drugs
Nurse practitioners, 37
Nurses' Health Study, 111, 128, 146
Nutrition and diet, 293–98; calcium in, 95–96, *97,* 99; cholesterol-lowering, 128; components of, 293; food as stress relief, 185–86; heart-healthy, 124–27, 332; hot-flash triggers, 28, 45, 56; low-fat, 95, 126, 292, 294–96, 332; migraine triggers, 227; osteoporosis prevention, 94–99, 106–8; pleasures from, 300. *See also* Dieting

Oatmeal, and calcium absorption, 99
Obesity, 116–17, 289, 333, 338
Olness, Karen, 220
Omega-3 fatty acid, 295–96
On Women Turning Fifty (Rountree), 35, 36, 223
Oocyte (egg), 27, 139, 357
Oophorectomy, 25–26, 237, 238, 355; alternatives to, 246–47; combined with hysterectomy, 235; depression link, 169, 240–41, 254; estrogen replacement therapy, 142, 144–45, 255; hot flashes from, 45, 46, 255; as ovarian cancer preventive, 241–42, 246–47
Oral contraceptives. *See* Birth control pills
Orgasm, 70, 240
Osteoarthritis, 90, 334–35, 357
Osteoporosis, 86–109; consequences of, 90–91; described, 88–90, 357; evaluation for, 93–94; low estrogen and, 139; prevention, 35, 88–89, 92, 93, 94–103, 104, 106–9, 140, 141, 146; risk factors, 91–93, 98–99, *107,* 142, 279, 284; treatment, 103–5
Ovarian cancer, 144, 241–42, 246–47, 338
Ovaries, 357; removal of: *see* Oophorectomy
Overweight. *See* Dieting; Obesity; Weight

Paced respiration. *See* Breathing techniques
Pain: back, 91, 330, 331; chest, 112, 129; intercourse-linked, 62, 71–72, 76, 79, 356; medication addiction, 287–88;

Drs. Landau, Cyr and Moulton founded Women's Health Associates, an interdisciplinary group practice affiliated with the Division of General Internal Medicine, Rhode Island Hospital, Brown University School of Medicine.

Correspondence can be directed to:

Division of General Internal Medicine
Rhode Island Hospital
593 Eddy Street
Providence, R.I. 02903
or telephone
(401) 273-2828 (Dr. Landau)
or
(401) 444-5344 (Drs. Cyr and Moulton)